Every Woman's Medical Guide

Every Woman's Medical Guide

PEERAGE BOOKS

First published in Great Britain in 1984 by
Octopus Books Limited
under licence from Whinfrey Strachan Limited

This edition published in 1989 by
Peerage Books
Michelin House
81 Fulham Road
London SW3 6RB

© 1984 Whinfrey Strachan Ltd

ISBN 1 85052 138 7

Produced by Mandarin Offset
Printed and bound in Hong Kong

CONSULTANTS

Dr Simon A. Smail, MA, BM, BCh, MECGP, DCH, D.Obst RCOG
Senior Lecturer at the Welsh National School of Medicine, Cardiff

Dr J. A. Muir Gray, MB, BCh, DPH
Community Physician, Oxfordshire Area Health Authority, Oxford

Dr Elizabeth Tilden, MRCS, LRCP, MB.B.CHIR., MRC.Psych.
Consultant Pyschiatrist, University College Hospital, London

CONTENTS

Tests and Operations

Medical Guide

CHAPTER 1

The Menstrual Cycle

Menstruation

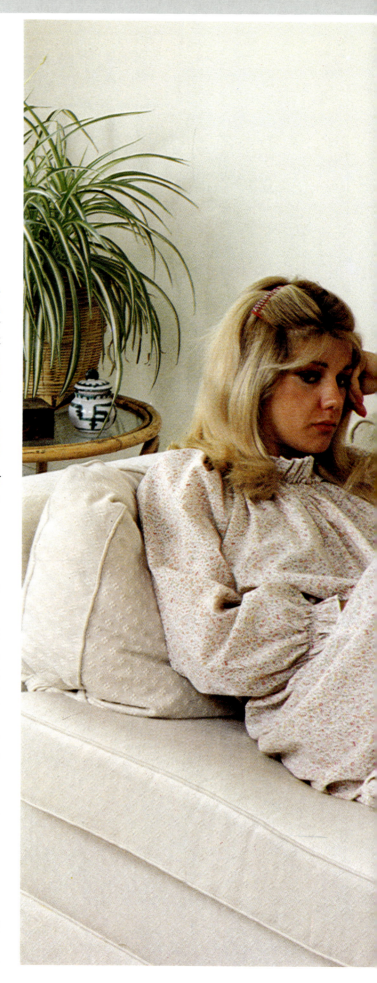

Menstruation has been described as the womb weeping for the pregnancy which did not happen. That's only one of the many bizarre things which have been said about women's monthly periods over the ages. The many myths and superstitions which surround menstruation still persist, and even today it's not always clear as to what is fact and what is fiction.

The average woman will probably experience about 400 periods in her lifetime. They spell misery to some women each month – heralded by stomach cramps, depression and headaches. To others they are a welcome confirmation of feminity and womanhood – and well worth any minor inconvenience.

Why do emotions influence a woman's period so much?

A woman's periods are governed by a sort of 'menstrual clock' located in the hypothalamus which is deep inside the brain. This control centre receives coded messages from the rest of the body and in turn feeds information to the pituitary gland which influences all the different production centres of the menstrual system – the ovaries, Fallopian tubes and the womb. The pituitary hormones and the two ovarian hormones oestrogen and progesterone regulate the entire process – and there's not a day when a woman is not subject to the ebb and flow of these hormones (see the box on page 11).

Given its location and the fact that it receives information as well as sending it out, it's hardly surprising that the hypothalamus will be affected by changes – both physical and mental – in the body. Illness, anxiety, fatigue, emotional disturbance, excitement – even changes in the weather – can all temporarily upset the hormone rhythm. It's a two-way process, with hormonal levels influencing emotions (notoriously in the form of pre-menstrual tension) and emotions also affecting hormone production. (Pre-menstrual tension

8

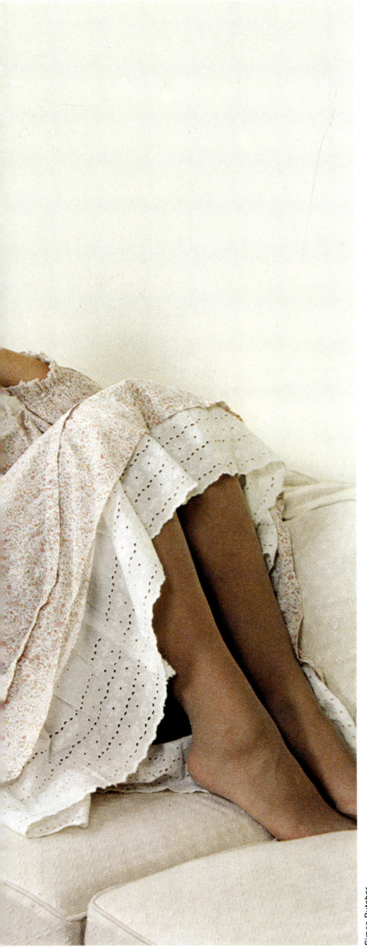

is covered in the next chapter).

The connection is well-established, but the exact nature is not clearly understood. What seems to happen, though, is that our conscious thoughts and actions relay impulses via the cerebral cortex in the brain to the hypothalamus. If the impulses are sufficiently intense, they can stimulate the hypothalamus to such an extent that the normal menstrual cycle is disrupted – as well as other body functions like sleep or appetite. In some cases, periods can be delayed, in others brought forward. So it's quite common for a young girl to find that her period starts on the same day as a big event she's been looking forward too – like a party or dance – or for another girl who fears she may be pregnant to find that her period is cruelly late in putting in its appearance. Because all the hormone glands are very closely interrelated, a disturbance in one can result in a change in the normal menstrual rhythm. The adrenal glands, for instance, are concerned with the body's natural defences against disease, as well as with the 'flight or fight' mechanism which stimulates the body's response to danger. A fright of some kind can affect periods – but so can a serious illness. Usually, once the cause for concern or excitement passes, the cycle returns to normal.

Emotions can affect periods more indirectly, too. Anorexia nervosa is a very common cause of loss of periods in adolescent girls. This 'wilful pursuit of thinness' through self-starvation seems to have a lot to do with a desire to negate their sexuality – in other words they are trying, unconsciously, to avoid growing up. Compulsive eating, often undertaken for similar motives, can have the same effect (in such cases, too much oestrogen is absorbed by body fat).

Why are some women called 'infertile' even though they have periods?

Just because a woman has periods, doesn't mean she's releasing an egg each month – it could be that the cycle is *anovulatory*.

A woman can have an anovular period at any time of her life, but it is most common for them to happen at the two extremes of her reproductive years. When a young girl first begins her periods, the ovaries are not yet ready to release their eggs. However, they are still capable of producing hormones which will cause the development of breasts, pubic hair etc., as well as building up the lining of the womb, but there won't be enough of the hormone to cause ovulation.

It can be quite difficult to pinpoint exactly when a young girl does begin to ovulate, though

Simon Butcher

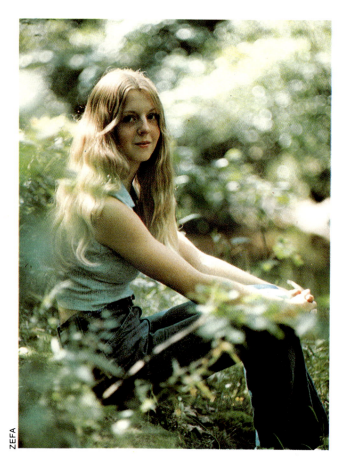

a few women do experience a sharp twinge in mid-cycle (around the 14th day after the last period) which coincides with the egg bursting out of the ovary. This is rarely strong enough to detect unless the woman is used to it, and usually the only clue for adolescents is that their periods start following a more regular pattern.

There is a theory that these anovulatory cycles are nature's way of protecting a young girl from becoming pregnant before she is physically or mentally ready. Even so, it's not something to rely on, and any adolescent embarking on a sexual relationship should always have adequate contraception.

Nature also seems to intervene in this way by stopping eggs from being released when women approach the menopause. Although their supply of egg cells (of which there are over 200,000 at puberty), will certainly not be exhausted they will certainly not be in prime condition either — and accordingly the chances of foetal abnormality are much higher.

But there are other times when a woman may be having periods, and still be infertile. There may, for instance, be some basic physical fault with the ovaries or a blockage of the Fallopian tubes, but also it may be due to some emotional disruption – often leading to a delayed period.

What has usually occurred in such cases is that

no egg has been released because the appropriate hormone messenger (LH) hasn't been discharged (see box on opposite page). What may have happened is that the hypothalamus – under stress – has failed to respond to the oestrogen signal, and so the oestrogen continues to stimulate the womb lining, but the egg stays in the ovary.

What is the normal pattern of periods?

Although all women have periods for the same biological reasons, this does not mean that all periods are the same. The process of the uterus shedding its lining in the form of a monthly bleed is not confined to the same time span for all women just as the amount of blood lost varies from individual to individual.

It's a mistake to assume that just because a 28-day cycle is *average* it's always the case. Perfectly normal, healthy women have cycles varying between 20 and 36 days.

Not only that, but the cycles may vary in one woman. Some have shorter cycles at certain times of the year (often in the warmer summer months) others notice that a short and long cycle alternate.

The bleeding may last for two days, or continue for seven. It may even stop or decrease for a day or two – and then start up again. It may be heavier at the beginning of each period, or it may start with only slight bleeding and gradually increase.

The amount of blood lost will be just as variable; it may be very slight, barely marking one sanitary towel – or it may be so heavy that it soaks three towels in an hour. There's absolutely no truth in the belief that if blood loss is scanty, it's because the blood is accumulating somewhere inside – ready to poison the body or be lost in

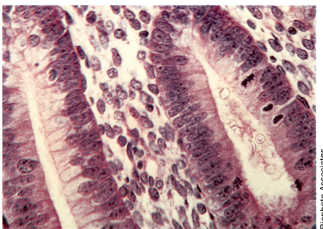

A magnified section of the uterus lining during the proliferative phase.

The cycle

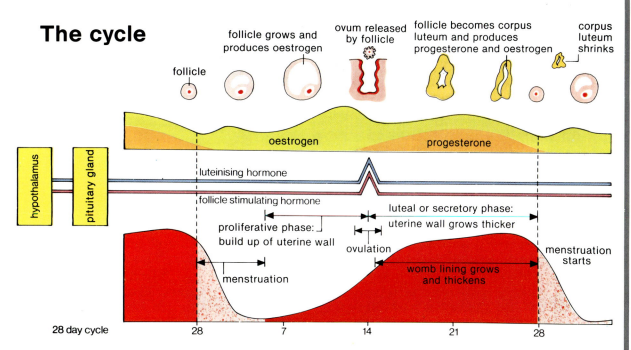

follicle grows and produces oestrogen

ovum released by follicle

follicle becomes corpus luteum and produces progesterone and oestrogen

corpus luteum shrinks

follicle

oestrogen

progesterone

luteinising hormone

follicle stimulating hormone

luteal or secretory phase: uterine wall grows thicker

proliferative phase: build up of uterine wall

ovulation

menstruation

womb lining grows and thickens

menstruation starts

28 day cycle

28   7   14   21   28

The complex circuit of hormonal stimuli and responses which is responsible for a woman's monthly periods starts, and ends, at the *hypothalamus* in the brain – the body's menstrual clock. If the circuit breaks, the monthly period is inevitably disrupted.

Phase one: menstruation
The hypothalamus sends quantities of FSH-releasing factor to stimulate the cells in the *pituitary gland*. This is the master gland considered to be the conductor of the orchestra of the body's other hormone-producing glands, responsible for controlling the ebb and flow of hormones. The pituitary then begins secreting minute quantities of FSH (*follicle stimulating hormone*) – and that's precisely what it does. This hormone stimulates the dormant egg cells which have been lying undisturbed in the ovary since before birth.

Phase two: proliferative phase
The egg cells now begin to develop, acquiring a fluid-filled follicle, like a protective sack, around them. Usually, only one of these follicles will go on to grow enough to force its way through to the surface of the ovary, where it forms a sort of bubble. (Occasionally, two follicles succeed and then twins are a possibility, provided both eggs are fertilized.)

As the follicles are developing in this way, they secrete *oestrogen*, adding to the quantity already being produced by the ovaries. This rise in the hormone level is a signal to the womb, and stimulates the *endometrium* (womb lining) to grow.

The lining is made up of narrow tubes, called endometrial glands, set in several layers of cells, called endometrial stromal cells. The oestrogen makes the glands grow, and the layers of the stromal cells increase or 'proliferate'.

Phase three: ovulation
When oestrogen output is six times higher than its starting level, about 13 days after the onset of menstruation, it has a 'feedback' effect on the hypothalamus/pituitary, causing the level of FSH-releasing factor from the hypothalamus to drop. Another factor – LH-releasing factor – is sent to the pituitary, stimulating the release of *luteinising hormone* (LH) which moves into the blood stream with a sudden surge on the 14th day. In combination with the FSH, the hormone induces the most mature follicle bubble in the ovary to burst – releasing the egg.

Phase four: the luteal phase
The newly released egg is caught in the finger-like fronds at the end of the *Fallopian tube* and is wafted slowly, and gently, into the tube itself.

The empty follicle it has left now undergoes its own transformation; it collapses, and, under the influence of LH, its cell walls turn yellow.

It is now known as the *corpus luteum* – literally the yellow body. The change of colour is, in fact, due to a change of activity. Now, not only does it secrete oestrogen, but also *progesterone* (or pro-pregnancy), whose main job is to preserve and modify the womb lining. Progesterone thickens the lining and stimulates the glands to secrete a nutritious fluid to nourish any fertilized egg arriving from the Fallopian tubes.

Phase five: pre-menstrual
If no fertilized egg embeds itself, the corpus luteum slowly shrinks and fades away, so that after 12 to 14 days the supply of progesterone is shut off completely, and the level of oestrogen drops back down.

As a result two things happen. First, without the oestrogen and progesterone to maintain it, the thick, juicy endometrium begins to shrink, and in doing so the tiny blood capillaries supplying it become bent – and so break. In the deeper layers of the lining, bleeding occurs, separating the lining above the blood. It crumbles and collapses into the womb cavity, along with the blood, eventually causing the womb to contract and expel its debris – a menstrual blood. Second, the restraint on the FSH-releasing factors (which followed the oestrogen surge) is removed (see phase one), FSH production is stepped up, and the cycle begins all over again.

one heavy haemorrhage. Nor does a heavy period mean you're losing too much blood. Most women quickly make up the loss, provided they're on a good diet – but if in any doubt, ask your doctor.

Even colour will differ – it may even change from day to day. In the first day or two, it's often pink and watery, but it could just as well be bright red, dark red, or almost black.

Is menstrual blood different from normal blood?

Yes. The menstrual flow is not just composed of blood, but also contains mucus and degenerated cells from the lining of the womb. You may notice dark shreds or even whole pieces of dark red membrane. Another difference is that menstrual blood is blood that has previously been clotted. The blood forms clots in the womb, then, to pass through the vagina and out of the body, the clots are dissolved and the blood is reliquified. Occasionally, though, you may see small clots of bright red blood.

Why are periods sometimes painful?

Not all women suffer from painful periods, some just sail through, as they would at any other time of the month, while others experience stomach aches, sickness, cold sweats, constipation and diarrhoea.

It is thought that hormones known as prostaglandins may be responsible since there are large increases in output just before menstruation. The sickness and diarrhoea, it is thought, may be caused by a particular prostaglandin which affects the muscles of the gut and the womb.

Because of this, drugs which suppress the build-up of prostaglandins can bring relief to many women. Aspirin is just such a drug, and many women find pain relief after taking a couple of these (see page 168.)

If pain is severe, or is accompanied by other symptoms such as headaches, depression or lethargy, it could be due to an oestrogen/progesterone imbalance – as is pre-menstrual tension. This may occur a week before and during the first two days of the period. Both PMT and pain during periods can sometimes be helped by hormone treatment, and it's well worth consulting your doctor.

Can using tampons be dangerous?

There is no truth at all in the belief that it is dangerous to collect menstrual blood in the vagina. Providing tampons are inserted correctly, they are a safe, trouble-free and comfortable way of dealing with periods. Many women prefer them to sanitary towels which can chafe, although for heavier days they may not give adequate protection.

Young girls just starting their periods might encounter a little resistance when first trying to use tampons, and a little petroleum jelly or a similar lubricant may help. There is no mystique involved with inserting them correctly and relaxation is usually the key to success. It is often the case that to begin with the hymen is not elastic enough to accept a tampon, but a few trial-runs when the flow is at its heaviest, or using towels for a few months until the cycle has had a better chance to establish itself, will both contribute to final success.

There are many different sanitary wear products on the market, all claiming to be more absorbent, hygenic or 'sweeter-smelling' than their competitors. Finding what suits you best is a matter of trial and error. Some women like to use a tampon and a pad during the heavier days of their period, while others will opt for a super absorbent product, either way it's best to change them very regularly – and at least twice a day.

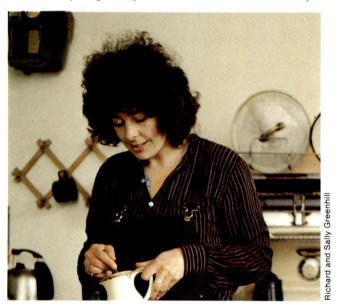

Richard and Sally Greenhill

Think carefully before choosing a super absorbent tampon, particularly if your periods aren't very heavy. You may think that you are saving yourself money by reducing the number of times you need to change them, but there is a possibility that the larger tampons may damage the superficial walls of the vagina.

Deodorized tampons are pointless. Menstrual blood has no odour until it comes into contact with the air. As tampons are worn inside the body, ones which boast the benefits of being perfumed are simply a marketing ploy. Indeed, the chemicals in these products have been known to cause allergy and may kill off the vagina's protective bacteria, allowing harmful bacteria to flourish.

If you have a vaginal discharge between periods don't use a tampon to absorb it because you could also be absorbing the vagina's natural secretions which are there to fight disease.

Always remember to remove your tampon when your period comes to an end. If a tampon is forgotten it can lead to a very offensive vaginal discharge and even to infection.

Is there any truth in the idea that menstruation is governed by the moon?

Menstruation is shrouded in myths and legends. For a long time it was regarded as something one didn't speak about – it was darkly referred to as the 'poorly time' when women would shut themselves away with smelling salts and cold compresses, to emerge five days later having 'recovered'. Even now with a greater social acceptance and scientific understanding, some bizarre beliefs concerning the subject still persist. Some are borne out by scientific investigation, others are mere superstition and their existence only serves to inhibit women from feeling easy about their periods.

The idea that the moon and a woman's cycles are linked has long been a favourite with old wives, but it has also found scientific credibility. A study in America revealed that more women ovulated during a full moon and menstruated during a new moon than at other times. This theory was further tested when women with irregular periods were asked to sleep with a light on during the nights of the fourteenth, fifteenth and sixteenth days of their cycles (when ovulation should occur in a regular cycle) in an attempt to 'bring on' ovulation by mimicking a full moon. Most of the women who took part in this experiment did find that they achieved a regular cycle by this method.

Another interesting theory which is receiving scientific attention is that of 'synchronized periods'. It is quite usual for twin sisters to start their periods at exactly the same time and it's common knowledge that women who live together or girls sharing dormitories also find that their menstrual cycles adjust to each other.

It is still not certain what causes this, but it seems very likely that the sense of smell has a lot to do with it. It seems that the body gives off *pheromones*, which have a faint odour of which we are not consciously aware but which the brain

---

How to cope with painful periods

1 Two *aspirin* taken with a hot drink will bring some relief.
2 By preventing ovulation *the Pill* also stops a build up of prostaglandins, the hormones responsible for painful periods.
3 *Avoid* very hot baths, these tend to make the blood flow more copious.
4 *Iron enriched* foods like watercress, liver and eggs will help to combat tiredness and that more general feeling of being run down which a heavy period can sometimes cause.
5 *Daily exercise* which helps to improve blood circulation and relax muscles will make stomach cramps less likely.
6 *Eat fruit,* vegetables and bran; this will ease constipation which often aggravates menstrual cramp.

---

registers. This odour is given off by each woman and may influence the hormone patterns of her friends.

For each theory which has a factual basis, there are many others which have none at all, but which have been passed down through the generations. Primitive tribes believed that loss of blood was the same as loss of life, it was therefore thought that a menstruating woman would have a dire effect on anything that was growing.

During her period she was kept away from crops and cattle, even from pregnant women. Even today some people still believe that a menstruating woman has the power to turn milk sour.

It's possible that all these theories stem from the fact that women who suffer from PMT (premenstrual tension) may be more irritable or haphazard at these times – so that their work suffers. Other common fallacies suggest that it is inadvisable to wash your hair during a period, or that a sexual relationship during menstruation is somehow wrong. Neither is true and, in the latter case, because of changing hormone level it is common for a woman to feel an increase in sexual desire during this time. Orgasms may even be a way of relieving painful periods for some women, because they increase the blood flow which reduces the pressure of pelvic congestion.

Current research, though, does indicate that women are more vulnerable to infection during menstruation, possibly due to the hormone link with the adrenal gland which is involved with the body's defence system.

Pre-menstrual tension

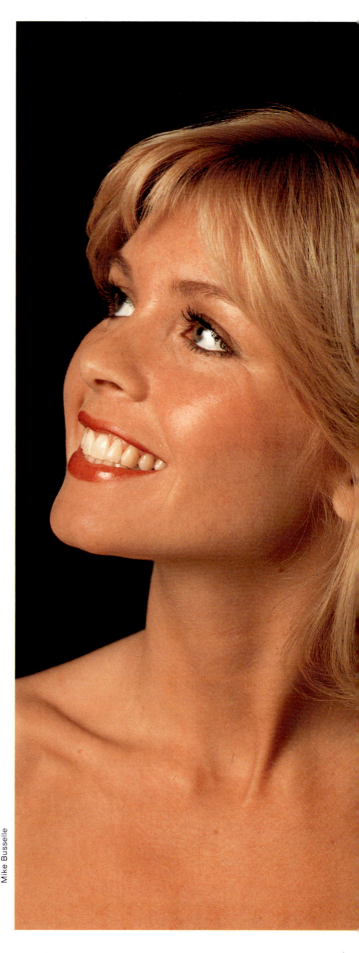

Mike Busselle

Pre-menstrual tension, with its symptoms of bad temper, impatience and fatigue, is now recognized as something that affects about 40 per cent of women every time they have a period. This is the strongest example of how the sex hormones – which control the monthly cycle – can upset the way you feel, although there are other events linked to hormone activity, such as pregnancy and menopause, which can also have a very powerful effect on your emotions.

What links hormones to changes in mood?

The experts know surprisingly little about why these sex hormones, which are after all quite natural body chemicals, should have such peculiar emotional effects. What they do know is that the 'menstrual clock' which controls sex homone production is a very delicately balanced mechanism, so that variations in normal hormone levels happen quite easily.

The way you feel depends on the messages your brain receives. It is a part of the brain known as the hypothalamus which controls your menstrual clock and co-ordinates your sex hormone activity, but it is also involved in regulating a number of other important things, including your water balance, appetite and mood. Because these 'control centres' are so close together, an upset in any one of these functions can affect the others.

The large diagram on page 16 shows you the usual pattern of hormone levels throughout a

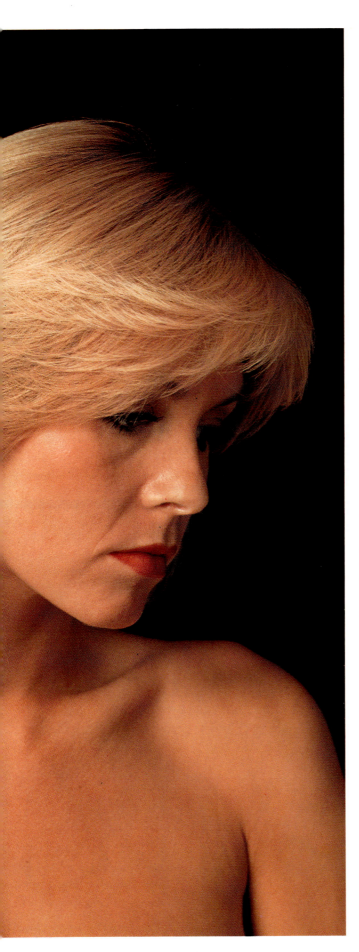

monthly cycle. Basically four hormones are involved, each of which has its role to play, in regulating the month's events – from stimulating the release of a new egg from the ovary through to the end of the cycle when, if the egg is unfertilized, the spongy lining of the womb is shed and the whole process starts all over again.

This all sounds very basic, but it actually involves a highly complex series of sex hormone messages acting upon the right parts of the body at the right times. It means that each hormone messenger goes through a variety of highs and lows throughout the month in order to do its job – and this is a perfectly normal pattern.

When you get a marked variation from the normal fluctuations it creates a *hormone imbalance*. Small differences may cause only mild changes in mood, but for some women their hormone production fluctuates so widely from the usual pattern that they regularly suffer emotional symptoms as a result – they become easily upset, annoyed, frustrated or even hysterical.

Which sex hormones are involved in pre-menstrual tension?

The two major female sex hormones are called *oestrogen* and *progesterone*. Pre-menstrual tension (PMT) sufferers tend to have lower than normal levels of progesterone and higher levels of oestrogen than normal. This creates 'difficult' feelings in the few days before menstruation (and sometimes during the period too) because those are the days when the hormone levels are changing rapidly and balance between them is very critical.

Some women who have never suffered from PMT start to experience it after having a child. During pregnancy, the placenta ('afterbirth') takes over production of progesterone and the ovaries stop supplying it altogether. After the birth of the baby the ovaries may have difficulty readjusting to produce sufficient amounts of the hormone again – leading to progesterone deficiency and all the unwelcome emotional upsets of PMT.

What types of upset do women experience through hormone imbalance?

The sort of feelings experienced, particularly in PMT, may often be no more than minor irritation, but for some women they reach truly nightmare proportions. Mood swings and unprovoked aggression are one kind of reaction; great tiredness, general lack of normal skills and efficiency are another. Just a few typical phrases from the many patients who have consulted a London specialist about these problems tell the story of this monthly misery:

☐ 'for the few days before her period she is sharp-tongued, impossible to live with. . . .'
☐ 'so nervy and irritable that I am sorry for any one who has to live with me. . . .'
☐ 'I do not batter my children but I do verbally, and I think that can be almost as damaging. . . .'
☐ 'I get so slow and stupid before my period. . . .'
☐ 'all I want to do is curl up in a corner away from all my responsibilities. . . .'
☐ 'it is as though there is somebody inside saying terrible things. I blame my son and tell him I hate him and hit him. . . .'
☐ 'the whole world gets on my nerves and I can only look at it with a jaundiced eye. . . .'

The tensions and depression in some cases are acute, verging on the suicidal, likewise the fits of temper can be so severe that they are very frightening. It may mean outbursts at home that involve smashing dishes, slapping the children or striking the husband, or it can end in serious crime.

Research in all kinds of areas now points to the 'hidden effects' of hormone imbalance during the four days just before a period, and in the first four days of menstruation itself. Here are just a few facts from the revealing evidence relating to these eight days of the female cycle:

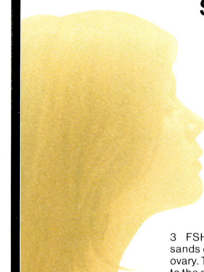

Sex hormones

1 FSH and LH are both produced by the pituitary gland and are responsible for setting the menstrual cycle in motion.

2 OESTROGEN is produced when FSH stimulates the ovaries. Among its many other functions, oestrogen starts to rebuild the lining of the womb.

3 FSH acts on one of the thousands of immature egg cells in the ovary. The egg matures and comes to the surface of the ovary, where it is contained in a small blister or follicle.

4 About 14 days later LH triggers the release of this mature egg cell, starting it on its journey to the womb.

5 LH stimulates the follicle to burst, releasing the egg from the ovary. This stimulates the production of PROGESTERONE which acts on the lining of the womb, preparing a soft, spongy surface to receive a fertilized egg.

6 If conception does not occur, menstruation begins, clearing out the womb for the cycle to start again.

The Image Bank

☐ schoolgirls' work deteriorates; they are more likely to fail important exams
☐ half of all female emergency hospital admissions to psychiatric, accident, medical and surgical wards take place
☐ half of all suicides in women are attempted at this time
☐ half of all female crime is committed, including crimes of violence and drunkeness.

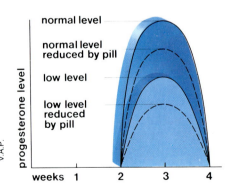

Above The pill's effect on progesterone levels. Reducing an already low level can make the symptoms of PMT worse.
Right Progesterone during pregnancy. Following the birth, the ovaries often have difficulty in readjusting to a normal level of production.

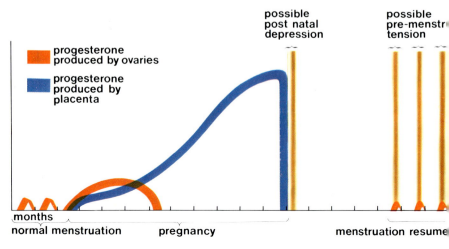

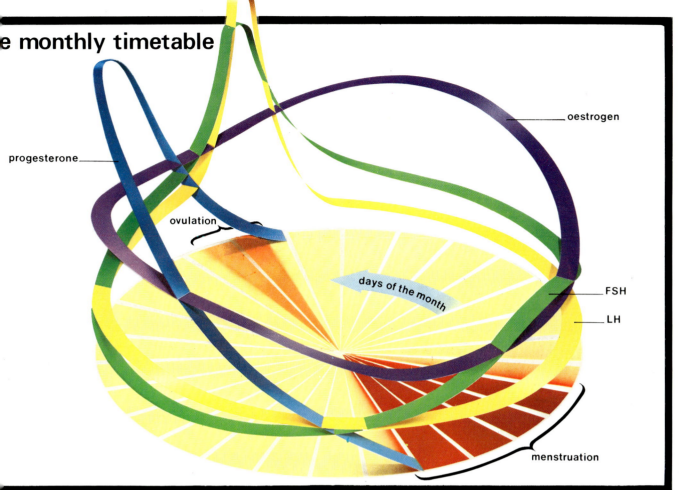

e monthly timetable

progesterone

ovulation

days of the month

oestrogen

FSH

LH

menstruation

V.A.P.

Are children affected by their mother's hormone cycle?

If a woman is suffering from the symptoms of sex hormone imbalance then her children are bound to be affected, however loving and caring a mother she is. Children find it difficult to accept the changing moods in their mothers. They cannot understand why some days she is ready for an energetic game of football yet on other days she only wants to sit on the park bench doing nothing, nor do they appreciate why one day when they spill water on the floor mother says 'Don't worry, I'll clear it up' and another day they get a spanking.

Studies of children under five attending a family doctor because of a cough or cold showed that half of the mothers who accompanied their child were themselves in the crucial eight days of their cycle, presumably suffering from tension, tiredness and depression, and felt they could stand the sick child no longer.

Further research into acute admissions to a children's ward at a big city hospital showed that half of all the children were admitted during the mother's 'bad' time of the month. Some of the children were admitted as a result of an accident, and it is difficult to avoid the conclusion that if the mother is accident-prone at this time, the child she is caring for will be more at risk too. She may be too lethargic to notice a child climbing a dangerous tree or running in the path of an oncoming car, or her own clumsiness could result in, say, the accidental scalding of the child.

Do men have any kind of hormone cycle like women?

The simple answer is 'no'. Whereas women only release an egg once a month, about half way through each menstrual cycle, men produce sperm throughout the month. The hormone that triggers the production of sperm in men is testosterone, and there are only slight variations in its daily level.

The research that has been done into certain behaviour patterns, such as the times when schoolchildren or prisoners act disruptively, has shown great differences between the sexes. While schoolgirls and female prisoners misbehave more at certain times of the month – clearly related to each individual's menstrual pattern – the behaviour of schoolboys and male prisoners fails to follow any cycle.

However, it's not uncommon for some men to show behaviour changes, such as lateness for work, on a monthly cycle, but these changes actually appear to be linked not to a cycle of their own but to their *wives'* menstrual pattern.

Husbands' and wives' body temperatures have shown a similar link. At ovulation a woman's temperature suddenly drops but is followed by a rise which remains constant until menstruation.

It's been demonstrated that a husband's temperature will rise at the same time as his wife's ovulation, then return to normal but, if the husband lives apart from his wife or she takes the Pill to stop ovulation, his temperature no longer shows this characteristic rise. As yet no one has been able to clearly explain this mysterious link.

Is it true that taking the contraceptive pill 'evens out' emotional ups and downs?

Among women suffering from the regular 'downs' of PMT, taking the Pill is much more likely to make things worse. Contraceptive pills contain varying amounts of a synthetic compound called *progestogen*. This is very different from the sex hormone *progesterone* which is produced naturally by the body. Progestogen has the effect of lowering the level of the *natural* hormone in the blood. Women suffering from PMT already have a hormonal imbalance, with too little progesterone, so the Pill is likely to make this worse.

In fact this kind of woman is the one most likely to stop taking the Pill early because of the increased depression, weight-gain and headaches – all of which are common reactions to taking oral contraceptives. And for those women suffering from PMT there is little to be gained in changing from one kind of Pill to another.

Are 'change of life' upsets similar to PMT?

The menopause is another time when sex hormone imbalance can affect the way you feel, and the types of emotional problems experienced by some women are in many ways similar to those of PMT. In fact, the women who suffer most from depression, fatigue and irritability at this age tend to be those who have been relatively free of PMT, while PMT sufferers at least have the consolation of looking forward to a fairly trouble-free menopause. This is because they have relatively high levels of the hormone oestrogen; it is oestrogen production which suddenly decreases in the menopause as the ovaries cease to function.

What kind of help is available for these hormone related problems?

If a woman is suffering seriously from tension or depression as a result of hormone imbalance – whether associated with the monthly cycle, with post childbirth problems, or with the menopause – a sympathetic doctor can certainly do something to help by prescribing hormone replacement treatment.

In terms of self-help for PMT sufferers, it has been found that eating frequent, regular meals during the 'difficult days', to stop the blood sugar level falling, is very effective. Simple avoiding action – not planning important events, parties, interviews etc. during the PMT days is a commonsense precaution.

Many women will find it reassuring to have these emotional problems out in the open: if you experience these feelings you know that you are not a freak, not cracking up, not falling out of love with your man, or turning into a bad mother.

It also makes a big difference if people around you, husband or boyfriend, children and parents, are aware of the problem. It may not make a sufferer any easier to live with, but at least everyone who is part of her personal life understands what is causing the trouble. If the effects become too upsetting, traumatic or impossible to cope with, then both the sufferer and her family know it is time to seek advice from a doctor.

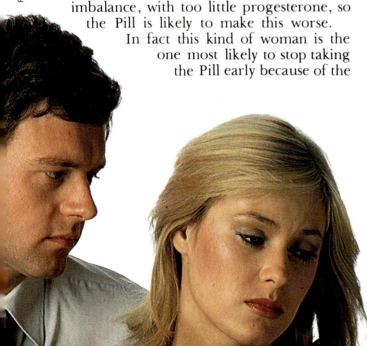

The menopause

The menopause simply means the time when a woman stops having her periods, but as any woman who has been through it will know, the change of life doesn't usually only involve this. There is a whole range of physical symptoms and emotional upheavals which may occur before, during and after her periods finally stop. It's for this reason that the menopause is more accurately known as the *climacteric*, which is derived from a word meaning the rung of a ladder. This word embraces all the changes, both physical and psychological, which a woman may be heir to once her ovaries stop releasing eggs and which eventually lead to a new hormonal balance.

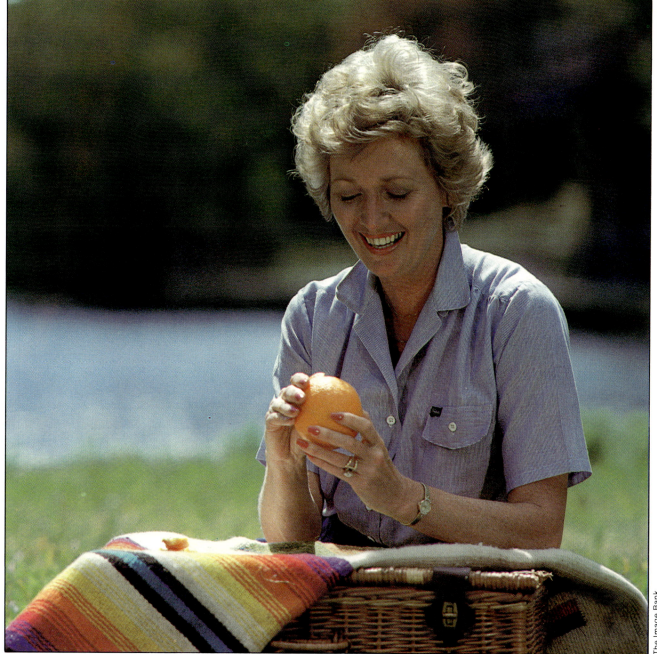

The Image Bank

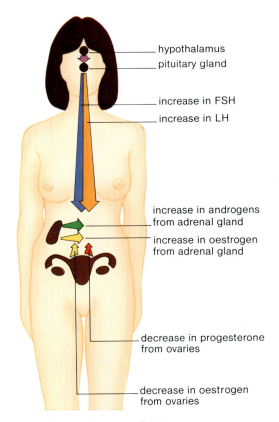

Changing hormone levels during the menopause

- hypothalamus
- pituitary gland
- increase in FSH
- increase in LH
- increase in androgens from adrenal gland
- increase in oestrogen from adrenal gland
- decrease in progesterone from ovaries
- decrease in oestrogen from ovaries

During the climacteric some of the hormones circulating in a woman's bloodstream increase while others decrease. It's these changes which account for the way a woman feels and the way her body reacts.

Bernard Fallon

started menstruating at 13 with those who had started at 18; in both groups there was no difference in the average age at which the women experienced the menopause.

At birth the ovaries contain millions of potential egg cells. Some die off, but thousands more become surrounded by cells to form *follicles*. During the fertile years only about 500 of these egg follicles will be used up – one for each month that a woman menstruates. The rest will simply degenerate. When this finally happens it will mean the end of a woman's periods and with it her ability to have children.

Not only does the degeneration of egg follicles mean the end of menstruation, it has repercussions on other parts of the body, too, most notably on hormone levels. It's the changes in the various hormone levels which account for most of the unpleasant symptoms of the menopause. But it's important to realize that after two years or so your body will have learnt to adjust to these new fluctuations – the symptoms don't last forever.

During the time of the climacteric, and in the years following it, there will be larger amounts of *follicle stimulating hormone* (FSH) in the bloodstream. This hormone, as the name implies, sets the follicles in action. Each month, combined with another hormone known as *luteinizing hormone* (LH), it stimulates one follicle to release an egg into the Fallopian tubes. Providing fertilization doesn't take place, menstruation results. During the climacteric, however, the few remaining follicles become increasingly less sensitive to FSH. In response, the pituitary gland then steps up production of this hormone in an attempt to stimulate the follicles into releasing their eggs.

Similarly, the degeneration of the follicles means that there will be lower levels of the hormones *oestrogen* and *progesterone* circulating in the bloodstream. Your body tries to compensate for this by stepping up production of oestrogen from other sources. The adrenal glands make more oestrogen, as well as *androgen* (the male hormone), which is converted into oestrogen in the liver and adipose tissues. But a majority of women aren't able to recreate the old balance.

How do you know when the climacteric has started?

The most obvious indication is when your periods cease, although, of course, this has to be coupled with your age. For most women the cessation of their periods is a gradual process and not something which happens abruptly overnight. Many women find the time between each period simply becomes longer and longer, while

Why do women have their menopause around the age of 50?

By the time you reach the age of 50 you'll probably be aware of certain outward signs of ageing; your hair may be going grey and your skin may have lost some of its suppleness. And, although you won't be aware of it, the same process will be making the internal organs, and in particular the ovaries, age and degenerate.

Ageing causes the ovaries to stop releasing their eggs. This is something which happens to every woman in middle age – sometimes as early as 45, sometimes around 50 and occasionally as late as 55. The age at which it occurs varies with each individual, and there are normal cases beyond these two figures.

There seems to be no truth in the idea that the earlier a woman starts her periods the earlier she'll experience her menopause. A study carried out some years ago compared women who had

Two typical menstrual patterns during the menopause

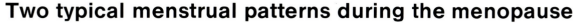

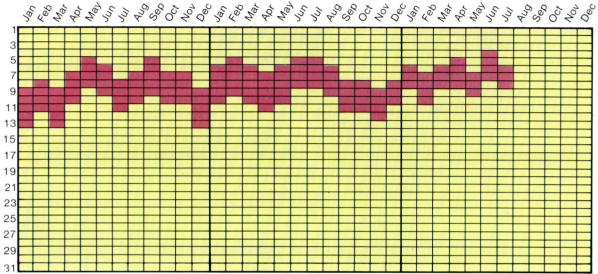

Periods continue to occur regularly each month. But the length of time each period lasts becomes shorter by one day, sometimes by two. Periods finally end abruptly, never to return.

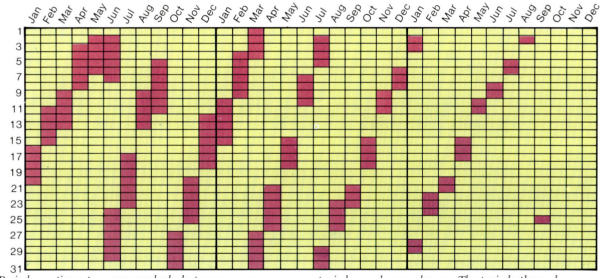

Periods continue to occur regularly but may go on longer than usual. Towards the end of the first year and during the second, the length of time between each period may become longer. The periods themselves gradually become shorter until finally, towards the end of the menopause, they may last for only one day.

the periods themselves may last the usual four or five days, or perhaps less. Others may experience the usual monthly cycle but with a scantier flow of blood each time, until the periods peter out altogether and finally cease.

Although the body is in a similar state of flux during this time as during puberty, any other menstrual pattern should be mentioned to a doctor. This is particularly important if the periods reappear after an absence of a year or if, after a year to 18 months of being fairly scanty, they suddenly become much heavier and last

longer. Either pattern could indicate an underlying condition which requires medical attention. Talk things over with your GP who will be able to establish whether or not your particular menstrual pattern is normal.

For some women the end of her periods may be the only outward sign of the climacteric. The other body changes, spread over several years, may be so gradual as to be barely perceptible. Such good fortune depends on your body's ability to convert large amounts of androgen into oestrogen.

A majority of women, however, will experience hot flushes at some time. These are sudden feelings of heat, often followed by cold, and sometimes accompanied by profuse sweating, particularly at night. The flushes usually start at the chest and spread upwards. Their actual cause is uncertain, but it would seem that the nervous control of blood vessels in the skin is disturbed either by the increase in FSH or by the reduction in oestrogen levels.

Another symptom which is caused by lower levels of oestrogen is the thinning of the vaginal lining. This lining, made up of 10 to 12 layers of mucous membrane may, during the climacteric, dwindle to as little as two or three layers. And since the thickness of the lining is a measure of its ability to protect the vagina from infection, many women find themselves more prone to infection after the menopause. Even without an infection, some women do encounter vaginal dryness and soreness or discomfort during intercourse.

Loss of calcium from the bones starts to occur during the menopause, although the effects are cumulative and may not be noticed for several years. This can eventually lead to *osteoporosis* – the thinning and weakening of the bones. This condition makes the bones, particularly those of the hips, wrists and vertebrae, more vulnerable to fracture. Even though the onset of osteoporosis coincides with the menopause, there is some contention over whether it's actually caused by reduced oestrogen levels. Although oestrogen therapy can help to alleviate osteoporosis, other factors such as smoking, heredity, being very underweight and a sedentary lifestyle are likely to play as large a part in causing it.

Is it true that a woman's breasts get smaller after the menopause?

Yes, this does often happen. The main factor in the development of breasts is oestrogen secretion from the ovaries. These become active just before puberty. Oestrogen not only causes the milk-producing duct system to develop, but also causes the number of fat cells between the duct tissues to multiply. It's these cells which determine the size and shape of a woman's breasts. The number of fat cells will be pre-determined by her genetic make-up and the size of the cells will depend on how much she tends to eat.

With the fall in oestrogen levels at the menopause the duct system within the breasts will decrease in size and the breasts may lose some of their firmness as a consequence. But the duct system only forms a relatively small part of the breasts; the rest is composed of fatty tissue formed by fat cells, so generally the amount of

The effect of oestrogen decline on the breast

ducts

fat cells

duct system decreases in size

number of fat cells may decrease

The changing profile of a woman's breast

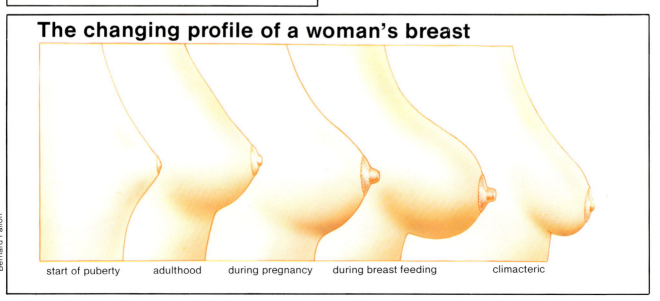

start of puberty   adulthood   during pregnancy   during breast feeding   climacteric

Bernard Fallon

How to cope with the unpleasant effects of the menopause

Symptom	What to do
Hot flushes	Try to avoid potentially embarrassing or stressful situations as these tend to trigger hot flushes. Taking vitamin E – found in wheatgerm oil – may help. Hot flushes are not always accompanied by blushing and often you may be the only one to be aware of them. They don't go on forever, generally only continuing for two to three years.
Facial hair	Electrolysis is an effective way of removing unwanted hair; bleaching will make hairs less obvious, and using tweezers on the occasional hair which crops up on the chin is effective, although only temporary.
Thinning of vaginal tissue	If you experience soreness or dryness while making love use a specially made lubricant. Oestrogen creams applied directly into the vagina improves this condition for many women.
Osteoporosis	Exercise and diet can both help to avoid this condition. Make sure you are getting enough vitamin D and calcium – the best sources are cod liver oil, halibut liver oil and milk or cheese. Exercise can be of any type; some women take up swimming, while others may prefer jogging or cycling.
Dry and thinning skin	Use a moisturizing cream day and night and avoid extremes of temperature.
Loosening of vaginal and pelvic muscles (may result in involuntarily passing water after coughing or sneezing)	Pelvic exercises can help to strengthen muscle control. Each time you wish to urinate, stop and start the flow of urine by tightening and then relaxing the muscles there.
Atherosclerosis (a thickening of the arteries feeding the heart, occuring in some women after the menopause once oestrogen levels are lowered)	Avoid smoking, and eat fatty foods in strict moderation. Exercise regularly and keep your weight down.

who don't have a sexual relationship, the vagina and *vulva* (the external genital organs) may shrink after the menopause. Once again, it's important to remember that these changes take place *gradually* over several years and don't occur suddenly when a woman reaches a certain age.

Many women seem to put on weight during their menopause. Is this avoidable?

Yes, it can be avoided. Weight gain around the time of the menopause has very little to do with changing hormone levels – it's due simply to the fact that a great many women become less active during this time. There is a tendency to blame the menopause for all sorts of changes, but it's unwise to put every new feeling or alteration in the body down to this.

If you do become less active but don't reduce your calorie intake to match, weight gain is inevitable whether you're going through the menopause or not. You may, however, experience a general alteration in your body's proportions even without weight gain. This is to do with ageing in general and not solely to the fact that you're experiencing the menopause.

The familiar 'middle-age spread', which tends to creep over the waistline and bottom but leaves the arms and legs relatively unaffected, is due to fat cells dying off from around the arms and legs. This makes the other parts of the body *look* relatively fatter, even though you may not actually have put on any weight. Remember though, that if you do put on weight, it will tend to accumulate round the waist.

You can avoid putting on weight by making sure that you're taking as much exercise as you were before the menopause; by reducing the amount of food you eat to match the decrease in physical activity; or by being more careful both to exercise and eat moderately. However, even the most rigorous attempts at keeping your weight constant can't guarantee that you won't get middle-age spread. The likelihood of this happening is governed by the genetic and constitutional make-up of each individual, and there's very little that can be done to influence it. But any type of exercise, even if it's only housework, will boost your physical well-being.

Do women develop facial hair during the menopause?

Yes, this may happen to some women. Superfluous hair, which is generally confined to the upper lip, is due to increased levels of androgen being secreted by the adrenal glands. The increase

shrinkage won't be very noticeable.

Oestrogen is also necessary to maintain the size of the womb. After the menopause this always gets smaller – sometimes shrinking to as little as a quarter of its former size. In women having regular sexual relations, the vagina itself won't decrease in size. But in the case of women in the levels of androgen has it's compensations, however. While some will be converted into oestrogen, the remainder, in its unconverted form, acts as a spur to sexuality. After the menopause, many women report an increase in their sex drive, something which is due, in part, to the increase of this hormone in the bloodstream.

If you do feel self-conscious about facial hair, it can always be removed by electrolysis or can be made less noticeable by bleaching.

As regards the general quality of your skin, it's almost impossible to tell whether an increase in the number of wrinkles and dry patches is due to the menopause and oestrogen deficiency or to general ageing and weathering. Certainly, if you've taken care of your skin all your life such changes will be less noticeable. If, on the other hand, you've been haphazard in the way you've cared for your skin, then skin problems in later life will be more obvious.

What sort of emotional changes are caused by the menopause?

Alterations in feelings and emotions at the climacteric are difficult to generalize about. One woman might not notice any upset in the way she normally feels. She may sail through the menopause with only the slightest physical discomfort. Another woman may experience anxiety and depression, or a mixture of the two. She may go through mood swings with feelings of being unable to cope or experience sudden uncontrollable urges to cry.

There is no doubt that shifting hormone levels can cause some emotional changes. The *hypothalamus* in the brain master-controls the endocrine system. But just as it can initiate changes in hormone levels throughout your body, so it can be affected when these levels change. When this happens the hypothalamus can trigger certain emotional reactions such as depression and irritability, and cause rapid changes in mood.

The way you feel about your own fertility will also have a profound effect on your emotional response to the menopause. It can be a tragedy for the woman whose family expectations remain unfulfilled, or a time of relief if she has had the family she desires.

It's unfortunate that the menopause coincides with certain of life's crises. It generally comes at a time when a woman's children are growing up and perhaps even leaving home – so she can't help but feel that her role as mother is changing. Her own parents will be ageing and may be declining in health. In this respect decisions may be needed as to who will look after them. Either

her husband's career, or her own, may have reached the stage where on the one hand, success is having a disruptive effect on family life, or, on the other, there may be the realization that ambitions will never be achieved. All these and other related domestic, social, and financial considerations will influence each woman's overall reaction to the 'change of life' apart from any of the physical effects that she may be experiencing at this time.

How can a woman best cope?

The simple answer is to regard the menopause not as a disease or an illness but to accept it as simply another aspect of maturity. It's important to remember, too, that a considerable number of women (one estimate puts it as high as 40 per cent) maintain similar levels of oestrogen after the climacteric as they had before it. So if you haven't been through the menopause already, don't automatically expect the worst.

Certain things can be a genuine help to a woman trying to cope. An understanding and sympathetic family, for example, can make a lot of difference. So, too, can a doctor who is willing to offer a listening ear and explanations of what's going on in your body rather than giving you a bottle of tranquillizers to 'calm you down'. Hormone replacement therapy (HRT), discussed in the next chapter, helps when there are upsetting oestrogen deficiency symptoms.

A job – part-time, full-time or voluntary – can give a purpose to life as well as giving a boost to morale. In this respect, one survey found that women who were employed full-time complained less of experiencing serious or unpleasant menopause symptoms. Boredom can be a terribly destructive state, especially to someone who is getting older.

As far as sexual activity goes, the menopause needn't signal any changes. Apart from possible vaginal dryness – and this can be temporarily improved by applying a lubricant before making love, or by treatments prescribed by your GP – you can continue to have sexual relationships well into old age. Your ability to enjoy sexual activity is not dependent on your ability to reproduce and, in fact, many women find that their enjoyment is actually increased once the fear of pregnancy has been removed.

Finally, it may help to remember that the climacteric doesn't go on indefinitely. Your body may be in a state of flux for two or three years. After this time it will have adjusted to the changing hormone levels, which themselves will also have settled into a more stable state.

Why does the body age?

Although no one really knows the answer to this, scientists have managed to isolate a number of different processes that contribute to ageing.

Our bodies are maintained by hundreds of millions of cells constantly dividing and reproducing exact copies of themselves. However, it seems that certain cells can only divide a certain number of times, after which they cease to do so. These cells have a genetically determined life span and die out when they have completed their total number of divisions. This happens even in a foetus. Early in its life, the foetus has webbing between its fingers and toes, but the cells of the skin web die out after a certain number of divisions, so that by the time the foetus is born the toes and fingers move as independent units.

One very obvious example of cells reaching the end of their life span is baldness. It seems that

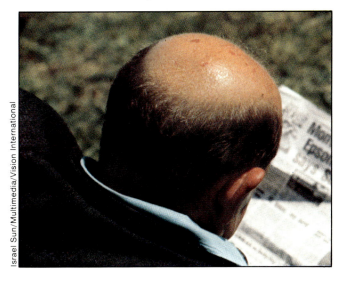

Israel Sun/Multimedia/Vision International

baldness is genetically predetermined and that the cells which make hair protein can only divide a certain number of times. In some people they die out much sooner than in others. The menopause provides another example of cell death: there is evidence that the reproductive cells of women can only divide a certain number of times and reach the end of their life span between the ages of 45 and 55.

A second process that contributes to ageing is the accumulation of cell 'mistakes'. It isn't surprising that out of the hundreds of millions of cells copied in the body each year, mistakes are occasionally made and some of them are flawed. If a mistake is very bad the cell will die, but in many cases it survives and goes on to make copies of itself, all showing the same flaw – rather like the scratch on a negative which is reproduced every time a print is made. An example of this is

white hair: a stage is reached when, because of an accumulation of 'mistakes', the hair cells alter and no longer distribute pigment in the hair follicle in the same way, and so white hairs begin to be produced.

The third aspect of growing older involves a change in the chemical structure of the body – particularly in the elastic tissues under the skin. The proteins that make up this elastic tissue alter, becoming more rigid and making the elastic fibres stiffer and slower to return to their normal shape. In youth, skin is held tight to the underlying tissues by elastic fibres, but as these fibres lengthen with age, so the skin becomes slack, just as when guy ropes on a tent come adrift, the tent itself sags. The chemical changes in the body mean also that the ratio of fat to protein increases, so that although a person may stay the same weight, he has more fat and less muscle.

Although the protein which makes up muscles continues throughout life to be broken down and rebuilt, with age, muscles tend to waste at a faster rate than they are remade – so that by about the age of 70 muscle accounts for 12 rather than 19 per cent of body weight. Apart from muscle shrinkage, the organs of the body lose some of their bulk in varying degrees – including the brain, kidneys, liver, uterus and pancreas.

Can ageing of the skin be prevented?

No. Many people apply oils and chemicals to their skin in the attempt to prevent ageing, but this is largely both time and money wasted, as nothing can reverse the process. Several important changes take place in the skin as a result of ageing. First, the skin becomes less elastic, which can easily be seen by taking a pinch of skin from the back of the hand, releasing it, and comparing how long it takes to return to normal with the skin of both a child and a much older person. At the same time, there is a decline in the amount of fat underlying the skin. This, together with the loss of elasticity, contributes to producing wrinkles.

Secondly, the sebaceous glands which secrete oils that keep the skin moist and soft emit less natural oil in old age, and the skin becomes drier.

Thirdly, the cells deep down in the *basal* layer of skin, which constantly divide and provide new skin cells, are prone to the types of error mentioned earlier. The mistakes lead to a change in appearance of the cells which come to the surface of the skin. For instance, the brown spots often seen on the skin of elderly people (especially on the backs of the hands) are due to errors in the distribution of pigment.

Hormone therapy

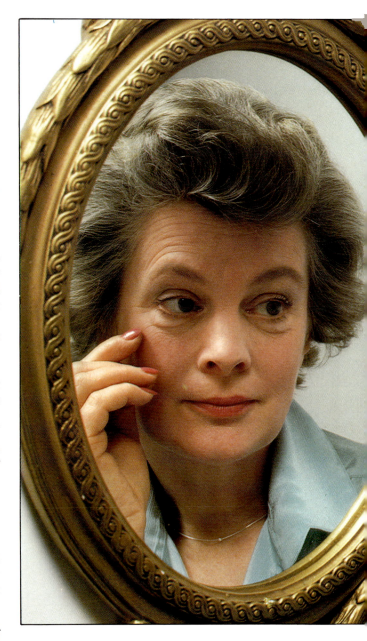

The search for the secret of staying young is as old as the fear of ageing itself, and many weird and wonderful treatments have been tried in the hope of finding a way to avoid the adverse effects of the passing years. Hormone replacement therapy (HRT) is one relatively recent approach which has some real scientific basis.

Primarily it is prescribed to minimize unpleasant 'change of life' symptoms, but there does seem to be evidence that it also postpones some of the general effects of ageing in women. Most doctors would stress, however, that HRT should not be taken casually, and any woman being treated with hormones has to have regular medical check-ups.

This seems to be a relatively new treatment – where did the idea come from?

It is now over 40 years since it was discovered that the ovaries, as well as producing eggs, secrete certain hormones which affect many different body functions.

From puberty to the menopause a woman's body is used to the repeated rise and fall of hormone levels. When an egg follicle is developing, it secretes *oestrogen;* this helps to prepare the lining of the womb for a fertilized egg, but it also influences many other functions, such as clotting mechanisms, fat and calcium metabolism, the skin and mucus membranes and bladder function. After the release of the egg, the burst follicle starts to secrete *progesterone* and some further oestrogen.

When a woman's periods stop, so does this regular production of ovarian hormones. The average age for a woman to have her last period is 50 years, but this varies a lot from one individual to another. The final period is usually preceded by months, or even years, of irregular cycles and therefore fluctuating hormone levels.

These facts about the decrease in hormone production in the menopause led doctors to look at how replacing the secretions of the ovaries

---

What happens at menopause

- hot flushes
- night sweating
- anxiety, depression and irritability
- sexual difficulties due to changes in vagina
- skin 'ages' as it loses elasticity
- bones weaken as calcium is lost

By alleviating the physical changes, hormone replacement therapy can lift the mind and help women to come to terms with the change of life.

might delay the effects of ageing. HRT was first used in the USA 35 years ago – it was slow to gain in popularity elsewhere, but there has been a gradual increase over the last 10 years. In the UK, the whole concept of this treatment has become much more 'respectable'.

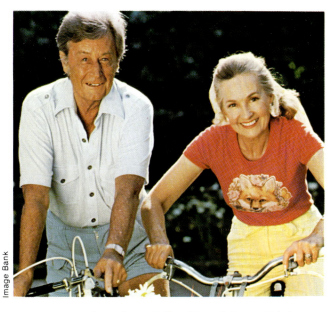

Image Bank

How does hormone therapy affect your sex life?

The reduction of oestrogen can make the lining of the vagina become thinner and less elastic – making sex uncomfortable or even painful. (This is known as 'vaginal atrophy'). Couples can find it very distressing when a previously enjoyable sex life becomes painful, and it can be a cause of great unhappiness and tension between them. Treatment with oestrogen soon restores elasticity to the vaginal wall and reduces discomfort, so that intercourse becomes a pleasure again.

On the other hand, difficulties that relate to *feelings* about sex, lack of enjoyment, not being 'bothered', are more often concerned with a woman's ideas about herself at this age. Her resentment at the inevitable signs of ageing is sometimes made worse by comparing herself with attractive daughters. Some older women begin to equate themselves with their own mothers, whom they never imagined enjoying intercourse, and feel that sex is inappropriate – 'I'm too old for that sort of thing'.

Each woman will have an individual reason for her sexual difficulty and only treatment which aims to help reach and understand the source of anxiety is really effective. If your own doctor does not know where you can find help, contact the Institute of Psychosexual Medicine who will be able to advise you.

Is it true that taking these hormones keeps you young?

Oestrogen does have a marked effect on the condition of the skin and connective tissues – just think about how the skin changes at puberty when oestrogen levels rise. When it is reduced during the menopause the skin becomes thinner and less elastic. This loss of elasticity may also mean that the breasts lose their shape. So the effect of oestrogen on the skin and connective tissue can help to keep a more youthful appearance.

However, it's worth bearing in mind that, until recently, most of the women who had HRT were those who had enough money to pay for it. They would also have had more money to spend on clothes, make-up, hair-care, etc., and have been more cushioned from the hard economic pressures of work and family raising which can contribute a lot to 'ageing'. Certainly the way a woman *feels* about herself is as important as her hormone status.

Decrease in oestrogen levels is also related to the gradual thinning of the bones which affects women as they get older; after the menopause calcium is lost from the bones at the rate of 1 per cent a year. This does not cause any immediate difficulty, but gradually makes women more likely to have fractures; which becomes more common around the age of 70.

HRT will stop the loss of calcium but only during the period of therapy. In fact, there can be an increased loss when treatment is stopped, so that the risk of fractures can only be reduced by prolonged therapy.

Can you get pregnant while you are having HRT?

It is possible to conceive while having hormone therapy. While a woman's oestrogen production may be sufficiently erratic to produce such symptoms as hot flushes, there may still be an occasional ovulation, which makes pregnancy possible. HRT does not suppress this. The oldest age of conception in the Guinness Book of Records is 57 years. It is always advisable to continue contraception until two years after the last period when this occurs before the age of 50, and one year when it is over 50 years.

There is no reason why an IUD cannot be left in the womb until contraception is no longer needed, provided there is no irregular or heavy bleeding, but it should then be removed. If a progestogen-only pill is used as a contraceptive, the doctor has to take this into account in HRT,

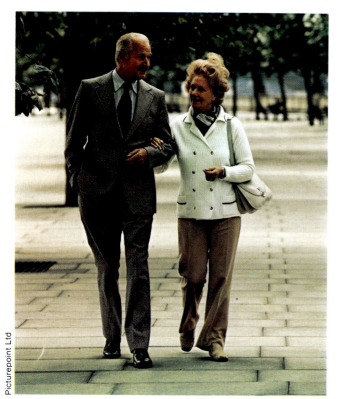

Picturepoint Ltd

On the other hand, women during the reproductive years, when oestrogens are naturally present, show a lower incidence of coronary heart attacks compared with men of the same age. After the menopause the rate rises to become equal, suggesting that natural oestrogens do protect against heart attacks.

For this reason it may be that HRT, in which *natural* oestrogens are used, protects against coronary thrombosis, because it restores a woman to her pre-menopausal state.

Does hormone therapy make the change of life easier, or does it only put it off?

Because hormone therapy can alleviate some of the acute symptoms of the menopause, it will help to restore a woman's confidence and prevent her from feeling at the mercy of her hormones. By gradually reducing the dosage, the treatment can often be stopped without the symptoms returning. But the caring attention that a woman receives during the treatment can often play just as vital a role, helping her to come to terms with the fact that some changes are inevitable as we grow older – and that, however regrettable, ageing cannot be put off forever.

So, although HRT can relieve the bodily symptoms, she may well need sympathetic counselling help with the more emotional causes of distress. It's interesting that studies have shown that single 'full-time' working women suffer from fewer complaints during the menopause, so it seems important for a woman to develop some new worthwhile occupations to hold her interest during these years.

because the therapy may contain a dose of progestogen in the second half of the cycle.

How safe is hormone therapy?

A doctor has to bear in mind some possible risks when prescribing oestrogen treatment – although in some areas the evidence is still rather confused.

Oestrogens are thought to affect the rate of growth of breast cancer, which is why the ovaries are often removed in those who suffer from this disease. HRT must *never* be given to a woman who has had breast cancer before the menopause, but there is no suggestion that HRT *causes* cancer of the breast in women.

There has been anxiety about the effect of giving oestrogen on the lining of the womb, especially when it is no longer shed at regular intervals during menstruation. This is why oestrogens are now usually given combined with progestogens for part of the cycle, to encourage a regular monthly bleeding from the womb. Any woman taking hormones should have tests to check that there is no abnormal thickening of the cells of the womb lining, which could later develop into cancer.

The connection between oestrogen and heart attacks is confused. Studies of patients taking oral contraceptives, containing synthetic oestrogens, have shown that they increase the risk of a coronary thrombosis, especially in the overweight woman, who is already liable to attacks.

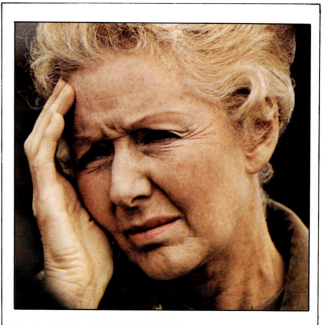

J. Allan Ltd

CHAPTER 2

Contraception

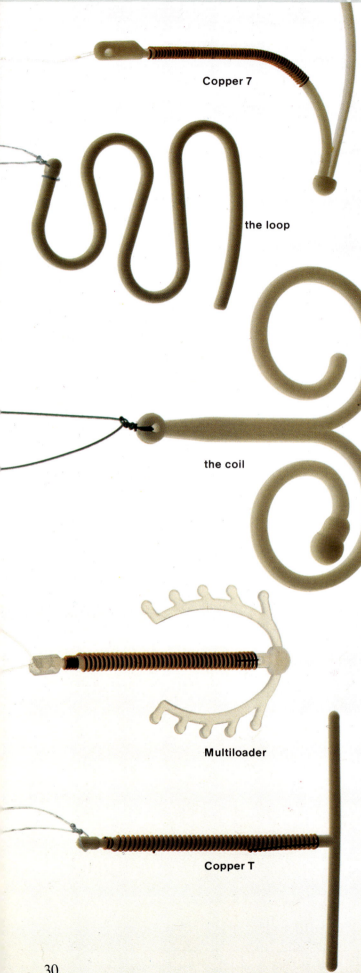

Copper 7

the loop

the coil

Multiloader

Copper T

The IUD

The IUD is the third most popular contraceptive after the Pill and the sheath. It's a small, flexible piece of plastic, between 2 and 4 centimetres long which sits in your womb. IUD stands for *intra-uterine device*, meaning a device inside the womb, but the more common names for it are the 'coil' or 'loop'. These were the original shapes of the IUD when it was first introduced.

Nowadays, they come in various shapes and sizes. Some have copper wound round the plastic, which is released into the womb in small amounts. These types are usually replaced every two or two and a half years, while the ones without copper can be worn indefinitely. They all have threads which hang down into the vagina so that they can be removed easily.

How does an IUD work?

The presence of an IUD causes the cells in the lining of the womb to change in some way; this change discourages a fertilized egg from embedding there. If an egg does manage to implant itself, the presence of the IUD usually prevents it developing very far.

No one knows precisely how the change is caused, but we do know that any foreign body in the womb produces the same response as an infection. The production of cells which fight unwanted organisms is stepped up and it may be these cells which make the womb lining unsuitable for the fertilized egg. Copper is used in some IUDs because it is thought to have an extra effect in making these cells accumulate.

The IUD may also cause change in the lining of the Fallopian tubes so that the egg travels down more quickly and misses the time when the womb is ready for it. Whatever its mode of action, it is effective immediately.

30

Is it true IUDs can only be used by a woman who has had a child?

This used to be true when only the larger IUDs were available. These were difficult to insert unless the entrance to the womb has been stretched by pregnancy. More recently, the smaller copper-wound types have been developed which overcome this problem.

But an IUD still may not be recommended as the first choice of method if you are young and have never been pregnant. Younger women are particularly fertile and some may feel they want greater protection than the IUD gives; in this case they are likely to prefer the most reliable method available – the combined Pill. Also, younger women who have a variety of sexual partners run a higher risk of pelvic infections, from which twice as many IUD users as Pill users suffer.

The IUD is most popular with women who have had at least one pregnancy and would not mind another child if the device failed. It's also popular with women in their mid-thirties who wish to come off the Pill and who don't fancy the idea of the cap or sheath. They are less fertile at this age so the risk of pregnancy is reduced. For young girls, who have no history of pelvic infection and who wish to use an IUD, the copper-wound types are more suitable than the all-plastic Loop or Coil.

How reliable is an IUD?

IUDs are considered to be 98 percent effective, which is about the same as the mini Pill and just a bit more reliable than the cap or sheath. These theoretical figures are based on each method being used perfectly. If, instead, you take into account lapses such as forgetting to take the Pill, or not using the sheath correctly, then the chances of becoming pregnant increases for every method except the IUD; once it's in, there's nothing you have to remember to do.

But the reliability of IUDs does vary. No one type is better than any other, but the skill with which they are inserted makes a difference. If the device is not pushed up far enough into the womb it won't be so efficient. IUDs also tend to be more successful with older women because they are less fertile and with women who have had earlier pregnancies, because their wombs are less sensitive and don't try to eject the device.

Sometimes the IUD comes out of the womb of its own accord. This 'expulsion' usually happens, if it's going to happen at all, within six weeks from the fitting, often during or just after your period. It's a good idea for a woman to learn to feel the threads or 'tail' of the IUD in her vagina.

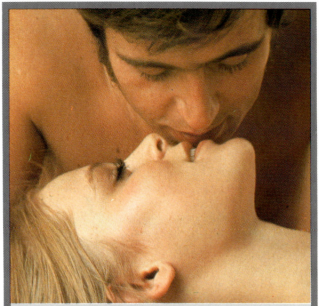

Facts on different types of IUD

The risk of pregnancy and the likelihood of an IUD being expelled or having to be removed due to pain or bleeding are very low, but the devices do vary in these respects, as trials have shown (see below). A doctor's recommendation will be based on this information in conjunction with a woman's medical background, whether or not she has children, and her age.

Multiload*

Low pregnancy and expulsion rates. Removal rate due to pain and/or bleeding also low.

Copper 7

Very easy to fit. Removal rate due to bleeding and/or pain lower than for most other devices, but pregnancy rate is higher than others. It has the highest expulsion rate for all IUDs.

Copper T+

Easy to fit. Has a very low expulsion and removal rate in comparison with all other devices. The risk of pregnancy is also low, but seem to increase with continued use. May need replacing after two years.

The Coil

Pregnancy rate lower than Copper 7, higher than Copper T but the same as the Loop. Expulsion rate, too, is higher than the Copper T, but can be compared with the Loop and Copper 7. The Coil has the highest rate of removal.

Loop (various types)

Has a low pregnancy rate – only the Copper T's is lower. Expulsion rates compare with the Copper T, but are higher than the Coil or Copper 7. Has a low removal rate.

★ information based on preliminary trials only
+ still relatively new, results may be revised

If you check this regularly it reduces the risk of losing the IUD without realizing – and possibly getting pregnant as a result.

How is the IUD inserted and taken out?

An IUD should be fitted by a specially trained doctor. It is usually done at a hospital or family planning clinic. Your own doctor may be qualified to do it, but if not he will advise you where to go.

You will probably be asked if your periods are regular, whether they tend to be heavy and whether there is any chance that you might be pregnant. Often doctors prefer to insert the IUD during your period to be sure that you're not pregnant. You should mention any history of infections in the pelvic area. The doctor will give you an internal examination and take a smear test and then your womb will be 'sounded'. This involves a thin feeler which is inserted into the womb to determine its exact depth and position so that the right sized IUD can be chosen for you. You may feel some general discomfort while this is being done, but you don't feel the instrument.

The IUD is then straightened into a thin tube which is pushed up through the cervical canal into the womb. The IUD is released and springs back into shape, resting against the walls of the womb. The tube is pulled out and the strings of the IUD are trimmed so that about three centimetres are left hanging down. The whole procedure only takes a few minutes.

Some women feel nothing at all, some feel the twang as the IUD is released and others find it uncomfortable but not painful. It is similar to having a smear taken – if you are completely relaxed, you hardly feel a thing, but if you are tense it can be a bit unpleasant. A little bleeding often occurs just after the fitting along with mild tummy cramp or back ache, but these don't last.

The IUD can be removed very simply by pulling the strings with a special instrument. This must always be done by a doctor – you should never attempt it yourself.

What are the benefits of this method of contraception?

These really depend on your own priorities and personal medical history. The great advantage of the IUD is that it is always in place when needed. You don't have to put a stop to lovemaking while you insert your cap or he puts on a sheath, neither do you have to remember to take a Pill regularly. Sex can be completely spontaneous. Although you should have regular check-ups, you don't have to worry about supplies. And,

because the IUD is effective from the moment it's fitted, you don't have to use some extra protection initially, as you do on the Pill.

A unique feature of the IUD is that it can be used to make sure pregnancy won't occur as a result of having intercourse without using any contraceptive. This will work if the IUD is fitted up to three days after intercourse.

Do many women have to give up because of pain or bleeding?

Each year, about one in 10 women fitted with an IUD abandons it because of pain and bleeding. The first six or 12 weeks after fitting are when problems are most likely to occur. You may bleed between periods and the periods themselves are likely to be heavier and sometimes more painful than before, although their regularity is not normally affected. You may suffer cramps and low back pain in the first weeks.

At your first check-up, which is usually about six weeks after the fitting, you should mention any pain and difficulties with your periods to the doctor. If increased bleeding is a problem he may recommend various treatments for reducing it. If these do not work or the pain continues, he may change the device for a different sort which is a better size and shape for you. Larger IUDs tend to cause more trouble than the smaller ones. But on the whole, periods settle down again and the pains disappear after two months.

Some women give up the IUD because they lose faith in it after it has been expelled once. The expulsion rates for the different types are all very similar but it may be that your womb particularly dislikes one shape or size, so a change may help. But obviously if you constantly worry about the possibility that the IUD has been expelled, you may find another method suits you better.

Can you use tampons if you have an IUD?

Yes you can. Your doctor may suggest not using them until after your first check-up, but after that there should be no problems. You may find you have to use the super-absorbant type. If you do, it's important to change them frequently.

What are the dangers of IUDs?

It's rare for IUDs to cause serious problems but any complications that do arise can be treated. The most common one is pelvic inflammatory disease (PID) — infections of the womb, ovaries, Fallopian tubes or cervix. Sometimes an infection is caught during the insertion of the IUD, or at a

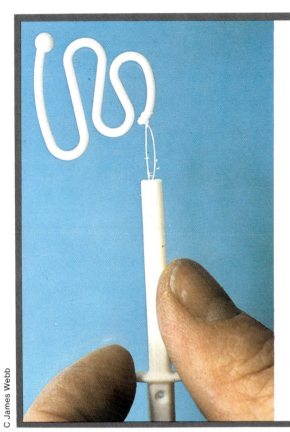

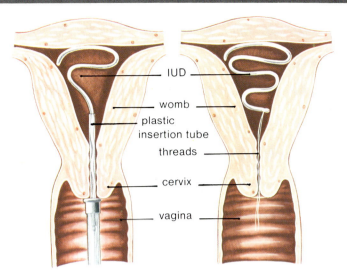

IUD
womb
plastic insertion tube
threads
cervix
vagina

For insertion, the IUD is housed inside a plastic tube fitted with a plunger. Holding the vagina open with a speculum, the doctor will first clean the area thoroughly, to make sure no germs get into the womb, and then push the tube gently through the cervical canal. Once the tip has reached the womb, the doctor gently pushes the plunger down to expel the IUD, which quickly resumes its true shape. The threads are left hanging through into the vagina. The whole operation takes only a few minutes.

later stage, an infection in the vagina can be drawn up into the womb via the IUD's threads. The problem seems to be more common with women who have several sexual partners.

PID can lead to abscesses developing in any of these organs and can result in sterility. Any unusual vaginal discharge, pain after intercourse or abdominal pain especially if it is accompanied by fever, should be reported to your doctor immediately. PID needs prompt treatment with antibiotics. If it does not clear up in a few days then the IUD will be removed.

Some women who have used an IUD for a long period catch a fungal infection, *pelvic actinomycosis*. This can have the same consequencies as PID but it doesn't always produce noticeable symptoms. If you notice any change, you should see your doctor who will take a swab.

Another rare complication is perforation of the womb or cervix by the IUD. This means that the device has been pushed through the walls of the womb, or very occasionally through the cervix, and an operation may be necessary to remove it. Perforation may cause pain but there are no definite symptoms. When it occurs the IUD user is no longer protected against pregnancy. The problem is usually discovered when the threads of the IUD cannot be felt in the vagina. This is one reason why you should always consult your doctor if you can't feel the strings.

There has been a great deal of publicity about one particular IUD which was withdrawn from the market in 1975. It is called the Dalkon Shield, and anyone still using one should have it removed even if it has caused no trouble. There have been a number of reports of serious risks associated with it. This may have worried many women about the safety of IUDs in general. But in reality IUDs carry very low risks to health.

What happens if you get pregnant while you still have an IUD?

If you are unlucky enough to become pregnant with an IUD in place there can be complications, so it is important to visit your doctor if you are ever 14 days overdue for a period. If a pregnancy test is positive and the strings of the IUD are visible, it may be possible to remove it if you decide to go ahead with the pregnancy. Miscarriages are more likely if the IUD is left inside the womb.

About one in twenty IUD pregnancies are 'ectopic'. This means that the foetus develops not in the womb but in one of the Fallopian tubes. Although it happens rarely, it is a dangerous condition, and one of the symptoms is acute abdominal pain. So any pain occuring after a delayed, light or missed period should be reported to a doctor at once.

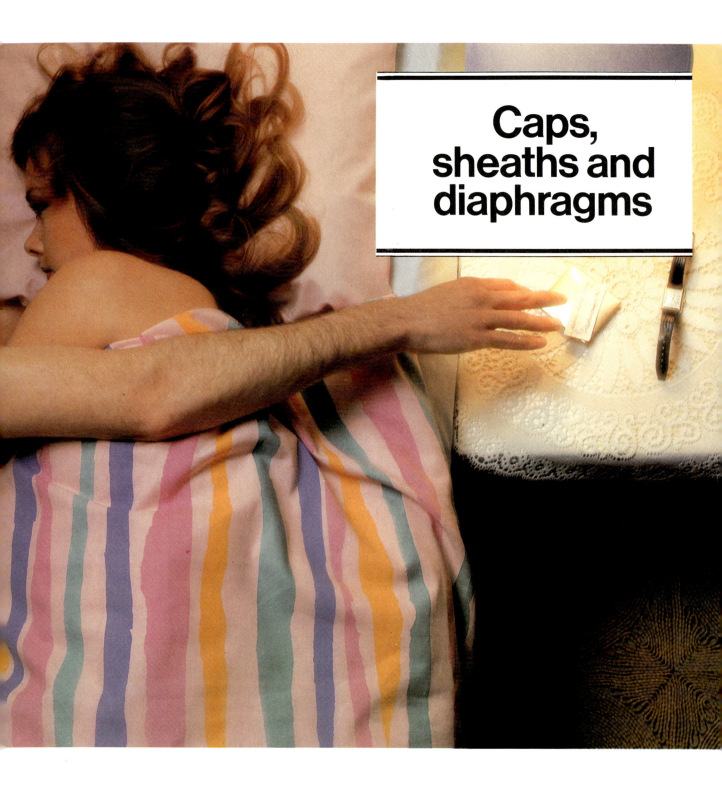

Caps, sheaths and diaphragms

Barrier methods of birth control are among the oldest practised. Certainly until the advent of the Pill some 20 years ago, the condom or sheath was, in fact, the most commonly used contraceptive device. Although the choice of contraceptives has grown enormously, the sheath is still an extremely popular method of birth control in Britain, and the diaphragm or 'cap' is widely used by women who cannot or do not want to use the Pill or IUD.

What is the proper way to use a condom? Are they safe to use on their own?

A condom, variously known as a sheath, johnny, french letter, rubber or durex, is a close-fitting covering which slips over the whole of the erect penis and collects the semen as the man ejaculates. Usually it has a teat shaped tip to hold the semen safely so that it doesn't seep down the sides and cause the sheath to slip off.

Family planning experts recommend using some sort of *spermicide* – a chemical which destroys sperms, but is otherwise not harmful – at the same time as a condom to give extra protection in case it should tear or leak at all. Some types of condom are sold together with spermicidal pessaries, and a few modern sheaths are covered in a lubricant which contains a spermicide.

There isn't total agreement among the experts about the need for spermicides or how effective they would be if the sheath did tear. One survey of condom users found sheaths were 96 per cent effective when used alone – among every 100 couples using this method for a year, only four pregnancies occurred. Many sheath users probably don't use a spermicide as well, but to be on the safe side, it is advisable to do so.

Although almost all modern sheaths are lubricated, it is a good idea to use some sort of additional lubricant to prevent the woman feeling sore from the friction of the rubber and to decrease the chances of the sheath tearing. Never use vaseline or any greasy non-spermicidal creams or oils – they can damage the rubber of the sheath, and tend to dry up the vagina's own natural lubrication. If a woman uses some sort of spermicidal foam or jelly it will also work as a lubricant.

Although properly tested sheaths (in Britain these can be identified by a kite-mark on the package) are usually very reliable, it's important to learn how to put them on before intercourse, and how to take them off afterwards.

Begin by holding the tip of the rolled up condom (they are packed already rolled) carefully between the thumb and forefinger to squeeze out any trapped air. Beware of those fingernails! If the woman is helping her partner to put it on she should do so from behind him, as then she's less likely to catch the sheath on her thumbnails from that position.

Next, place the condom's opening on the head of the erect penis and unroll it all the way to the base. If by any chance the sheath does not have a specially shaped tip, then leave about half-an-inch of sheath loose in front of the penis head to collect the semen.

After intercourse, the man should withdraw as soon as possible after actual ejaculation so that no semen leaks into the vagina when his erection subsides, and he should hold the sheath against the base of the penis (to prevent it from slipping off as he withdraws). The sheath is then disposed of; never try to use one twice. Also, be sure to keep sheaths away from heat as this will cause the rubber to deteriorate and weaken.

Are sheaths really one of the most reliable methods of contraception?

Properly tested sheaths used carefully with a spermicide have a success rate of 96 to 97 per cent – about the same as the success rate of the diaphragm, and just under the reliability rate for the IUD or mini-pill.

Tested sheaths are available shaped and unshaped and in a variety of colours. When they bear a standard mark to show that they have been carefully made and tested, they are reliable; but similar devices (usually sold as sex aids to stimulate the woman) are not effective contraceptives. Neither are the short condoms, sometimes called 'American tips', which only cover the head of the penis.

Sheaths come in packets of three, six, or more – but there are no special sizes made for fit. Always check the date they were made on the packet. If left unopened in a cool place, sheaths should be good for about two years.

What are the advantages of condoms?

Many people prefer to use condoms rather than other methods of birth control because they have virtually no side effects, and are no risk to health. Unlike hormonal methods of contraception and IUDs, condoms don't interfere with the body's internal chemistry, nor do they have to be used continuously, but only when needed.

They don't require any prescription, fitting or medical examination, or any discussion with doctors or nurses about intimate sexual details.

Furthermore, they are easy to obtain, and not too costly. They can be bought at chemists, by mail order or from special slot machines. They should also be available free from family planning clinics, but GPs do not supply them.

Further benefits of using condoms are that they can give some protection against sexually transmitted diseases, such as gonorrhoea and genital herpes, and that they may protect women against cancer of the cervix.

Are there any drawbacks to using sheaths? Does it lessen pleasure for both partners?

Naturally every method of contraception is apt to have drawbacks for some people and sheaths are no exception. A very few people will be allergic to the rubber from which they are made. But today, it's quite easy to buy special non-allergy sheaths – a chemist can advise you. A few women may be allergic to the lubricant with which the pre-packed condoms are coated. Changing to

TYPE OF CONTRACEPTIVE	Diaphragm & spermicide	Cervical cap & spermicide
Rate of success	97 per cent	96-97 per cent
Advantages	Not felt during intercourse. May offer some protection against cancer of the cervix.	As for diaphragm & spermicide.
Disadvantages	Cream needs to be applied before each act of intercourse. Needs to be fitted professionally and should be checked regularly for fit. Occasionally people are allergic to rubber and there is a greater chance of suffering from cystitis.	As for diaphragm & spermicide, but not as easy to position as a diaphragm.

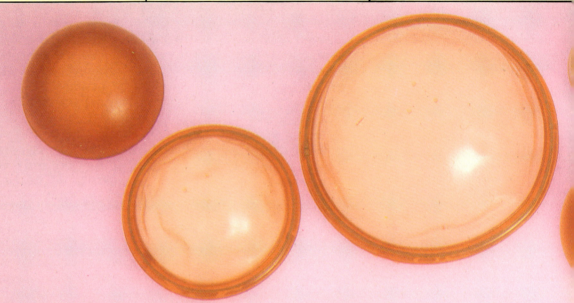

un-coated ones, and using a separate lubricant may cure this problem.

For the remainder of people, the drawbacks are mainly a matter of habits in love making and aesthetics. Some couples say that they feel embarrassed or 'turned off' by having to stop during foreplay and have the man put the sheath on. If the method is otherwise suitable, you may overcome this disadvantage by making the process part of love play with the woman putting the sheath on the man before he enters her.

Another complaint from both men and women is that the need for the man to withdraw immediately and carefully after he has ejaculated spoils their sense of contentment and well being after orgasm. A few men find that they tend to lose their erection when the sheath is rolled on. Even if they can be stimulated to erection again, the method is not a good one for them.

Many couples dislike using sheaths, no matter how fine in texture, because they complain that they dull sensation. However, a new 'ribbed' condom is now available which, some people report, increases sensation and is still an effective contraceptive.

It's also worth noting that some men who have a tendency to premature ejaculation actually prefer to use a condom because the reduced sensitivity they experience delays their climax, and so gives the woman more time to reach her orgasm.

What you feel about the loss of sensation and how important it is to you is very personal, and will decide your own attitude to the sheath.

What is the cap or diaphragm?

Caps come in a variety of types, but they all perform the same function – of forming a barrier across the opening of the *cervix* (neck of the womb), to keep sperms from reaching the womb and fertilizing the egg in the fallopian tube. Again, as an added precaution, a spermicidal preparation *must* be used.

Is it complicated to fit a cap?

Since all types of caps must fit correctly to be effective, you will need to consult a doctor or family planning clinic for an individual fitting and for instructions on use.

At a clinic the doctor or trained nurse will examine you, and probably try fitting one or two caps before finding your size. Diaphragms are

...heath	Sheath & spermicide	Spermicide in various forms
...5 per cent	96-97 per cent	80 per cent
...ves some protection against sexually ...ansmitted diseases and is easy to ...rry around with you.	As for sheath on its own but not as convenient to carry around. Gives added protection.	Easy to use.
...eeds to be put on during full erection ...hich can disrupt lovemaking and puts ...me people off. Felt during intercourse ...d can be uncomfortable. Man needs ...withdraw immediately after ...tercourse.	As for sheath on its own.	Not recommended from a reliability point of view. Can be messy.

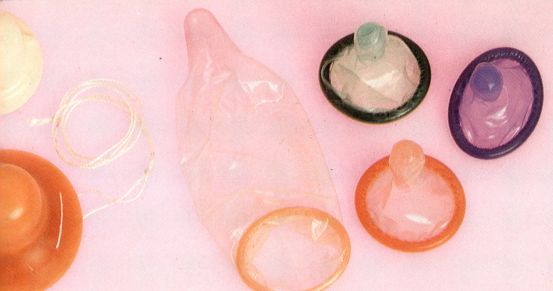

Simon Butcher

probably the easiest to use, and are by far the most common. You will be shown how to use them with a spermicide, and then asked to practice the method at home – using additional means of birth control during this time.

You will be asked to return after a week with the diaphragm in place when a check will be made to be sure you are putting it in correctly. After that you'll need to return about every six months for a check on size and for weaknesses. If you gain or lose more than seven pounds in weight, have a baby, a miscarriage or a termination, you must have a check-up to see if you need a different size. Most women can use a diaphragm, even those who haven't made love before.

How do you insert a diaphragm? Do you have to use a spermicide with it?

Yes, you should always use a spermicide with the diaphragm or any cap as the 'fail-safe' precaution to avoid pregnancy. You will need to remember that the spermicide only stays active for a limited time. Inserting a diaphragm takes a little practice but it is not hard to do. Always use a recommended spermicidal cream or jelly. Apply two one- or two-inch strips of the spermicide on each side of the cap, and with your finger spread it so that it covers the cap. Smear a little around the rim of the cap to make insertion easier. Then squeeze the diaphragm into a long, thin shape, and either squat, or rest one foot on a low stool, to make insertion simpler. With your free hand, open the lips of the vagina and slide the cap up until the rim rests behind the pubic bone at the front and the rubber dome covers the cervix at the back. If you have a bath before intercourse, you should put in your cap after your bath rather than before it.

You can put in the cap and spermicide any time before making love – many women do so every evening as a matter of course. If you have intercourse more than three hours after inserting the diaphragm, you need to put more spermicidal cream, jelly, foam, or another pessary into the vagina before doing so. Moreover, before each additional time that you have intercourse, you must add more spermicide – and, most importantly, you must not remove the cap for *at least six hours after* the last intercourse.

You can leave a cap in place for up to 24 hours. After taking it out, you should wash it in warm water with mild soap and dry it carefully. Check it for tiny holes periodically.

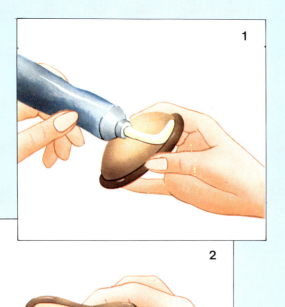

Creams, caps and diaphragms

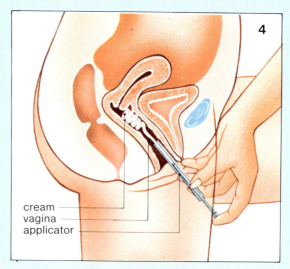

cream
vagina
applicator

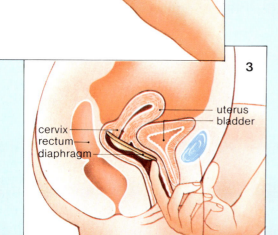

uterus
bladder

cervix
rectum
diaphragm

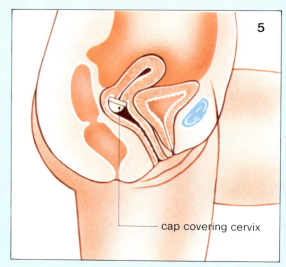

cap covering cervix

Dee McLean

1 *Before insertion, two strips of one to two inches of spermicidal cream should be smeared each side of the diaphragm or cap.*

2 *Squeezing a diaphragm into the correct shape for insertion.*

3 *The diaphragm should fit closely against the cervix so that sperms are blocked from entering the uterus.*

4 *Make sure to insert cream deep into the vagina so that the cervix is covered.*

5 *A cervical cap covers the cervix and works in the same way as a diaphragm but, being much smaller, some people find it more difficult to position.*

Types of caps available

The most common variety of cap is known as the *Dutch cap* or *diaphragm*. It consists of a shallow rubber bowl (or dome depending on how you look at it) with a flexible rim that allows the device to 'spring' back into shape once it is placed in the vagina. When it is in position, it fits above and behind the pubic bone with the dome covering the cervix and the spring rim fitting smoothly against the walls of the vagina. As women vary in their internal size and shape, different sizes of diaphragms are made, and an individual fitting is required.

The *cervical cap* cap is much smaller than a diaphragm and looks a bit like a thimble with a thick rim. It fits snugly over the cervix rather than across it. Although it is flexible, it has no spring in the rim as does the diaphragm, and so is harder to insert and remove. Two long threads can be attached to the rim to make withdrawal easier.

Other caps, namely the *vault (Dumas)*, *Prencap* and *vimule* are held in place by suction; to remove them you must insert your fingers under the rim to break the suction, which again may be awkward for some women to manage. Each of these types has a slightly different shape and are often recommended to women who have either lax vaginal muscles – perhaps after childbirth – or cannot retain a diaphragm because of the position of their cervix. All of these other types of caps require careful individual fitting by a doctor or a trained nurse.

What are the advantages of the diaphragm?

The main advantages of the cap are its reliability (97 per cent when used with spermicide) and the fact that almost any woman of any age can use it without suffering side effects or long-term medical risks. Also, there is some evidence that, like the sheath, it gives a woman some protection against cancer of the cervix.

If you use it properly there will be no chance of infection, irritation or smelly discharges. But these could happen, just as with tampons, if you leave the cap in for too long, or do not wash and dry it carefully.

Neither the woman nor the man should be able to feel the diaphragm during love-making, and it is very rare for it to become dislodged – even in the most vigorous love-making. If you or your partner do feel any discomfort, you should check whether you have put the cap in correctly:

if not, and your cervix is uncovered, you should insert some spermicidal cream into your vagina at once. You should also return to your doctor or clinic for the fitting to be re-checked.

One further advantage of the cap for some couples is that you can use it safely to hold back the menstrual flow during a period, and so make intercourse at this time more pleasant.

Are there any drawbacks to this method?

The main drawbacks to using the diaphragm are having to be more calculating about your love-making – remembering to put it in ahead of time, and then adding more spermicide every time you have intercourse – and you can't be squeamish about your body. Putting in and taking out a cap can be a rather messy business, and many a new recruit has found herself chasing a jellied diaphragm across the bathroom floor, despairing of every mastering it! But large numbers of women *do,* and in a pretty short time, so you must weigh carefully the drawbacks and the advantages, and not give up in a hurry.

Of course, some women will not find the cap suitable — those who suffer from the very rare rubber allergy, for instance, or those who suffer from regular, serious bouts of cystitis (see later chapter). There may be a greater chance of suffering from cystitis if you wear a diaphragm, either because it presses on the outlet from the bladder, or because you can't ensure that it is completely sterile, although one of the newer kinds, the 'arching spring' diaphragm is reputedly less likely to provoke cystitis attacks.

An allergy to spermicide is much more likely to occur than one to rubber, and the symptoms may appear to be very similar – soreness and sometimes a rash or redness. This is usually caused by the cream or jelly in which the spermicide is contained, so changing to another recommended brand solves the problem for most women, but if you are allergic to the spermicide ingredient itself, you may be unable to use this method.

Can you use spermicides safely on their own?

No. None of them is reliable as a contraceptive if used alone – the rate quoted is a failure of about 20 in 100 users per year. However, if you discover after intercourse that a sheath has leaked or torn, you can cut down the risk of pregnancy by *immediately* placing fairly generous amounts of spermicidal cream or foam or a spermicidal pessary high up in your vagina. However, this is by no means foolproof.

39

Natural family planning

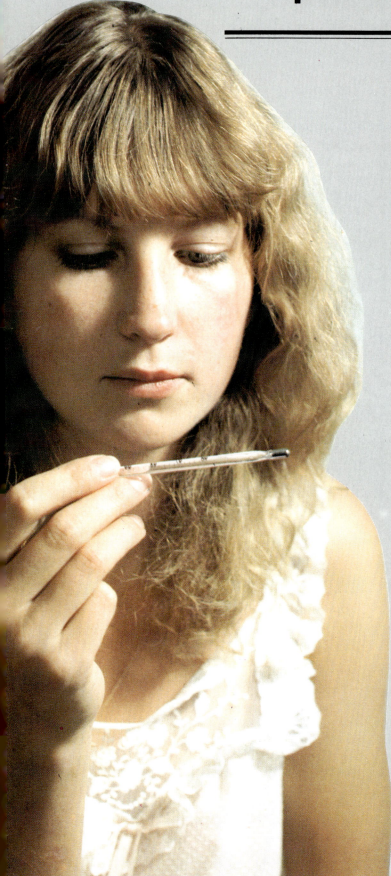

Natural family planning is more than a method of birth control – it's a way of life based on the biological fact that women are only able to conceive on certain days in the month. Its success depends on a couple avoiding sexual intercourse during the fertile days of the woman's cycle. Its main drawback is that predicting the precise time of fertility is extremely difficult and involves some rather complicated calculations.

Although there are today several more effective methods of contraception readily available, some people will still choose to use natural methods of family planning. They include those with religious objections, those who dislike interfering with their natural bodily functions (either with hormones or mechanical aids) and are not too worried about becoming pregnant, and those who find that other methods produce unacceptable complications or side-effects.

One further feature of NFP is that both partners can share control over their fertility – and the method is unique in that it can help couples wishing to conceive, by indicating the best times to have intercourse to achieve a pregnancy.

Anthea Sieveking/Vision International

What is natural family planning? Is it different from the 'rhythm method'?

The traditional terms 'rhythm method' or 'safe period' used to describe types of birth control based on periodic sexual abstinence have been replaced in recent years by the term 'natural family planning'. The overall aim of NFP is to teach couples to recognize the beginning and end of the woman's fertile days so that they only have intercourse during the 'safe' times when pregnancy is unlikely to occur.

In a typical menstrual cycle (which varies between 20 to 36 days from woman to woman) the ovary releases one egg about 12 to 16 days before the next period is due. This is the fertile phase – called ovulation – when sexual intercourse is most likely to lead to pregnancy. The egg remains in the fallopian tube ready to be fertilized for about two days, and the man's sperm can survive in the woman's body for up to five days. It can be seen, then, that to avoid getting pregnant, you must not have sexual intercourse for several days before and after ovulation. However, the precise times will differ depending upon which of the four main NFP methods a couple chooses to use: the *calendar* method, the *temperature* method, the *Billings* (or ovulation) method, or the *sympto-thermal* method (combining different techniques).

How effective is natural family planning?

While the various methods may sound fine in theory, actual clinical trials have shown that in practice, failure rates can be high indeed. As with any method of contraception, some failures must be expected, but with NFP methods, the rates are rather higher than with the chemical or mechanical methods, probably for two main reasons. First, there is still a great deal that is unknown about the precise workings of the reproductive system, and predicting the exact times of fertility is still not accurate. As you will notice, the 'safe' times in the month even differ slightly according to the method you are using – calendar, temperature or Billings. Secondly, both partners need to be highly motivated to avoid pregnancy as the various methods can be complicated to work out and, of course, mean that a thoroughly spontaneous sex-life is impossible.

Statistically, reported failure rates using the Billings method alone vary widely – from 15 to a staggering 39 per cent per year. This means that if you use this one method alone, you risk between 15 and 39 chances out of 100 of becoming pregnant in any one year. In contrast,

clinical trials using the sympto-thermal method show a much-reduced failure rate – an average of 8 per cent. There is no doubt, then, that combining methods will considerably improve protection against conception.

What effect does NFP have on a couple's sex life?

Defining the effects of natural family planning methods on a couple's relationship is nearly as difficult as trying to generalize about how to practise the methods for large numbers of

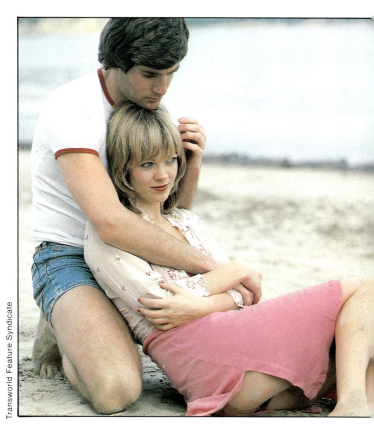

Transworld Feature Syndicate

women – the individual holds the key to success.

As mentioned earlier, a spontaneous or casual sex life is simply not possible, as long periods of sexual abstinence are required to make the methods work. Although both partners take equal responsibility about when they need to abstain, inevitably there'll be times when desire conflicts with this. The strains on both partners, if this occurs often, will soon be evident.

Some studies of female sexuality have suggested further, that women reach their peak of sexual desire around the time they ovulate. If this is so in your case, you may well find it is just too inhibiting to have to limit your sexual fulfilment to such an extent. Anxiety about becoming pregnant, even on 'safe' days, may also interfere with sexual fulfilment.

On the other hand, some people will find that by having to be closely in tune with one another physically, they may grow closer in other aspects of their relationship, and learn to express their love without full intercourse by exploring other ways of giving and receiving intimate sexual pleasure. Some advocates of NFP claim that periods of abstinence can lead to a greater appreciation of the quality of sexual intercourse that they do enjoy. And, of course, since you do not have to use any form of mechanical device during actual love-making, you may feel a greater sense of sexual freedom.

Are there any dangers or side-effects as with some other contraceptive measures?

One big advantage of NFP methods over other chemical, hormonal or mechanical means of contraception is the absence of physical side-effects. However, it must be noted that recently scientists have been conducting more detailed studies of NFP methods in a search to perfect them and to determine more specifically if there are any possible long-term side-effects.

One factor which has come to light concerns the occurrence of an unplanned pregnancy. It appears from studies of animals, and from birth statistics in largely Catholic countries where NFP

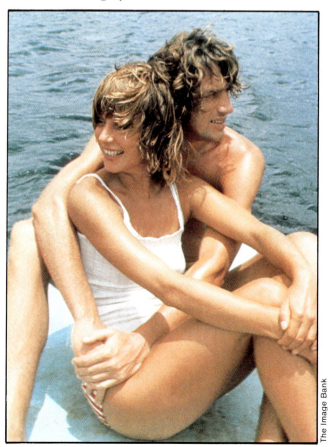

The Image Bank

is widely practised, that the birth of a congenitally abnormal child might be more apt to occur if conception happens between an ageing ovum or a deteriorating sperm. However, many doctors disagree with this theory. Certainly, at this stage it is merely an interesting speculation with no conclusive evidence yet found to back it up. Research into NFP methods continues all the time.

How can you decide whether NFP is suitable for you? How can you learn to use it?

If you are trying to find a suitable method of contraception and are in general good health, most experts would not recommend NFP methods to you as a first choice – the scope for error with them is still fairly great. However, if you have found that other methods really do not suit you and if you can realistically accept the higher risks of pregnancy involved, then these methods may be just right for you.

An older woman with perhaps one or two children already who feels she wants to stop taking the Pill as the risks to her health increase, may find that she and her husband can use NFP without much difficulty – especially if a further pregnancy would not be a disaster for them.

However, a young, single woman could find them practically impossible to implement, and an older woman beginning to go through the menopausal changes would most likely find it difficult to use the normal indicators – i.e. temperature shift or mucus change – with any certainty. Women who have recently given birth will find difficulties for similar reasons – their bodily functions are likely to be very changeable. If you have very irregular periods or unusual difficulties with menstruation, you would be better advised to try another method of contraception if possible.

For those who do choose NFP, learning how to practise the methods requires individual tuition and cannot be done solely by following instructions in a book. Most local family planning clinics now can provide some of the necessary advice and information, but are likely to refer you to special tutors.

These tutors, who are available in many areas, can give each couple specific training – especially in interpreting mucus changes and temperature charts. They are helpful in providing moral support for both partners, and are essential for those women who must use NFP, perhaps for religious reasons, and who have various irregularities in their reproductive functions – after childbirth, menopause, etc.

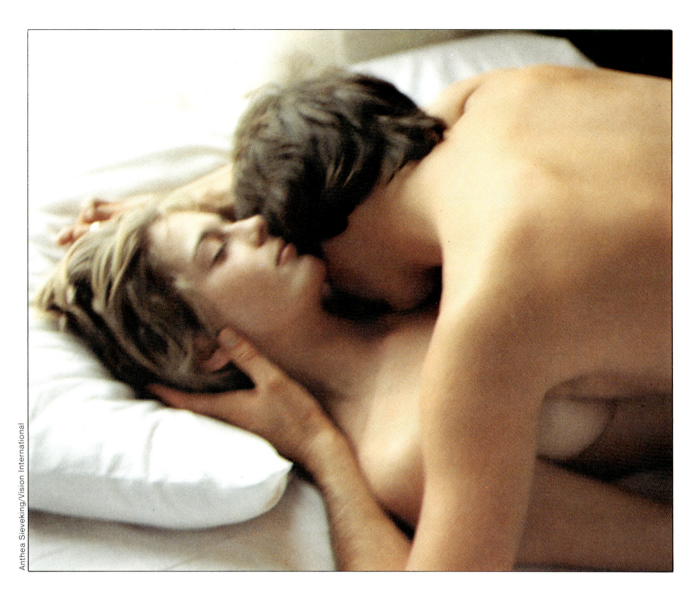

Are there any new NFP methods being developed for the future?

With the growing awareness of the possible long-term effects in other birth control methods – namely the Pill and IUD – scientists have been working much more on trying to find an aid that will accurately predict when a woman ovulates and becomes fertile. Many developments have come about as a result of studies done to help infertile couples. By and large they are still confined to the laboratory.

One such aid is known as a urine 'dip-stick'. This test involves dipping special paper into your urine daily. The colour of this paper will change as the amount of *luteinising hormone* in the urine increases. This hormone is one of several which are essential in the female reproductive cycle, and it is known that its level of production rises sharply just before ovulation. To date the test only detects when you have ovulated; it has not been proved accurate in predicting it. Home-

kits based on this finding are being investigated.

Another aid which has been developed, is known as an 'intelligent' thermometer. Basically it incorporates a computer memory bank so that a woman using the basal body temperature method need not rely on charts. She merely takes her temperature in the usual way and the machine will store the information and give her a green light go-ahead when three successive days of a temperature rise are noted and she is safely past her fertile phase. It includes a fail-safe mechanism for bouts of illness.

While in the future these devices may undoubtedly help users to practise NFP more effectively and scientifically, critics would question just how 'natural' it is to use a method that relies on abstinence for about half of each menstrual cycle, and requires daily observation and recording using calendars, charts, thermometers, graphs or other implements. But that aspect must be for couples to decide themselves, weighing the benefits against the disadvantages.

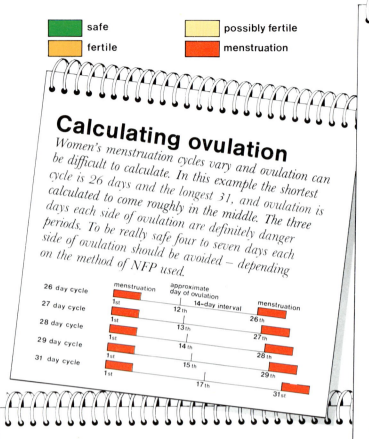

	safe
	fertile
	possibly fertile
	menstruation

Calculating ovulation

Women's menstruation cycles vary and ovulation can be difficult to calculate. In this example the shortest cycle is 26 days and the longest 31, and ovulation is calculated to come roughly in the middle. The three days each side of ovulation are definitely danger periods. To be really safe four to seven days each side of ovulation should be avoided – depending on the method of NFP used.

26 day cycle	menstruation	approximate day of ovulation	menstruation
27 day cycle	1st	14-day interval	26th
28 day cycle	1st	12th	27th
29 day cycle	1st	13th	28th
31 day cycle	1st	14th	29th
	1st	15th	31st
		17th	

The calendar method

The calendar method attempts to predict the time when a woman is fertile by noting the dates of her monthly periods and then predicting that ovulation will occur 14 days before each period begins. Needless to say it is the least precise of all methods, as no woman can be certain that her periods will follow a completely regular pattern and always begin at the time expected! The method can't be used until a woman has kept a record of her menstrual cycle for at least six, but preferably 12, months.

A further disadvantage with this method is that, since it is difficult to be precise, most advocates recommend that you do not have intercourse at all for at least seven days on either side of the time you ovulate. The reasoning is that since the man's sperms can live inside the woman's body for several days, intercourse should not take place for at least three days before ovulation, or they may still be able to fertilize the ripe egg. In addition you must allow at least two days after the release of the egg for it to pass out of your body (as it is microscopic in size, it passes out unseen through your vaginal secretions). To allow a safety margin for the actual time of ovulation, several days again are added either side of the predicted date – making a total of at least six days before and five days after your expected day of ovulation. For ease of calculation these are rounded up to seven days either side. If you find intercourse during actual menstruation unpleasant, that only leaves about eight or so days a month when intercourse is considered 'safe'!

Since the method uses a calendar to mark out the dates in a cycle, it is useful to give a woman a clearer picture of her menstrual pattern and, as such, it can be combined with other methods. However, you shouldn't use it as your only means of detecting fertility.

Sun		7	14	21	28
Mon	1	8	15	22	29
Tues	2	9	16	23	30
Wed	3	10	17	24	31
Thurs	4	11	18	25	
Fri	5	12	19	26	
Sat	6	13	20	27	

menstruation starts   ovulation

This shows a 28-day cycle with ovulation calculated as occuring 14 days after menstruation starts. The day you ovulate and the days crossed out – that is seven days before and after ovulation – are unsafe.

The temperature method

The temperature method is widely used; with it you learn to identify the small but definite drop and then immediate upward shift of body temperature which occurs when you ovulate. The reason for the temperature rise is thought to be due to the effect of the hormone progesterone which is released into the bloodstream in greater amounts around and after the time of ovulation. Since your temperature varies throughout the day, the basal body temperature (the body's temperature at rest) is measured. Ideally, a woman should record her temperature in the usual way, under the tongue, at the same time immediately on waking each morning – before getting out of bed, having a cup of tea or any other activity. An ordinary clinical thermometer can be used, although a special fertility thermometer, marked in tenths of a degree, is easier to read. Results are marked on a special chart. When charting the temperatures, it may be difficult to identify the very slight drop which occurs just prior to ovulation, so it is the temperature rise – only about 0.2°C (0.4°F) – which you must watch closely. It has been found that this rise occurs just after ovulation and stays at this higher level for 10-14 days, when it falls again just before the next menstrual period.

The rule of thumb is that you chart three consecutive daily temperatures at the higher level, before intercourse can be resumed on the fourth day.

Unfortunately, although this method is fairly accurate in helping you to know when ovulation has passed, it is of no help in predicting when it will take place. This means that you and your partner must wait until the second half of the cycle before you can safely have intercourse. Also, you have to be extra careful if you become ill or if you have a late night, drink alcohol, go on a holiday or become emotionally upset – as all these factors can cause a temperature shift which may lead you to think you have safely passed your fertile time.

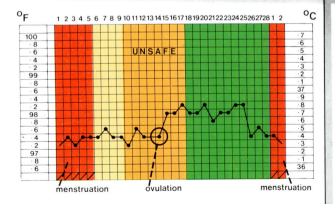

This shows a 28-day cycle with normal changes in temperature after ovulation.

Trevor Lawrence

The Billings or ovulation method

This method, named after the Australian doctor who developed it in its present form, teaches women how to examine their daily vaginal secretions to detect changes in the quality and quantity of cervical mucus. To date it provides the best means for a woman to predict when she is due to ovulate.

As a woman's monthly cycle progresses, the quantity, colour and consistency of the mucous secretions, the cervix alter – probably as a result of changes in the hormone levels of oestrogen and progesterone in the body. At the start of the month (that is the first day of menstrual bleeding) there is more oestrogen in the bloodstream; after ovulation, more progesterone.

In the earlier stages of the cycle, just after menstruation, there may be one or two 'dry' days with very little secretion evident. The normal discharge is thick and sticky during this time, forming a kind of plug in the cervix which impedes the passage of sperms. As ovulation approaches, the mucus increases in amount and becomes slippery and stretchy – rather like the texture of egg white. At this time a woman may notice a definite sensation of wetness or 'openness' in her vaginal area and she will be able to see this stretchy mucus quite easily. This clear, thinner secretion allows easy passage for the sperms to reach the egg. It will increase in amount up to what is known as the last, or peak day, which indicates that ovulation is imminent, before returning to a cloudier, thicker consistency and then to dryness up to the next period.

As soon as you detect any sign of this clear, stretchy mucus, you must abstain from intercourse and continue to do so until four successive days after its 'peak'. It's important to remember, if you're using this method, that the term 'peak' does not refer to the amount of this stretchy mucus, but to the last day on which you can detect any evidence of it – no matter how small the amount.

From the fourth day after the 'peak' until menstruation (in a 28-day cycle, this would be about 10 days) a woman is considered to be infertile and can safely enjoy intercourse without risk of pregnancy.

However, when using this method, it is not considered safe to have intercourse during menstruation because if you should ovulate early in the cycle, the identifying mucus could pass unnoticed in the bleeding. Intercourse is allowed on the 'dry' days after menstruation, provided it is on alternate nights only. This is because you must make sure the vagina is 'dry' before having intercourse and so you must wait 48 hours after intercourse to ensure that the semen has drained away completely, so that there is no danger of confusing mucus with semen.

Without doubt, there are potentially serious drawbacks to the accuracy of the Billings method; any change or increase in vaginal secretions will invalidate it. But trials have shown that most women can learn to recognize their mucus symptoms.

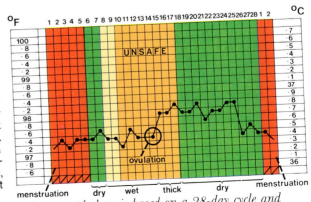

DAY OF CYCLE																												
1	2	3	4	5	6	7	8	9	10	11	12	13	14	15	16	17	18	19	20	21	22	23	24	25	26	27	28

menstruation — dry — wet — UNSAFE — ovulation — thick — dry

With the Billings method the infertile days are taken as being those when there is no vaginal secretion – but intercourse should only take place on alternate days to be on the safe side.

The sympto-thermal method

This method, also known as the muco-thermic or double-check method, combines three different methods of NFP in order to increase effectiveness and predict more accurately the number of 'safe' days. For example, by combining the Billings and temperature methods, you can predict the start of your fertile time by observing the mucus, and confirm the end of it by noting the temperature rise and the further change in mucus secretions.

With careful training and observation, you can also learn to be aware of various symptoms which indicate ovulation in great numbers of women. You might, for instance, become aware of a slight sharp pain in the back and lower abdomen accompanied by a 'crampy' feeling. This is known as *mittelschmerz*. Or you might notice a very slight blood loss known as 'spotting'. Breast discomfort, headaches and depression occurring at specific, fairly regular times in each cycle may also be signs that you are about to ovulate.

Some of these changes can be very subtle, and naturally they will vary considerably from woman to woman. But if you choose to practise natural family planning, you will need to become more aware of such bodily changes, as there is no general rule which can be applied to everyone.

The example here is based on a 28-day cycle and uses a combination of temperature chart with vaginal secretions. This is particularly useful in the safe period where it provides a double check.

The Pill

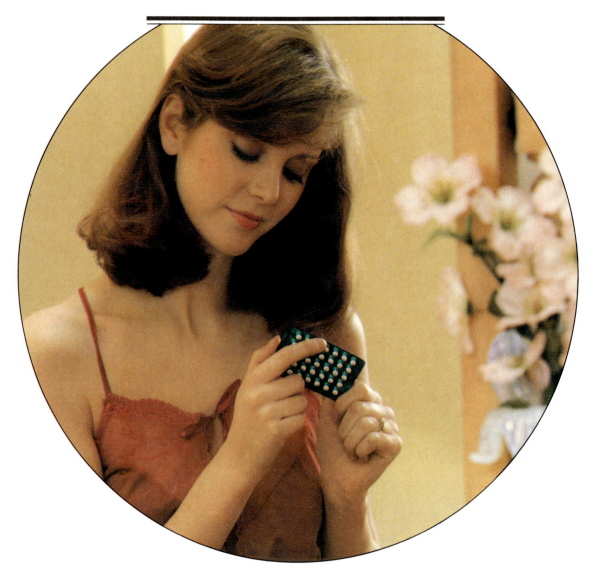

Belinda Banks

As long as you follow the instructions on your packet, the Pill can be considered 99 per cent effective in preventing unwanted pregnancies – higher odds than any other form of contraceptive.

Why is the Pill such an effective contraceptive?

The Pill's effectiveness is so high because it depends not just on one contraceptive action but on *three*, each of which takes place in different parts of a woman's body. In contrast, other methods – the diaphragm, the IUD and other rival methods – have only one, or at most two, contraceptive actions.

Briefly, the Pill contains two synthetic hormones – oestrogen and progestogen. Oestrogen is similar to the natural hormone involved in your monthly cycle, but progestogen is not the same as your natural progesterone. These synthetic hormones interfere with the body's natural sex hormones and effectively 'trick' the body into believing it is pregnant.

If you are on the Pill, the synthetic hormones impose their own pattern on your monthly cycle. Firstly, they stop the ovary from releasing and expelling an egg. Secondly, they act on the lining of the womb, so that instead of developing its usual rich lining – ready for a fertilized egg – it remains thin and poorly nourished, so that no egg can embed itself or be allowed to develop.

Finally, the synthetic hormones affect the womb's natural secretions. Normally, at the time

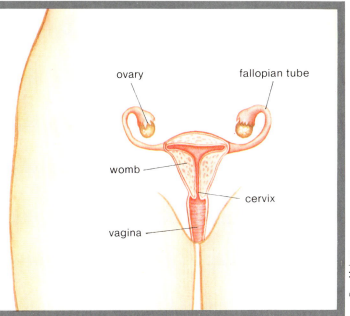

How the pill works

The *hypothalamus* in the brain controls menstruation, sending hormone messengers (LH and FSH) to stimulate the production and release of an egg.

1. The *oestrogen* and *progestogen* in the Pill prevent the hypothalamus from releasing the LH and FSH hormones, so no egg cell is released from the ovary.

2. Progestogen lowers the levels of the body's natural progesterone. The natural hormone is involved in building up the rich lining in the womb which nourishes a fertilized egg. The progestogen prevents this from happening.

3 The progestogen acts on the entrance to the womb – the cervix – making the normal mucus thick and sticky and impeding the progress of any sperm along the vagina to the inside of the womb.

ovary

fallopian tube

womb

cervix

vagina

Dee McLean

of the month when the egg is mature, the womb releases a clear fluid, rather like the white of an egg, which enables the sperm to move easily along the vagina. The Pill inhibits this mucus, and, instead, a thick sticky fluid effectively plugs the entrance to the womb, so that the sperm cannot pass through.

Why do some brands have 21 pills and others 28 in each packet?

Because of the changes brought about by the Pill, the periods you have when you take it are not 'true' periods. Although the womb sheds its lining, the lining itself is slightly different from normal, partly because no egg has been released.

In fact, the lining is shed because you stop taking the Pill. There is no need to have a period at all on the Pill, but the scientists who developed it found that women preferred to retain a monthly cycle, with the added advantage of being able to predict exactly when their period was due. Most brands therefore contain just 21 pills, giving you a seven-day break when bleeding occurs.

The reason that some brands have 28 pills is that manufacturers have included an extra seven 'blanks' which contain no hormones at all. This allows you to keep up the habit of taking the Pill each day, but still gives you seven days 'off'.

Because you don't need to menstruate each month, you can take up to three of the 21-day packets in succession, without a break, so that your period comes at a time which is convenient to you. Although it cannot harm you, doctors

usually advise against a longer stretch. Remember, though, that when you first start on the oral contraceptive you should always use some other form of contraception while taking the first 14 pills from the first packet. This does not apply to those on the new *triphasic* pill which gives you immediate protection.

What body changes or symptoms can you expect when taking the Pill?

Many women experience some side effects from the Pill, but usually they are not serious and will probably settle down with time. Some of them may be positively beneficial.

One of the things you may notice when you start taking the Pill is that your periods are not only more regular, but also shorter and lighter than before. The blood will be dark, rather than bright red, with no clots. If you previously suffered from period pains, you may also find that these lessen. Although the reasons for this pain – known as *dysmenorrhoea* – are not clear, it seems probable that they are linked to ovulation and consequently disappear when ovulation doesn't take place.

The changes vary from woman to woman. Some find that their skin actually improves once they start taking the Pill, while others find that it aggravates a tendency towards acne. The vagina may become more moist and the discharge may increase. This can raise the chances of contracting 'thrush', a common vaginal complaint. So if you find the discharge is accompanied by irritation, see your doctor. On the other hand, very occasionally you may find that vaginal dryness becomes a problem.

Weight gain is a common source of complaint and often continues to rise in spite of dieting. Many women feel irritable, depressed or even nauseous when they first start taking the Pill; sometimes the breasts also become very tender.

What causes these changes?

These side effects are usually the result of the new hormone balance in your body and the changes in your general body chemistry. The alterations in your blood chemistry, for example, can account for weight gain, and may also increase your blood pressure, although if this is the case, your doctor will suggest you come off the Pill straight away. The acidity or alkalinity of your skin will also be altered – and this may make you more prone to thrush.

Some of the changes are due to the indirect effects of the Pill hormones on the part of the brain called the hypothalamus which monitors menstruation. The hypothalamus controls many other functions, including your water balance, appetite and mood: changes in one group of hormone messengers sometimes affects the hormone messengers relating to these other functions, so you may find you are retaining more body fluid, for example.

Many of these symptoms disappear after the first three months, but sometimes they persist, and your doctor may suggest that you change your brand or suggest that you come off the Pill.

Why are there so many different forms of the Pill on the market?

Different Pills not only contain varying amounts of oestrogen and progestogen, but also different forms of these chemicals. Some women do better than others on the various types, according to their natural body make-up and hormonal balance. A doctor will try to prescribe the Pill which will suit you best, and you may have to try several different brands until you find the best one for you.

For example, if your periods are normally heavy, prolonged or frequent, you will probably respond best to a Pill which contains low oestrogen and high progestogen. Conversely, infrequent or painful periods will probably improve if you try a high oestrogen/low progestogen type. Women with acne, a poor sex drive, small breasts or a rather dry vagina will find that they benefit from a high oestrogen Pill while if your breasts become tender, or if you have varicose veins, your doctor will either prescribe a low-oestrogen Pill, or the mini-pill.

Of course, if you develop any of these symp-

What your doctor may recommend

Your personal characteristics and medical history may affect the choice of Pill your doctor recommends, or symptoms developed on a certain Pill may suggest a change of brand/type is advisable. For some women, doctors usually advise an alternative contraceptive to the Pill.

Natural characteristics	or	Symptoms developed on current brand	Start on or change to
Acne Dry vagina Low sex drive Periods painful Periods light and infrequent Small breasts		Acne Break-through bleeding No periods	High oestrogen/low progestogen
Breast feeding Periods heavy and prolonged Tender breasts Varicose veins		Brown patches on skin Contact lenses uncomfortable Fibroids Nausea Tender breasts Thrush (recurrent) Weight gain or bloatedness	Low oestrogen/high progestogen or Mini-Pill
Diabetes Epilepsy Heart disease High blood pressure Kidney disease Menstrual cycle unstable Pre-menstrual tension Cigarette smoker over 30		Aching veins Breathlessness Chest pains Depression Headaches High blood pressure Migraines Sex drive reduced	Other form of contraceptive

toms on one type, they may be relieved by swapping to a different Pill which contains the opposite balance of hormones.

What is the mini-pill?

Unlike the standard 'combination' Pill, the mini-pill contains only one hormone – progestogen. This has the advantage of avoiding those side effects which are due to oestrogen. A woman who is breast-feeding, for example, and who does not want to change to another form of contraceptive will probably be prescribed the mini-pill because it does not reduce milk-production; indeed, it may increase it. It also avoids side effects like nausea and vomiting, 'bloatedness' and breast tenderness.

The mini-pill does have disadvantages, though. Since it contains no oestrogen, it's not so effective in preventing ovulation, and it is vitally important to take it each and every day, at the same time, for month after month, or you may risk becoming pregnant. Because the mini-pill has a higher failure rate, a few doctors recommend that a spermicidal jelly should also be used. Irregular bleeding is another problem – your periods may come at any time, or not at all for long spells.

Can the Pill have more serious side effects?

Oestrogen can interfere with the body's blood clotting mechanism, making it clot more easily. If a blood clot forms, this can lead to a stroke or a heart attack.

When researchers discovered this link, the dosage of oestrogen in the Pill was immediately lowered. Today, no brand is allowed to contain more than 50 micrograms of oestrogen and many contain a good deal less. As a result, the chances of a woman on the Pill dying as a result of a blood clot are less than 4 in 100,000.

There is no evidence that taking the Pill can cause cancer, but doctors will not usually pre-scribe the Pill for anyone who has had cancer of the breast, ovaries or womb.

It's worth remembering that the Pill is one of the best-researched drugs in the world and the risks lower than in pregnancy and childbirth.

When is taking the Pill not advisable?

Because of the links between the Pill and heart problems, there are certain obvious circum-stances when a woman will be advised not to take the Pill – if she has any history of heart disease, for example. Smokers, too, are encouraged to stop taking the Pill when they reach 30, and in any case, since the chances of heart problems increase with age, anyone over 35 should consider switch-ing to one of the other contraceptives.

Anyone suffering from diabetes or diseases of the liver, kidneys or gallbladder are also excluded, and doctors avoid prescribing the Pill for any woman found to have raised blood pressure, since it may raise it still further.

If you have an irregular cycle, with long gaps between periods, you may risk seriously upsetting the cycle permanently by going on the Pill. If your periods aren't regular, but you want to go on the Pill, doctors normally recommend that you try the Pill for one year, and then come off for a break of three months or so, to make sure your natural cycle reasserts itself.

Finally, women who suffer from pre-menstrual tension (PMT), or those who develop it after having a baby, usually find that the Pill aggravates the condition. This is because the progestogen suppresses the production of the natural hor-mone progesterone; PMT is actually a result of too-low levels of progesterone.

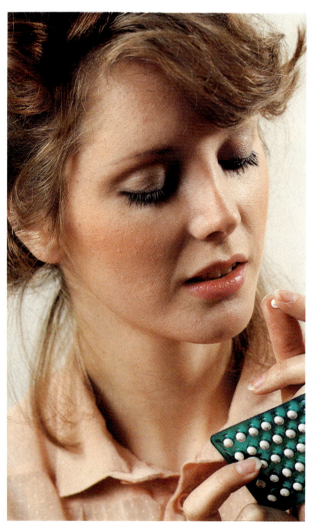

Why are regular check-ups necessary?

Anyone who takes any drug for a long period of time should always have a regular check-up, and Pill-users are no exception. Introducing extra hormones into the body, gives it more work to do; the oestrogen and progestogen have to be broken down in the liver and this can mean that it is less efficient in clearing the blood of other, potentially harmful chemicals. Such changes in the blood chemistry are responsible for some of the Pill's more serious side-effects. Build up of some chemicals can increase blood pressure, for instance.

Regular check-ups make sure that the body is coping with the changes in the hormone pattern and with the waste disposal of oestrogen and progestogen. It also gives the doctor the opportunity to assess how well the type of Pill is suiting the patient.

As a matter of routine, your doctor will ask about your general health to ensure that no side effects have developed, and if necessary, either change the type of Pill or advise that you switch to a completely different type of contraceptive.

Blood pressure and weight checks are particularly important but the doctor will also examine your breasts, and give you an internal examination as well as taking a cervical smear (samples of cells from the entrance to the womb). He may also ask for a urine sample.

You should always tell your doctor about any side effects, however harmless they may seem. If your contact lenses have been bothering you, for example, or if your skin has developed brownish patches. These are not serious, but may indicate to the doctor that you should switch to the mini-pill.

Should you develop severe headaches, migraine or painful veins or if you have any pains in your chest or suffer from sudden breathlessness, you must consult your doctor straight away. They are signs that you should change to another form of contraception.

Can the Pill cause loss of interest in sex?

Yes. Sexual desire is created by a combination of many different hormones. If the hormones in the body cannot adjust to the hormonal changes brought on by the Pill a woman may find that she no longer reaches a climax or enjoys lovemaking. When this happens, she should use a totally different form of contraception – just changing to another type of Pill will probably not be enough. The Pill's side-effects may also cause problems – thrush can make intercourse painful, for instance.

Psychological factors can play a part too although these can be complex and difficult to pinpoint. For some women on the Pill, sex loses its appeal because having intercourse when there is a risk attached adds to the excitement. Others may feel that the Pill makes them less feminine, and this can also affect their sexual desire. At the opposite extreme, there are women who find that the Pill actually increases their sexual pleasure because it removes the fear of pregnancy.

Should you 'come off' the Pill at regular intervals, to give your body a rest?

Opinions vary as to whether you should come off the Pill regularly but all agree that there should be some break just to make sure that your system is in good working order. Recommendations range between once every year to once every three years, but naturally each case is judged on its own merits and many factors will be taken into consideration – your medical background, age and any other circumstances.

How to live with the Pill

- *Don't* forget to take your pill every day. If you have forgotten one pill, take it as soon as you remember, even if you have already taken one that day. If you have missed more than one day, take two pills daily for the next two or three days until you have caught up, and remember to use other contraceptives for the rest of the month.

- *Do* take extra precautions for the first two weeks of the first cycle when you start taking the Pill.

- *Do* take extra precautions if you have had diarrhoea or vomiting for more than one day, as this will have prevented the Pill from being absorbed properly.

- *Do* take the mini-pill every day at the same time, or you risk pregnancy.

- *Do* consult your doctor if you start suffering from severe headaches, chest pains or breathlessness.

- *Do* consult your doctor if your monthly periods stop. You may need to come off the Pill for a while or change your brand.

The whole point of contraception is to be able to enjoy your sex life without becoming pregnant. So it's important to feel happy that the contraceptive you choose will not spoil your love making, as well as being a suitable method for your health and age.

Who decides about a contraceptive – a woman or her doctor?

When you go to consult a doctor about contraception, his job is – as far as possible – to give you the kind of protection that you want. Most family planning courses for doctors lay great emphasis on helping every couple to use the method that is

How to choose a contraceptive

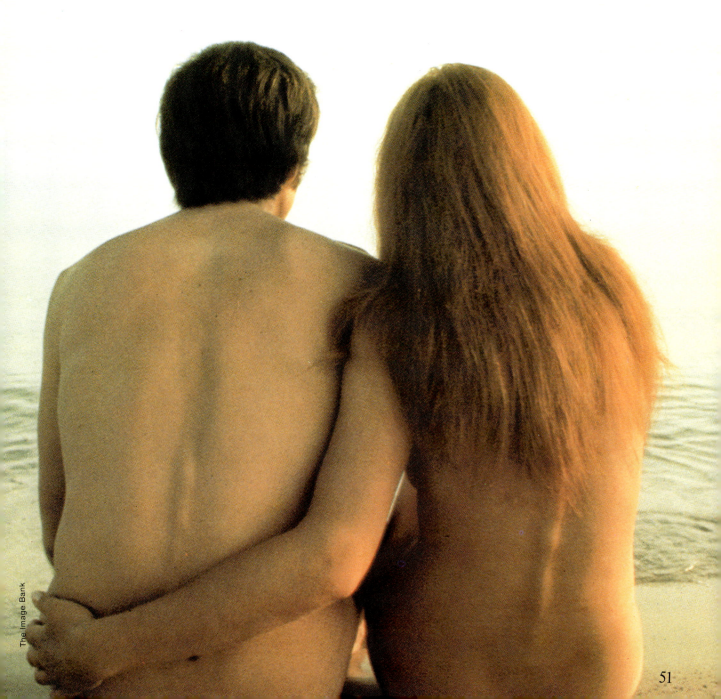

The Image Bank

right for them personally. So, if you already have a strong preference, a doctor will try to go along with your personal wishes – unless he can see a good medical reason why not.

The potential health risks are always something your doctor has to take into account. Before prescribing the Pill, for example, he will take a medical history and examine you – because high blood pressure, liver disease or a history of thrombosis would mean the Pill is not advisable. If you request an IUD ('coil') but have very heavy periods, the doctor may advise against this method, as it may increase the blood loss.

Of course, it may not be as clear cut as that. With the Pill there are some 'marginal' medical factors such as migraine, epilepsy, being overweight or in the 35-plus age group (especially if you are a smoker); these can lead the doctor to say an alternative to the Pill would be *preferable*. But he may well still prescribe it if you insist it is the most convenient method – perhaps with the proviso of more frequent check-ups. The doctor here is really making sure you *understand* the possible risks of problems. (Detailed discussion of side effects and medical considerations will be covered in separate articles on each method).

If you're less sure about the type of contraception you want, or perhaps want to change to another method, the doctor will be able to discuss with you the pros and cons of different contraceptives. Don't be afraid to bring up your feelings about a particular method, even if you think perhaps they sound trivial. If you don't want to have a cap because you think it's a real nuisance to put it in before you have sex – then say so; if you're worried about the Pill making you put on weight or giving you varicose veins, then discuss it.

There is no point in having a contraceptive you dislike or that makes you feel anxious; in many cases the doctor will be able to reassure you about a particular worry. Most family doctors are very helpful when it comes to contraception, but remember there are alternatives – specialist family planning and birth control clinics – where you can go for advice and contraceptive supplies.

How does a husband's or boyfriend's opinion count as far as contraception is concerned?

In a regular relationship, it should certainly concern both partners that they can make love without fear of an unwanted pregnancy. Often it's a case of discussing it together, then the woman coming along to a doctor or clinic. But if a man wants to know more about any of the methods available, the doctor will be happy to

How effective is your contraceptive?

These figures are based on surveys conducted amongst women using the various products. In clinical trials the figures are even higher.

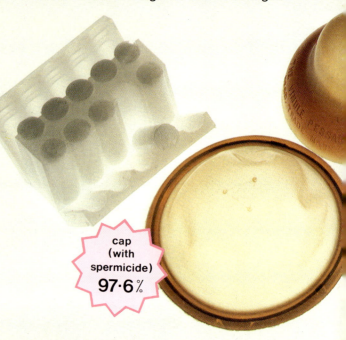

cap
(with
spermicide)
97·6%

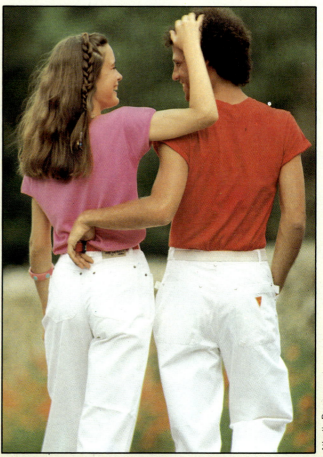

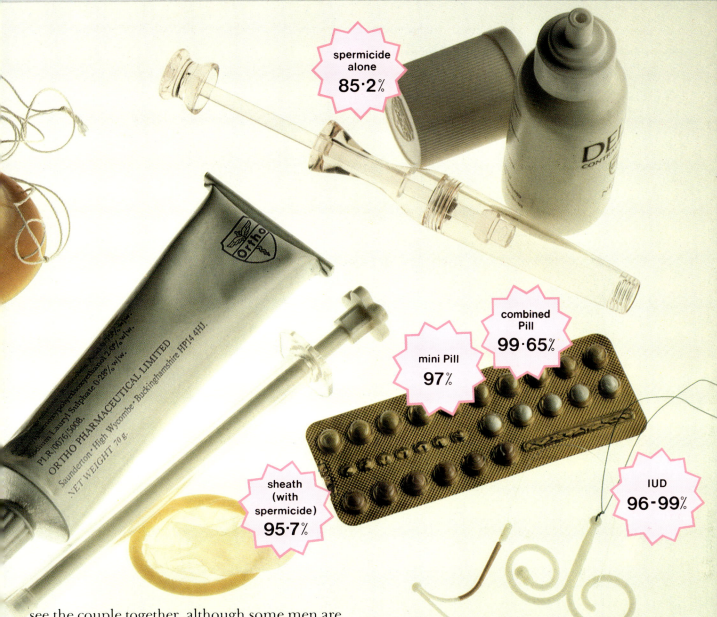

spermicide alone
85·2%

combined Pill
99·65%

mini Pill
97%

sheath (with spermicide)
95·7%

IUD
96-99%

see the couple together, although some men are a bit daunted by the predominantly female clientele in the waiting room at a clinic.

Sometimes a couple's attitudes towards having children diverge a lot, which can make contraception and sex in general an area of conflict. If a man wants more children but the wife refuses to embark on another pregnancy, then it may be a question of a wife reluctantly seeking contraception. She really wants another baby, but her husband is insisting the he doesn't want, or can't afford, another child.

This kind of conflict about contraception can have a real effect on a couple's sexual feelings. Some women who blame the Pill for the fact that they have 'gone off sex' are actually reacting to the fact that it is so *safe*. They enjoy the risk of conception as part of the experience of sex or perhaps, despite practical considerations, deep down would like a child.

If this is causing sexual problems, perhaps the most important thing is for the couple actually to acknowledge their feelings and manage to talk through the difficulty with their doctor. But, besides this increased understanding, a change of contraceptive method may help too. If a woman feels sex is futile without *any* chance of conception, she may feel happier even with the very slightly increased risk associated with an IUD, while an anxious husband can still be reassured that she is continuing to use a reasonable contraceptive.

What is the most effective method of birth control?

Absolute safety is an important factor in choosing a contraceptive for many women – particularly when they are young, unmarried, training or pursuing a career. The figures above show you the figures on effectiveness – but these are based

What contraceptive do women choose at different stages in their lives?

Although there is no 'most suitable' method for different age groups, there are some considerations – like absolute reliability, effects on fertility or breastfeeding, various health concerns – that have a different emphasis at various stages of most women's lives.

These case histories are loosely based on the experiences of a doctor at one family planning clinic (of course, anything you say to a doctor is strictly confidential). They show how these factors can operate – but they also demonstrate how very *individual* are the needs and preferences of every woman.

Young women

Most women want the maximum protection when they first start having intercourse, perhaps they are still students, interested in their career, buying their own flat or are just not ready for children. At this time, the health risks of the most effective and carefree method, the Pill, are also minimal, so this is often a very sensible choice. But individual feelings and personality may mean some other method is preferable.

■ Sonia had recently returned from travelling abroad when she came to the clinic. Although she wanted an effective method of contraception she would not consider the Pill, as she disliked the idea of anything which would affect her natural hormones, and she rejected the idea of having 'something foreign' inside her uterus. She was very content with the cap, had no difficulty in fitting it correctly herself, and I explained that if she used it conscientiously there was only a very small failure rate.

■ Sally had already had an abortion six months before coming to the clinic. When contraception was discussed afterwards she did not like the idea of any of the methods and they had decided that they would use sheaths and pessaries, but they sometimes ran out, or became too absorbed in their love-making to bother to use them, and had often taken a chance. This month her period was late, and she had been in a state of panic until last night when she had started. Now she felt she would like a reliable method, but was doubtful whether she would remember the Pill.

on surveys taken from a group of highly motivated women who used their contraceptives conscientiously.

The combined Pill, containing oestrogen and progestogen, is the most effective reversible method – pretty well 100 per cent effective if taken regularly. Only very rarely, when taking other medicines such as anti-epileptic drugs or antibiotics, is there a failure. Sterilization and

I suggested that the coil, though in theory less effective, would give her better protection because once it was fitted she would then have nothing to remember. As she was menstruating I could fit

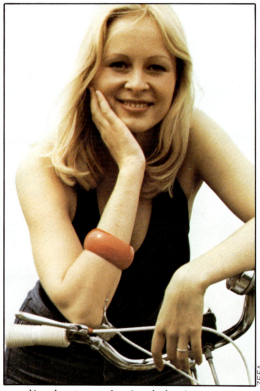

ZEFA

her immediately. I emphasized the importance of coming back to the clinic regularly for her check-ups, or at any time she had low abdominal pain, because although the coil has no effect on fertility in a healthy woman, there can be a more rapid spread of pelvic infection to the Fallopian tubes in a woman fitted with an IUD, and this can occasionally lead to sterility.

■ Susan was in the second term of a 2 year commercial course when she came to the clinic, by appointment. Although she had already had sex a few times, her boyfriend had always used a sheath; she wanted to be really safe as she was determined to finish her training. As she had no medical problems she was given the Pill, being the most effective reversible method.

vasectomy are the only other methods that offer complete protection but they must be regarded as irreversible so you should feel absolutely convinced that you don't want more children. Even when an operation is done to join up the tubes which carry the sperm or the egg, it does not often restore fertility.

The progestogen-only Pill (mini-Pill) and the IUD both have a failure rate of about 2-3 per cent, but it is important to realise that this drops as you get older and fertility declines, so that it is less than 1 per cent over the age of 35 years. The effectiveness of the cap and sheath depends on how carefully they are used. For a woman who is highly motivated (who has completed her family, perhaps), and therefore always remembers to use the cap, the failure rate for this method can be as low as 1 per cent.

First married

Although most couples want to continue to use contraception when first married, they may want to reconsider the methods that they are using. If they plan to start a family in the near future, a woman may now be more concerned about any likely effect of the various types of contraceptive on her future fertility.

■ When Judy first started the Pill the doctor warned her that, because she had irregular periods, there may be a delay in return to regular menstruation when she stopped the Pill, and this would mean that it would take her longer to conceive. Judy wanted to wait a little longer

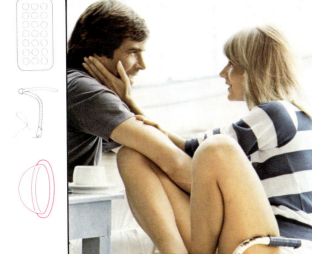

before she started a family but had decided to stop the Pill in plenty of time. I agreed that this could save her anxiety later on, and she said she would like to use a cap, as this has no effect on the rest of the body. I felt she would use it reliably until she was ready for a baby, and that she would not be upset if she *should* conceive – although the chances of this were still very low.

■ Jane had been advised to stop the Pill by her doctor because, though she was only 29 she had now taken it for 10 years. They had been using a sheath but she was very worried because she had had no periods since stopping the Pill. I explained that this could happen after stopping the Pill, and a test confirmed that she was not pregnant. She was very anxious not to conceive; her husband was retraining and she supported him, but she also wanted to be able to start a family as soon as he was earning again. We decided that, even when the periods returned, she would be unwise to take the Pill again until her family was complete. She did not like the idea of the cap, so she chose to be fitted with an IUD.

After a baby

Some women prefer to use a different method of contraception after childbirth; while spacing children, they may be content with a method that is less than 100 per cent effective. Breast feeding affects the use of the Pill, but it is easier to insert an IUD after childbirth.

■ Margaret came back to the clinic six weeks after her baby was born; she had just had a post-natal examination and everything was all right. She had been on the Pill, quite happily, until she

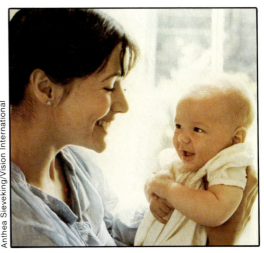
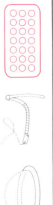

stopped to start a family and now she wanted to start taking it again. I explained that we did not advise taking the combined Pill while she was breast feeding. She told me she preferred to take a tablet, so that she was safe all the time. The idea of anticipating intercourse by fitting a cap put her off altogether. When I told her that the mini-Pill, containing progestogen only, was quite effective while she was lactating she was very pleased. I asked her to return as soon as she stopped breast feeding, so that she could go back to the combined Pill if she still wanted to.

■ Mavis had always been quite happy to use a cap. Now she had a baby she found she was often tired with all the extra housework and disturbed nights, and felt using the cap was too much bother. A previous attempt to fit a coil, before the baby, had been given up as the neck of the womb was too tight, but now I could insert one without any difficulty.

35 plus

In their late thirties many women become very anxious about the risk of conceiving; they feel they are too old to cope with a baby, so that the effectiveness of a method is again very important. A more careful assessment of the woman's health is necessary, as the risks of the Pill increase with age. One helpful aspect is that the failure rate of the IUD and mini-Pill is reduced as fertility declines. Also, sterilization is usually an easier decision at this age, after a family is complete or the woman has definitely decided against having children.

■ Barbara was 37 years old, had been on the Pill without any side effects for eight years, and asked if she could continue. I saw that she had recently

gained weight, her blood pressure had gone up slightly since her last visit, and she was still smoking 20 cigarettes a day. I had to tell her that I felt it unwise to continue the Pill but that she could change to the mini-Pill, if she preferred to take a tablet. As she was anxious to be as safe as possible she agreed to use this while she discussed sterilization with her husband.

■ Beryl was also 37 years old, and had been on the Pill five years. Her husband had recently lost his job, and she was supporting the family; they had a frequent and enjoyable sexual relationship but, although she wanted to be absolutely sure of

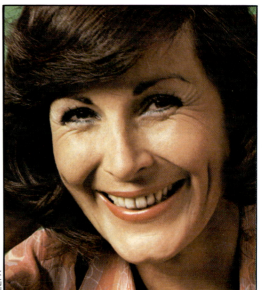

her contraception, she did not want to be sterilized, as she felt it would reduce her femininity. She was slim and healthy, her blood pressure was normal and she did not smoke. I agreed that she should continue to take the combined Pill, but asked her to come more frequently for a check on her blood pressure.

■ Edna was 46 years old and rather upset when she came to the clinic. Her doctor had stopped the Pill, telling her that now she was only having a period every few months there was no need to bother with contraception; if she should conceive — which was unlikely – he would recommend a termination at her age. She could not bear the thought of termination and so had avoided intercourse, and her husband was getting irritable. I said that policy in the clinics was to continue contraception until two years after the last period because there could always be an occasional ovulation. We discussed the possibilities open to her, and she decided on the mini-Pill.

CHAPTER 3

Your
Sexual
Needs

Sexual techniques

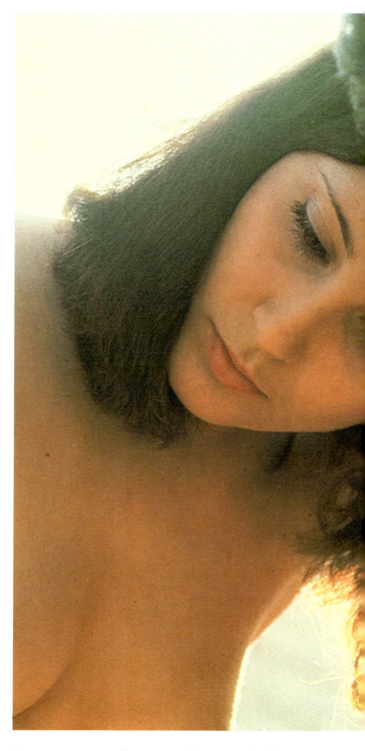

There are many myths about differences between men and women in the area of sexual arousal. It used to be thought that women are very slow to be aroused compared with men, and that a man who was a successful and considerate lover would spend a lot of time on elaborate foreplay to arouse a woman before they had intercourse.

Whether or not particular lovemaking techniques improve arousal is a debatable point. A great many words have been spent in books and magazines promoting the idea that a woman needs a lot of arousal in the form of manual or oral stimulation – usually directed towards the clitoris – before she will achieve an orgasm. Many couples do find a long period of foreplay is a very pleasurable and sensual experience, and certainly many women find stimulation of the clitoris an effective way to reach an orgasm. But there is no set of rules or magic formula.

The whole cult of 'sex technique' can be rather damaging if it produces a mechanical approach to sex. Too often it leads to an anxious and self-defeating exercise in which the man may feel himself to be in a test situation, where a mutual and simultaneous orgasm is the goal and anything else 'scores low marks'. In the end, there is no substitute for a couple having a relaxed and frank approach to their sex life, regarding sex as a way of giving whatever kind of mutual pleasure they choose, rather than a 'performance'.

Is it true that women respond to sex more slowly than men?

Arousal response in women and men is basically very similar, though there are a few obvious physical differences. The male response – developing and maintaining a firm erection – is clearly noticeable. It can occur in a few seconds in a young man, but may take several minutes to develop fully in an older man.

In women, sexual arousal is not signalled so dramatically. The lips around the opening to the vagina swell to some extent and in states of high arousal they 'open' slightly. Internally, the walls of the vagina secrete a lubricating fluid – and the upper part enlarges considerably. At high levels of arousal the lower part of the vagina swells slightly to form a kind of 'cuff' called the orgasmic platform. While all these changes are

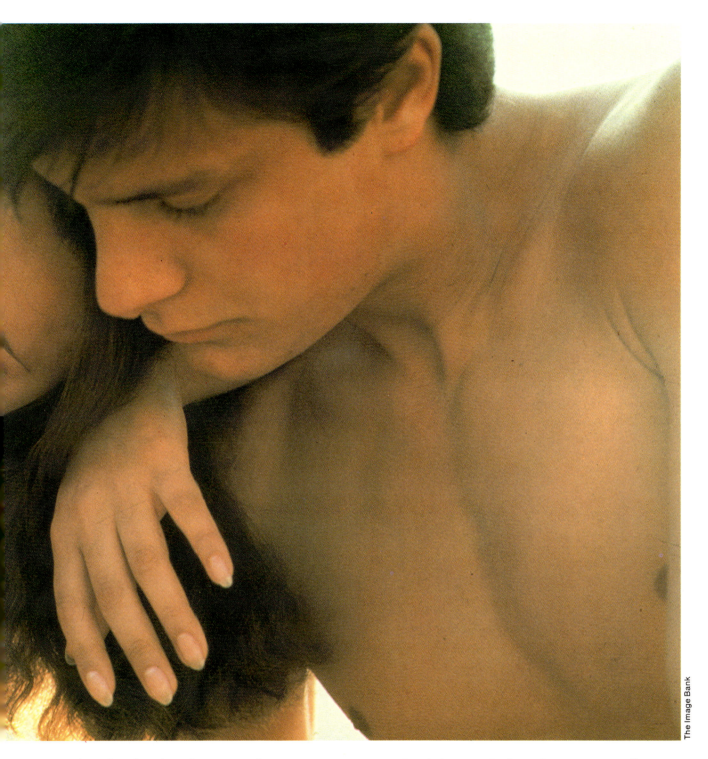

occurring the clitoris enlarges, as do the two tiny folds of tissue that surround it.

All this sounds rather complicated, and one might imagine this response would take some time to build up, but experimental studies have shown that full physical arousal can easily occur in women within a minute or two of being stimulated sexually.

After orgasm there are once again slight differences in the male and female reactions. In men as the sexual excitement level falls, the erection is lost, and what's known as a 'refractory phase' occurs – when they are not able to experience another orgasm. In a young man this period may last just a few minutes, sometimes hours in an older man.

In women, however, orgasm does not lead inevitably to a refractory phase. Some women find that if the partner continues sexual stimulation they can experience repeated orgasm – hence the much-quoted phenomenon of the multiple female orgasm.

Do certain people really have a higher or lower than normal sex drive?

When it comes to sex drive, the idea of what's *normal* covers a very broad range of behaviour. It differs tremendously from one person to another.

One way to measure the average sex drive is to look at the frequency of having sex – a number of different surveys have done this. These all show a slightly higher level of sexual activity among men than women, and a gradual decrease towards middle age, but it's interesting that they also suggest that the sex drive has actually changed with the times. A survey of married men in 1953 showed an average weekly figure for intercourse of 2.45 for 16–25 year olds, and 1.95 for 26–35 year olds. This compares with 1974 figures of 3.26 and 2.55 for similar age groups.

How large a part does fantasy play?

It's not possible to explain in any precise way the various 'triggers' that initiate sexual desire. The sex drive is quite a complex mixture of biological urges and external triggers, and the kind of real images and mental pictures that can act as sexual 'turn ons' are very varied.

What has come to light, however, is the important part which fantasy plays as a stimulus to sexual activity, and the wide variety of erotic fantasy that most people experience. Sexual fantasy questionnaires have been used to work out a way of broadly grouping people as having high, 'normal' and low sex drives.

The survey indicated that someone with a low sex drive is more likely to fantasize about having intercourse with a single partner, whereas someone with a higher sex drive tended to have more varied erotic fantasies, such as having oral sex, being forced to take part in intercourse, or having sex with more than one partner.

How does an unsatisfactory sex life affect the sex drive?

It's a fact that lack of sexual satisfaction often leads to a *loss* of sex drive. It's largely a psychological process – the man or woman concerned may initially have had a normal sex drive but will soon lose interest in sex if they have a continued problem with intercourse.

One of the commonest sexual problems in men is the failure to achieve an erection and this can affect men who have had no sexual difficulty of this kind before. Whatever the underlying cause – it may be some kind of depression, emotional upset, a physical problem or any of several possible reasons – unless the condition resolves itself or is successfully treated, the victim very quickly loses interest in sex.

In women, a similar type of reaction may develop. Unlike a man, it is quite possible for a woman to take part in sexual intercourse while in a very low state of arousal. But if her experience of sex repeatedly fails to arouse her to orgasm, she may eventually come to view intercourse as a mechanical business, totally lacking in interest.

A low level of sexual desire is sometimes linked with another quite common sexual problem in men – premature ejaculation. This means the man finishes his sexual activity too soon for his partner, coming to orgasm and losing his erection too quickly for her to be sufficiently aroused. In this case, the female partner may herself eventually lose interest in sex, because it continues to be an unsatisfactory experience.

It's natural enough to avoid any activity which causes pain – and sex is no exception. Intercourse for women can become painful or difficult for a number of curable physical reasons. Unless the problem is properly resolved, a turning away from sex and even a complete dread of it may result.

When the sex drive has been 'switched off' for some reason to avoid intercourse, it may be that the man or woman is not aware of feeling frustrated. Nevertheless, the damage to a relationship can be very great. A sexually-frustrated partner, a personal feeling of guilt, resentment or rejection may cause severe emotional problems. In such cases, it is always worth seeking advice from a doctor.

Some people find it very difficult to talk about sexual needs. Is there an easy way to start?

Starting to communicate about sexual needs can be a problem. In the early days of a relationship a couple often find it difficult to talk about sex; this may be a barrier that is gradually broken down – but it can unfortunately become a 'taboo' area for discussion. There is really no easy solution, but it's surprising how, if one person plucks up courage to talk about their sexual needs, the other partner, too, will often be eager to have the opportunity to talk.

On this score, it is well worth remembering that sexuality is an area where almost everyone feels a degree of vulnerability, despite the fact that it is a very natural and pleasurable activity. In most cases, provided sexual problems are worked out against a back-drop of love and respect, the differing needs slowly resolve themselves.

Sex therapists and counsellors often find that

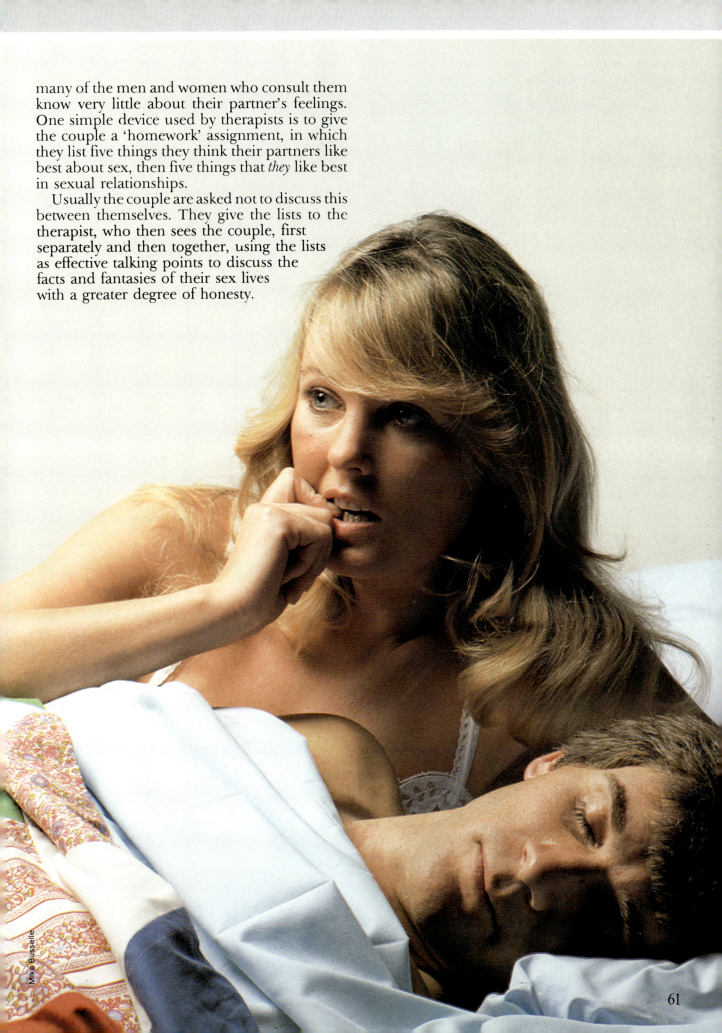

many of the men and women who consult them know very little about their partner's feelings. One simple device used by therapists is to give the couple a 'homework' assignment, in which they list five things they think their partners like best about sex, then five things that *they* like best in sexual relationships.

Usually the couple are asked not to discuss this between themselves. They give the lists to the therapist, who then sees the couple, first separately and then together, using the lists as effective talking points to discuss the facts and fantasies of their sex lives with a greater degree of honesty.

Mike Busselle

61

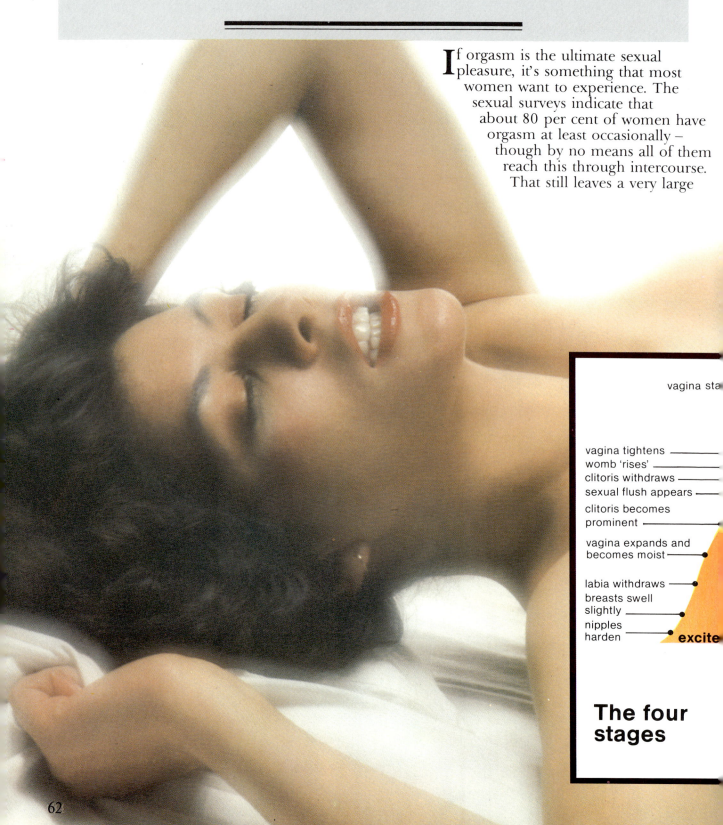

The female orgasm

If orgasm is the ultimate sexual pleasure, it's something that most women want to experience. The sexual surveys indicate that about 80 per cent of women have orgasm at least occasionally – though by no means all of them reach this through intercourse. That still leaves a very large

vagina sta

vagina tightens ———
womb 'rises' ———
clitoris withdraws ———
sexual flush appears ———

clitoris becomes
prominent ———

vagina expands and
becomes moist ———

labia withdraws ———
breasts swell
slightly ———
nipples
harden ——— **excite**

The four stages

number who have never had an orgasm – but just how much that matters is up to the individual concerned.

There's been so much discussion about female sexuality in terms of 'the orgasm' that some women may feel there is something desperately lacking in their make-up if they never have a climax – and that something is really wrong if they never particularly *want* to. That's certainly quite unnecessary.

Some women get a great deal of emotional and physical satisfaction from making love without having an orgasm; their feelings of well-being afterwards are very intense, and they can imagine no greater pleasure from a more physical reaction. Such women are genuinely not frustrated by lack of orgasms and do not feel in any way deprived or inadequate.

But others are continually upset by an unfulfilled desire to have an orgasm, which can lead to them becoming more and more tense and unhappy about sex. It can also be physically uncomfortable: arousal creates a build-up of blood in the tissues in the genital area and without an orgasm there is no immediate release of this. There's no physical reason why any healthy woman should not experience orgasm; it's more likely that emotional factors intervene to prevent fulfilment.

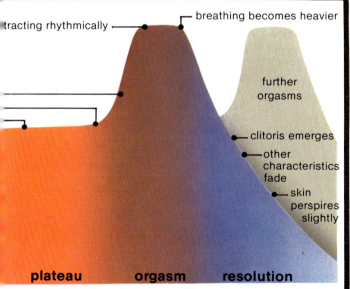

breathing becomes heavier

tracting rhythmically

further orgasms

clitoris emerges

other characteristics fade

skin perspires slightly

plateau   orgasm   resolution

Although each woman will experience orgasm in a different way, she will go through four well-established stages. Things happen at different rates on different occasions – the rise to orgasm may be swift or extended, and may or may not be followed by others (the multiple orgasm). Of course, not every woman experiences all the physical changes, but this is a typical example.

Bernard Fallon

What happens to the body during an orgasm?

Orgasm is a reflex action of the body – it's way of releasing the physical tension built up by concentrated sexual stimulation. The *kind* of stimulation that brings a woman to a climax is still the subject of some controversy (see question below) but the actual body changes that happen during orgasm can be described quite precisely. Four 'stages' are involved, though naturally when someone is experiencing an orgasm these stages merge into a continuous feeling.

The first phase, of *arousal* or excitement, brings a number of physical changes as the woman's body prepares for orgasm. Firstly, the vagina lengthens and widens and secretes a lubricant to make lovemaking easier. There tends to be a pleasant ache or feeling of fullness in the genitals as they fill with blood – just as a man's penis does when it swells to erection. The breasts may also swell and become more sensitive, and the nipples stand out.

As she moves into what is called the *plateau* phase, the woman's breathing and heart rate increase, as does the general muscular tension. The colour of the labia (lips around the vulva) deepens, and the clitoris tends to retract within its hood which prevents it becoming painful from too much direct contact. Some women also sweat and experience large variations in temperature, and some develop a flush or rash.

Providing stimulation continues and there are no other distractions, the plateau phase eventually evolves into the orgasm itself. This is felt as a series of rhythmical contractions centred round the vagina, but they may be felt elsewhere in the body as well – the uterus, anus, stomach, limbs, even the face.

Reactions during the climax vary a great deal; some women hold themselves very still and quiet, while others groan and move with the contractions; a few even briefly lose consciousness. The final stage is the *resolution*, when the body gradually returns to its unaroused state – muscles relax, breathing is slower and deeper, blood pressure and heart rate fall, and generally a feeling of fulfillment and repose takes over.

What's the best way for a woman to reach a climax?

The simple answer is that whatever works is best. Sexual response involves a complex mixture of emotional and physical triggers, and it's not possible to be dogmatic about it. However, there has been a lot of discussion about the 'vaginal' and 'clitoral' orgasms – in other words about

63

where the main focus of sexual stimulation lies in a woman. The clitoris is a tiny organ, swathed in a protective hood, situated at the front of the genitals. Most of the research that's been done explodes the myth that there are two 'types' of orgasm, in that it suggests any orgasm depends on clitoral sensation to stimulate it.

Sexual pleasure can come from stimulating other areas of the body but the majority of women – however much they enjoy the full range of love play – only achieve an orgasm as a result of continuous stimulation of the clitoris or the area immediately around it. The vagina is in fact relatively sparse in nerve-endings, and therefore not particularly sensitive except around the entrance and just inside. The actual contractions, however, are felt in the vagina, and this feeling may be intensified when the area is filled by a penis.

Despite the fact that there is only one physical definition of orgasm there are differences in the way women experience it. Sexual surveys in the Seventies showed that many women felt a difference in sensation, depending on whether or not their partners' penis was inside them. Reaching an orgasm by masturbating, or by a partner stimulating them by hand, can sometimes create a more intense and specific sensation, while orgasm during intercourse may lead to a kind of sensual experience which some women find more satisfying. However, the idea that there are two types of orgasm, vaginal and clitoral, is quite misleading, and there is no basis for thinking that any particular way of climaxing is better than another.

Is there something wrong if a woman can't reach orgasm during intercourse?

There can't be anything wrong with something that is in fact normal for a large percentage of the population. Studies concur in their findings that fewer than 30 per cent of women regularly come to orgasm with intercourse alone. Very few couples have the physical 'fit' which assures the clitoris is sufficiently stimulated during the thrusting of the penis in the vagina; in any case, actual intercourse may not last long enough to bring the woman to orgasm.

The action of the penis pulls the labia which in turn moves the clitoral hood – and actual pressure on the clitoris may be exerted by the man's pubic bone. If a woman has been sufficiently aroused before penetration, this may be enough. However, she may continue to need more direct stimulation and that is easily supplied by continuing to use her own or her partner's fingers at the same time as having intercourse. Sometimes a couple may choose for the woman to have her orgasm before they move on to intercourse, or afterwards. *When* really does not matter in the least so long as both of the partners are happy.

Simultaneous orgasm, where both partners climax together, is not necessarily the 'right' way to come and it is not some sort of great sexual achievement; scoring it as 'top marks' and anything else as less is nonsense.

Is it true that some women reach orgasm more easily than others? If so, why?

Yes it does seem to be true – but no one knows precisely why. There is a very wide variation in the kind of sexual response that both men and women experience; for any individual the feeling can be quite different from one occasion to another in either intensity or range of sensation experienced.

Some women are very easily aroused and can reach an orgasm quickly in just a few minutes; others arouse much more slowly and the sensation only builds up from much caressing and stimulation. However, sexuality is at least as much of the mind as of the body, and for most women the psychological factors are crucial too. The fantasy element – the mental pictures that are happening – can contribute a great deal to the intensity of excitement, and every individual has a particular kind of mood setting and partner which combine to make the right components for arousal and satisfaction.

The contractions felt in orgasm usually only last a few seconds. A few women experience several orgasms in a row, either merging in to one-another, or punctuated by brief returns to the plateau phase. But one orgasm is more usual, and the kind of sensation it creates can be anything from merely pleasant to exquisite. Surveys asking women to describe their orgasms reveal all sorts of sensation from 'total bliss', 'delirious' or 'out of control' to 'a feeling of warmth and love'. As long as a woman feels happy and satisfied, there's little to be gained by wondering how her experience of orgasm compares with someone else's.

Some women complain that after being aroused, they don't actually reach a climax as it 'goes wrong'. Why does this happen?

The female orgasm is rarely something that happens automatically the first time a woman has sexual intercourse. It is a reflex, but in order to get the body to the pitch at which it can happen, there needs to be a certain series of events. It's usually a question of both her and her partner exploring the sensations and the timing that this sequence involves – then it's much more likely to become something natural and assured.

The last steps from the plateau to the orgasmic phase is one which many women find very difficult indeed. Physically, a woman needs to have discovered the kind of touch and stimulation she needs to achieve that last step. She may be very lucky and have a partner who instinctively gets it right, but as each body is different in its needs it makes sense for the woman to be prepared to encourage and guide her partner.

Many men (and women) do not realize how long it may take for a woman to reach the orgasmic stage, and they may give up or move on to intercourse long before the woman is ready. Alternatively, in an excess of zeal, a man may over-stimulate the very sensitive clitoris, which can be an altogether painful and very unerotic experience.

Sometimes, even with a sensitive and co-operative partner, a woman cannot move into orgasm, usually because of some emotional problem. This may be an expression of something wrong in the relationship, or it may indicate a block in the woman's emotional attitude to her own body, and to having an orgasm. Many women are still brought up in ignorance and embarrassment about their bodies, if not actual dislike and disgust. As well as understanding how her genitals work, a woman has to learn to accept that this part of the body – and the range of sensations it can offer – are there to be enjoyed.

Learning to love your own body when you may have been brought up to think its functions dirty can take a long time. Gaining the confidence and insight to overcome emotional difficulties may go against a lifetime's behaviour. No-one would pretend that such change is easy, but it is possible and there are people who can provide professional help.

Faking orgasm is no answer – having done it once it almost inevitably becomes the norm and meanwhile makes orgasm itself more and more elusive. It can put you off sex completely. If you don't want an orgasm there's no need to pretend, and if you do, faking will only hinder it.

What kind of help can a woman get if she has difficulty reaching an orgasm?

Perhaps the greatest boost towards learning to have an orgasm is for a woman to realize that she is not unique in having a problem – thousands of others share her frustrations. Some women gradually get over their difficulties, either by themselves or with the help of a loving partner but, if anyone wants to seek professional help, it is available.

There are many clinics specializing in this kind of counselling or therapy – you could ask your doctor or a local family planning clinic for details. Any woman can seek advice – it doesn't matter whether she is single or attached. The counsellor's approach will depend on the problem the woman is experiencing, and what kind of emotional factors are involved.

Learning to have an orgasm must begin with learning to enjoy your own body – the sight, touch, taste and smell of it. Some orgasm therapy tends to start with exploration and explanation of how the genitals work and moves on to teach a woman to enjoy her own sensuality. Learning to give herself an orgasm by masturbating, perhaps with a vibrator if her fingers are not enough, has given many women sensations they thought they were never going to experience.

This may help many women, especially if they can go on to apply their new awareness in the context of their relationship with a loving and co-operative partner. But it's important to realize there is no 'rubber stamp' approach to sexual therapy – it will always depend on the individual involved and the therapist's understanding of her special problems.

Is it true that a woman can lose her ability to achieve orgasms?

Most women get better at orgasms as they become more mature. They are more self-assured, more assertive and they've had more practice. There are, however, bound to be occasions when things don't work out, and this is quite normal. In addition, alcohol or some drugs can have a temporarily lowering effect on sensitivity which may make orgasm difficult. Ill health or just plain tiredness can interfere. Taking the contraceptive Pill or being pregnant may affect the secretions which lubricate the vagina, but this can easily be offset by using a lubricating jelly – available from most chemists.

Worrying about failure to orgasm sets up a vicious circle, as it inhibits the chances of success next time. Sometimes it may help break the circle to return to masturbation techniques or to massage and other pleasures not specifically aimed at orgasm. Certainly, to demand orgasm as the outcome of every sexual encounter is unrealistic and may simply be inviting problems.

Sexual inhibitions

People are generally more knowledgeable about sex today than ever before. So much so, that many things which were considered undesirable 30 years ago are now seen as quite healthy aspects of sexual experience. Masturbation for example, used to be seen as something dirty and unhealthy. But now it's regarded as a very normal activity, which helps teach young people to achieve and control orgasm, and a useful way for a highly sexed person to adjust to a partner with less sexual desire. Similarly, there is now a lot of new information available about women's sexuality, including such basic facts as the importance of the clitoris in the female orgasm.

It takes time, however, for radical changes in thought to filter through and affect general attitudes. Even though anyone today can read about a wide variety of sexual experience in books and magazines, there are many reasons why people still have inhibitions about experimenting with sex.

Why is it that people have such different views about what's normal in sex?

Everybody has their own idea about what is normal sexual behaviour. At one end of the scale there's the relaxed attitude that 'anything goes'; at the other there is the easily disgusted individual who thinks sex is a 'necessary but dirty' activity. These two cases encountered by a sex therapist illustrate just how different are people's views on what is normal. While one of his male patients complained that he could 'only' make love for 45 minutes at a time and three times in any one session, a female patient said she thought it 'kinky' when asked to help her husband (who suffered from premature ejaculation) to do some therapy exercises with him at home. These involved taking off her clothes so that he could give her a body massage – she explained that they rarely touched and never allowed themselves to appear naked in front of each other.

Social scientists have always argued about what is normal in any form of human behaviour. Looking at things in terms of statistics doesn't really help us decide what is natural or right; just because a small number of people enjoy a particular form of sex doesn't automatically

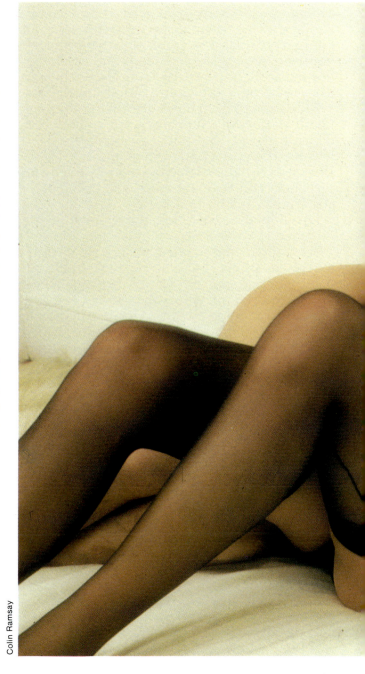

Colin Ramsay

make them weird or perverse, even though statistically they are 'abnormal'. Most sex therapists would say that any form of sexuality is acceptable if both partners enjoy it, provided it doesn't cause any real emotional or physical harm.

Just why people grow up with such conflicting views about sex is a fairly complex matter, but it is generally accepted that parents and early home life have a very strong influence. If you are brought up in a relaxed, affectionate atmosphere where people talk quite freely about sex, and nudity is not something shameful, you are likely to feel quite differently from someone whose parents considered sex to be an embarrassment

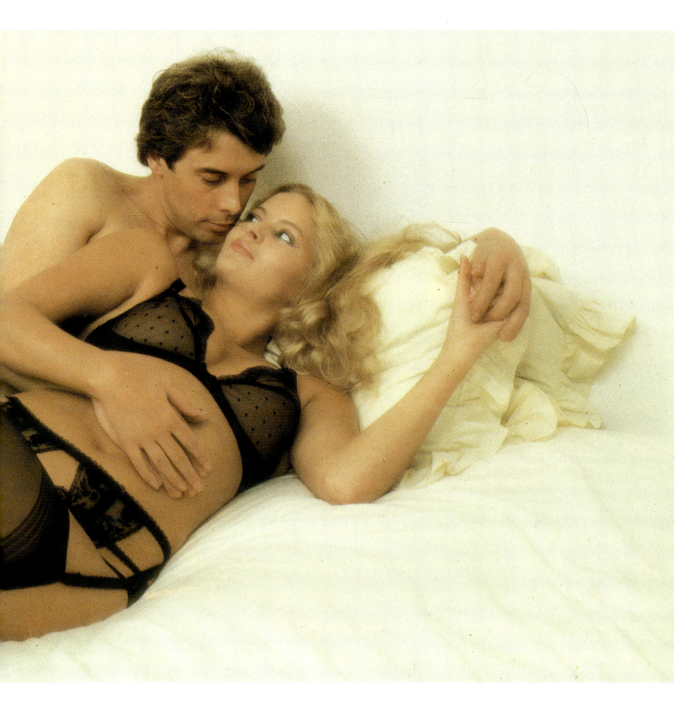

and the human body something to be hidden. Even if their inhibitions were never mentioned, the conspiracy of silence about sex gets the message across with great force.

When and how someone learns the facts of life may also colour their attitude, as will their first sexual experiences. If these are happy and successful, that person is more likely to have a relaxed and optimistic attitude – and be interested in exploring sex and the sexual needs of their partner.

In growing up, we all meet a lot of different sexual attitudes – from our families, our friends, television, newspapers and other media. At the same time, we're trying to come to terms with

having adult sexual feelings. It's only natural to have some fear about new experiences – and sex is no different in this respect. Given all the conflicting needs and pressures people encounter, it's hardly surprising that they end up with some doubts about what's 'acceptable'.

Should people feel guilty about experimenting with sex?

It's not uncommon for a person to suspect their partner of being unfaithful if they suddenly introduce a new sexual technique into their love making. Somehow they think that once the pattern of their sex life has been established, any change in it must indicate that something is wrong in the relationship. But people are naturally inquisitive and imaginative and require a variety of stimulations. Sex is like any other activity – if it becomes repetitive it can become boring, and when people become bored it is better to start looking for new experiences in sex than for a new partner.

It's all too easy to get into a sexual rut – you find a formula which guarantees successful results and play safe rather than explore other techniques. But in fact sexual boredom is a common cause of infidelity and a major factor in the increasing divorce rate. So, rather than feel guilty about experimenting with sex, you could regard it as a positive part of lovemaking, essential to a developing relationship.

Just how adventurous people want to be is up to them, but even something as simple as making love in a different room, or with the light on if you're used to a darkened bedroom, can make quite a difference. If one of the partners is shyer or less enterprising, trying to enliven a stale sex life overnight could come as quite a shock, so don't be too ambitious at first.

The most important thing about exploring new ways of giving and receiving pleasure is for both partners to be able to communicate what they do – and don't – like. Most people have a rich sexual fantasy life which unfortunately they rarely share with their partners, because they think it will be embarrassing, and perhaps shocking. The only way around this is to take direct action and find a way to talk over your needs and feelings. Whatever anyone else says, you're *not* unusual in having sexual fantasies, and when you come to discuss them you may well find that your partner shares them. There's no reason why the woman shouldn't take the initiative in this. Tell your partner what you enjoy most, ask him to do different things, or reverse roles and take the lead where he is normally the active partner.

As well as talking about your sex life, you can communicate your needs in other, more subtle ways. Try leaving a book or article about sex around where he will see it; or see what reaction you get to wearing a sexy nightdress or suspender belt and stockings. If nothing else, it should create the opportunity to talk about trying something new in your sex life.

Why do so many sex manuals stress experimenting with positions?

Making love face to face with the man on top is still the most common position for intercourse.

While in many ways it allows for a lot of intimate and loving contact, it is by no means the most natural or satisfying for everybody. And, like other aspects of sex, if a couple always use the same position it's quite likely to become tedious.

The shape and size of the genitals varies from one person to another, and the only way to discover which position is most satisfying is to experiment. Many women find that in the 'usual' position there is not sufficient pressure on the clitoris to achieve an orgasm. Positions with the woman on top can improve this and a variety of positions, such as the man entering from behind, give greater penetration. Occasionally a woman finds a certain position uncomfortable because of the shape of her vagina, but it's just a matter of experimenting to find out what works for a particular couple. Trying out something new is simply a way of making lovemaking more exciting and satisfying.

Why do some people think that oral sex is distasteful?

Many people still have the feeling that contact between the mouth and genitals is 'not quite nice' because it involves kissing parts of the body which urinate. These doubts may be deeply seated if someone was brought up to think of their genitals as something to be ashamed of, but sometimes people simply think it's rather 'unhealthy'. Such fears are quite groundless as there are normally fewer germs around the genitals than there are in the mouth. And providing the couple wash regularly, there needn't be anything distasteful about the act. In fact genital odours produced during sexual arousal can be very stimulating. There is no harm in the woman swallowing semen, although some women prefer to remove the penis just before ejaculation.

It helps if a couple can show each other the positions each other likes most; some men prefer to have all their penis stimulated, some just the tip; some women prefer direct stimulation of the clitoris, others around the edge. Oral sex can be an exciting part of foreplay, or the main sexual activity – it's interesting that a recent American study has shown that a majority of women have their most intense orgasm during oral stimulation.

Is it wrong to have violent or masochistic feelings during sex?

Sex should be fun and, as with many other 'games', it's likely sometimes to involve a certain amount of roughness. For many people playful biting, slapping or scratching is a natural part of

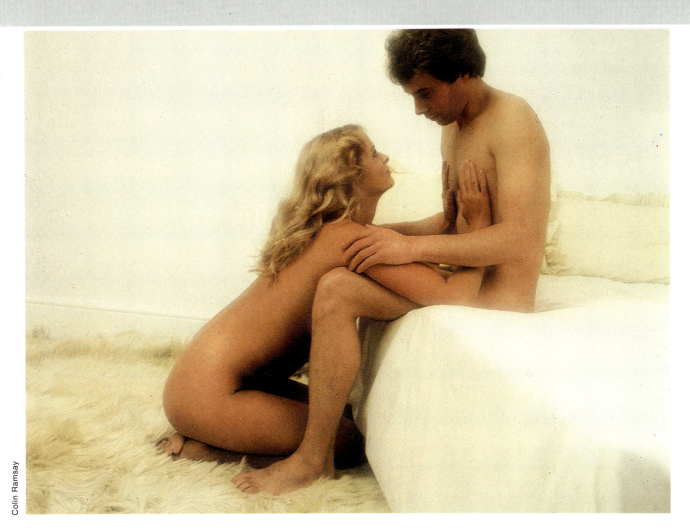

Colin Ramsay

lovemaking. Even if they don't do it deliberately, it often happens unconsciously in the heat of the moment. People vary in the amount of pain they are prepared to inflict and receive but, so long as no one comes to any real harm and both partners are enjoying themselves, some roughness is perfectly normal.

There's only need for concern if one partner is making demands which the other finds unacceptable or distressing. There are some individuals who believe they can only enjoy sex if it involves a strong element of pain; they may become very violent, and inflict severe pain and physical injury. Obviously this is a dangerous situation which shouldn't be allowed to continue and either one or both of the people involved should seek professional help.

Is there anything wrong in using sex aids?

For many people, sex aids are synonymous with the weird and wonderful array of clothing and gadgets displayed in the windows of sex shops. They tend to be dismissed as objects needed to satisfy the flagging sex lives of lonely people and sexual misfits. Yet we all have our own individual 'turn ons' – things which stimulate our sexual desires and enhance our lovemaking – even if

they are simple things like the satin sheets or silky underwear that are readily available in department stores.

It is surprising how often couples are not aware of the particular preferences of their partners. Discovering what these are can add enormous pleasure to lovemaking. Some couples find that pictures or prose, ranging from romantic poetry to the harder porn material available in sex shops, can act as a strong sexual stimulus; so can perfume, music, flowers and food. Some people are very susceptible to particular types of clothing, from saucy underwear and nighties to more exotic leather and rubber wear.

More direct sex aids such as vibrators and various attachments for the penis (which are designed to increase physical contact) can be used to intensify pleasure during sexual intercourse. Many women who have trouble reaching orgasm have found that they can first achieve one using a vibrator and are then able to achieve it during normal sexual intercourse – although it's arguable that this could often be achieved just as well by learning to masturbate.

Sex aids can become a bore if they are used as 'mechanical' turn ons, but certainly there is nothing wrong in using them if they increase arousal and add novelty to lovemaking.

Why sex can be painful

It's not unusual for a woman to experience discomfort with intercourse at some time – but often it's a temporary problem which clears up. Some women do have more serious difficulties – perhaps they have enjoyed a good sex life for years but find they develop a problem after childbirth or during the 'change of life', while others find intercourse painful right from the start. Both the woman and her partner may try hard to improve the situation but she continues to experience pain. This can be so severe that the couple find they cannot achieve full penetration, and sometimes none at all.

Women with this type of experience often turn up fairly early in the course of their relationship, but others wait until quite a long time has elapsed – perhaps when their relationship seems on the point of breaking up, or they have finally been forced to realize that it won't just 'go away' if they wait long enough.

Or it may be a doctor who first brings up the subject; if a woman turns up for an examination – say, related to a cervical smear or fitting a contraceptive – the doctor may find she has such a tense, tight or dry vagina that he can't examine her at all, so naturally he will want to ask whether she is having problems with intercourse as well.

Can a woman ever be 'too small' for sex?

Some women who find attempts at intercourse difficult and painful tell their doctor that they think they are 'too small'. Occasionally this can be due to a tough hymen which has a rather small opening (the hymen is the 'maiden head', a membrane which partially closes the lower end of the vagina in a virgin).

There is usually a perfectly normal vagina behind the hymen, and the doctor can show the woman how to use a simple lubricating jelly to gradually stretch the opening themselves, gradually inserting one, two or even three fingers. More rarely, if the hymen is very thick and has a tiny opening it has to be stretched and incised by the gynaecologist, under a general anaesthetic; it heals quickly.

The 'smallness' some women complain of is nearly always due to tension, apprehension and some underlying fear of penetration. Many have the idea that the hymen is not at the entrance to the vagina but is a membrane stretching across some way inside; they are terrified that the thrusting of the penis would mean a 'breaking' through the membrane – and dread that this will be a painful and bloody experience.

In fact, nowadays, with the kind of active life young girls lead, and with tampons so widely used for sanitary protection, it is much more usual to find that there is no hymen at all. Any pain or tightness a woman experiences is more likely to be caused by a spasm of the muscles at the entrance of the vagina. This spasm happens when a man tries to penetrate her during intercourse, or when the doctor tries to examine her. The vagina itself when relaxed is not 'small'; in fact it is extremely rare to find a vagina so small that it affects or prevents enjoyable sex.

Is it true that poor 'technique' can make sex painful?

Intercourse may sometimes be painful if the man penetrates the woman very quickly, without any preliminary caressing or lovemaking; she may be still quite unaroused, perhaps tense and certainly dry, because the natural 'lubrication' is only secreted in the vagina when the woman feels sexually excited. If the man also has a very quick climax, this increases the difficulty, because she doesn't even have time to experience arousal from the movement of the penis once the man has entered her.

This kind of difficulty is often something that a man experiences at the start of a new relationship when he is nervous and over-anxious – and in this case it's likely soon to get much better. But, if it is a more serious potency problem, in which the man can only achieve intercourse by rapid penetration and climax, then the woman's frustration may lead to her becoming 'frigid'; intercourse then continues to be painful because she is dry and tense.

Rough and violent intercourse is another cause of pain, although some women do find this kind of lovemaking very exciting and enjoyable. More often, it's a question of an inexperienced or

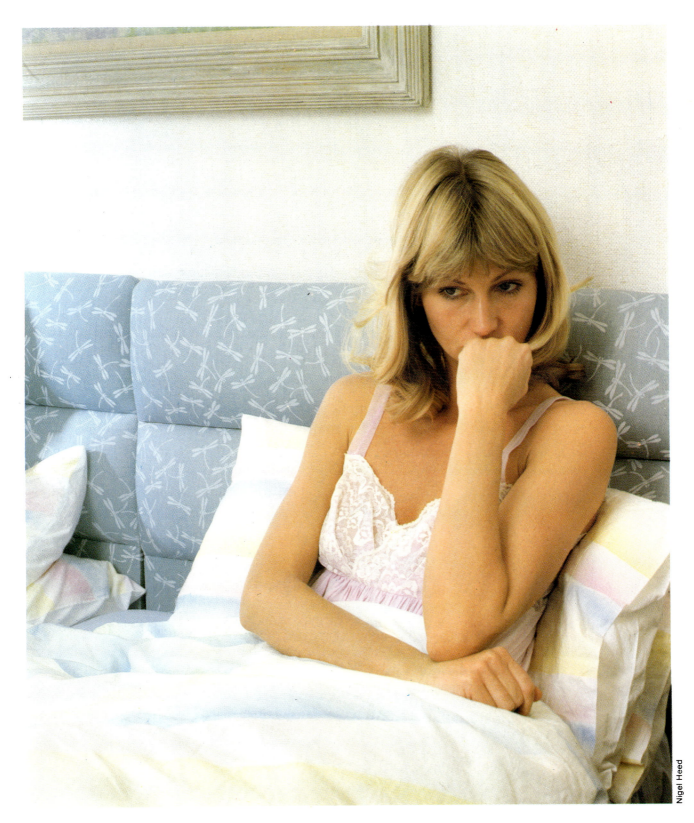

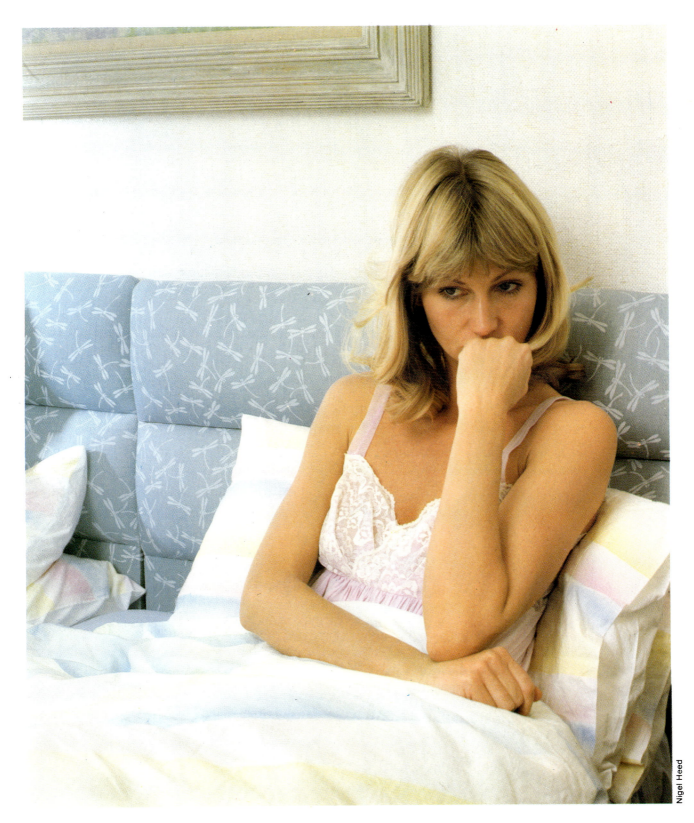

Nigel Heed

nervous man being rather clumsy and, if the woman herself is more confident, she can do a lot to teach him a more relaxed and skilful approach.

There is another kind of pain which can occur when a man penetrates a woman very deeply; in some women the position of the womb and the cervix (neck of the womb) means that deep penetration exerts a lot of pressure on sensitive areas. In this instance, the doctor may be able to give advice on different positions for lovemaking which will avoid the sensitive areas – or the couple themselves could try experimenting with different positions.

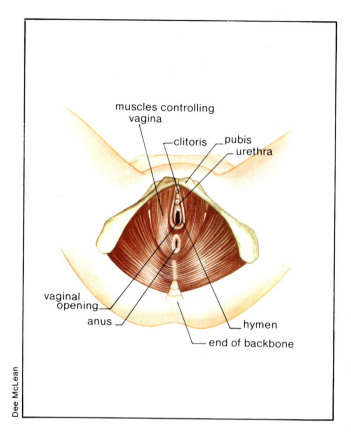

muscles controlling
vagina

clitoris — pubis
— urethra

vaginal
opening

anus

hymen

end of backbone

Dee McLean

*How can a fear of sex make intercourse painful
– can you do anything to overcome this?*

The tensing of the whole vagina, and a spasm of
the muscles around the entrance, may well be
due to some kind of fear of sex. This condition is
called *vaginismus*. When any kind of penetration
is attempted, the woman may also arch her back
and draw her knees together, so that it's quite
impossible even to make any kind of near
approach.

With some women, the doctor can in time
encourage her to explore her own vagina, so that
gradually she finds out it is roomy and long
enough to take three fingers fully without any
pain. Once she's able to accept the reality of this,
she is usually able to relax enough to enjoy
intercourse without finding it painful.

But there are some women who find all this
quite impossible; despite a very patient and
skilled approach by the doctor, he cannot succeed
in getting her to insert even the tip of her own
finger, let alone allow him to give her a vaginal
examination.

She could be said to have a 'fear of sex', but this
is just one aspect of a set of complex, often deeply
unconscious, emotional conflicts. She may feel
any attempt at penetration 'inside' is a threatening,
perhaps dangerous, and 'forbidden' activity. Her
problems are nothing to do with the physical
nature of her vagina, so it's a question of her

acknowledging this fact and seeking help from a
skilled psychotherapist.

*Why do some women find problems with sex
after having a baby?*

Some young women who have always found sex
easy and enjoyable find, after childbirth, that
intercourse has become uncomfortable and even
painful. It's generally quite well known that these
difficulties – as well as the post natal 'blues' – do
often occur, as a passing phase.

But this doesn't always reassure a new mother;
sometimes she has a deep underlying fear that
the baby's birth has really damaged her physically,
especially if she has had a rather long labour and
stitching afterwards. She may be afraid she has
been stitched too tightly or think the tear might
'burst' if there is full penetration. Like someone
guarding a 'wounded' place she is likely to tense
up and dry up with apprehension when she and
her partner try to have intercourse.

A woman's womb and vagina are all 'inside'
her and she cannot have a good look and
reassure herself that all is normal. Tiredness and
anxiety over caring for the new baby is likely to
make her rather pre-occupied and unlikely to
feel very 'sexy'.

The doctor may be helpful in two ways.
Providing a post-natal check up six weeks after
the birth and getting the woman to explore her
own vagina, can help to reassure her that she has
not been 'damaged'; showing her how to relax
and use a good lubricating jelly to overcome her
present dryness can ease the whole situation. He
can also give her the opportunity to talk about her
feelings and any anxieties she may have about
caring for the baby and relating to her husband.
After all, this can be a time of maximum
uncertainty about herself, not only as a woman,
but as a mother and a wife.

Temporary discomfort, itching and perhaps
some pain in intercourse can be caused by the
dryness which accompanies vaginal infections –
in particular the fungal yeast infection known as
thrush. Pregnant women often develop this
owing to the change in their vaginal acidity
brought about by the pregnancy. It may also
develop following antibiotic treatment for some
other illness. This condition is quite easily treated
by the doctor.

How can the menopause cause painful sex?

In the menopausal years, many women who
have never had any sexual difficulties before,
may develop discomfort and increasing pain

from intercourse. This is due to a lessening output of oestrogen, the hormone which in her fertile years has nourished the vagina, keeping it comfortably moist and supple.

This can generally be easily helped with applications of an oestrogenic cream onto the vaginal walls, to restore them to their previous condition. The use of a good lubricating jelly in the vagina during intercourse is also very helpful. It is important that older women should understand that painful intercourse at this age does *not* indicate that she is 'too old' for intercourse and should give it up. On the contrary, it is important for both partners that they should cherish their sexual life together, so that they can continue to have satisfactory intercourse throughout the years ahead.

Is intercourse ever painful for men?

Whatever the reason, if a woman is suffering from a dry, tight vagina then her male partner is obviously affected too. Penetration and movement are bound to be painful for him if the vagina is not open and well-lubricated. But there are other possible causes of discomfort (for example, an infection or inflammation of the penis) and a few men have a foreskin which is too tight; this can be put right with a simple operation. If there is no obvious physical cause, then the problem is likely to be an emotional one – perhaps excessive fear about the 'vulnerability' of the penis. A skilled psychotherapist may be able to help overcome this, and your doctor should be able to recommend you to one.

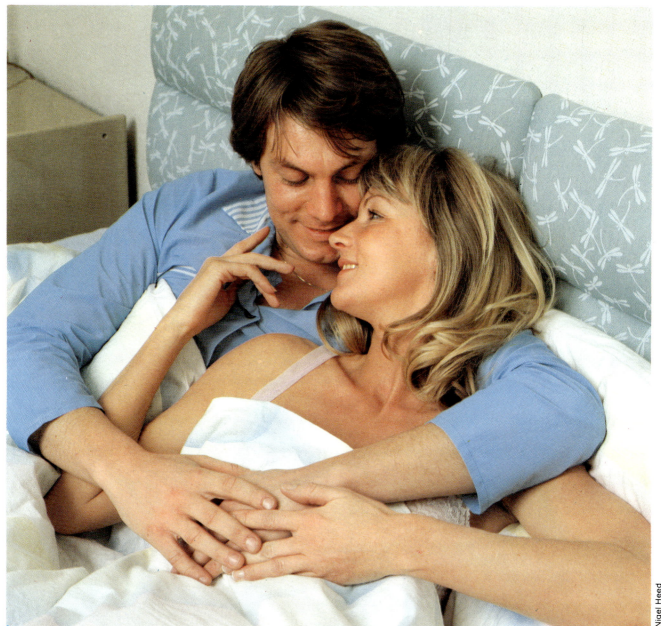

Nigel Heed

Sexual fears and worries

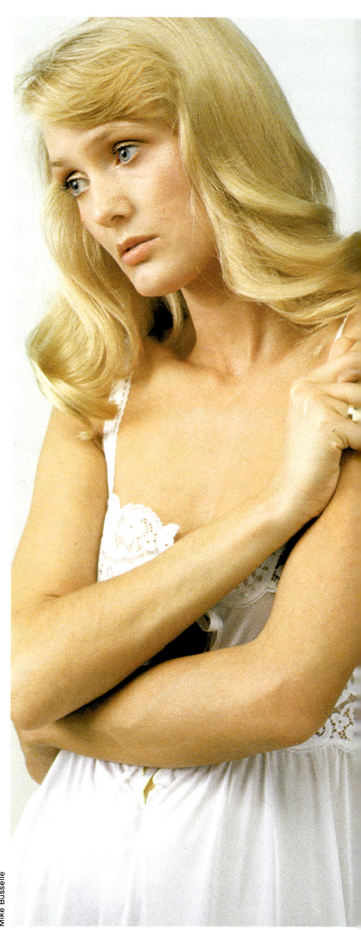

Mike Busselle

Frigidity might almost be called a dirty word these days. No woman likes to be labelled as 'frigid'; it's a strange contrast with our great-great-grandmothers' times, when the ideal woman was held to be the complete opposite – innocent of all sexual desire and 'pure as the driven snow'.

What does being 'frigid' really mean?

Although there is no precise medical meaning, frigidity implies that a woman, during love-making with a man, has some degree of inability to achieve a passionate release of sexual excitement, culminating at some point in an orgasm. But, in fact, the women who turn up in the consulting room saying they are 'frigid' have all different kinds and levels of sexual problems.

Sometimes a woman is simply uncertain of herself and of just what *is* normal in sexual relationships. She may in fact experience orgasms, but worry that the timing does not coincide with that of her partner; or it may be that she just doesn't want sex as much as her man. On the other hand, the woman may have a partner who, inexplicably, hardly ever wants to make love to her. He may defend himself – by blaming her and implying there is something about her sexual behaviour which fails to arouse him; so the woman comes seeking advice to find out whether she is frigid and it's 'all her fault'.

The *way* a woman has an orgasm is another common cause of worry. There are many normal women who only climax through their partner caressing their body and clitoris, and don't reach an orgasm through the movement of the penis in the vagina. A few women do get hung up on the **idea of experiencing a 'vaginal' orgasm** and believe, quite unnecessarily, that they have some serious defect.

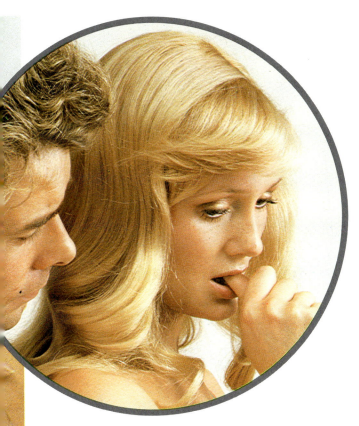

Women who are really anxious about these problems are usually lacking in self confidence in their own sexuality, and tend to measure their performance against some idealized and quite unreal notion of what sex should be like.

She and her partner may try and follow what they read about better techniques for the sexual 'mechanic', as if sex like cars, can be compared. And when she finds no improvement this simply increases her certainty that there is something wrong with her.

Do some women never have a climax?

In contrast to the type of problems about frequency or quality of orgasm, there are some women who seek advice because they don't achieve *any* kind of climax. It may be that they do get very aroused during lovemaking, but cannot find a way to resolve their excitement naturally by coming to an orgasm. They may actually think of themselves as passionate rather than frigid and blame their partners for lack of skill.

Some go seeking other lovers with better techniques, or, if they do seek help from a doctor, they find it hard to acknowledge that the difficulty may have something to do with their own inner emotional problems. Then they blame the doctor's lack of skill too, thinking he should be able to offer some easy secret which will solve their problem.

Then there are other women who seem quite unable to feel desire or excitement from the actual experience of lovemaking. Sometimes they will describe this as if they were not in their own bodies during intercourse, but up in the corner of the ceiling looking down at themselves on the bed. It's as if they cannot let themselves feel the experience to be 'real' at the time, so they are totally blocked from having any warm sexual reaction.

They may actually have quite strong sexual feelings and fantasies when they are by themselves. One such woman told her doctor that travelling home from work in the train she would feel such desire that if, at that impossible moment, her husband was to make love to her she would enjoy it; but when he was really there in bed with her and available, she would feel nothing.

Other women appear *never* to have any sexual desire or pleasure from any form of lovemaking. They may feel affectionate, happy to give their man a kiss and a cuddle in bed; they will sometimes talk of their husbands as being 'good' to them when they really mean that their husbands do not often ask for sex. Some do regard intercourse as distasteful, repulsive or dirty, and submit to their husbands out of a sense of duty.

Among this group of women, there are some who do come for help – not because they want to experience sexual pleasure for themselves, but because they'd like to please their husbands by having an orgasm. 'I don't want it for myself, but I do want him to be really satisfied.'

In fact, they may be very loath really to talk about their own deeper feelings; 'Leave me alone' they imply; 'Just retune the mechanism; that's all I have come about'. Perhaps these women are the most difficult to reach with any effective help, since it means somehow getting behind the fortifications they have carefully built around their own vulnerability.

How can your upbringing affect your feelings about sex?

In a general way, every woman starts life equipped with the potential to have sexual feelings and satisfaction. But she may encounter some unlucky experience or deficiency in her emotional environment that has a severe effect on this. Somewhere, somehow, in the years from birth to womanhood her experiences lead her to exclude sexual feelings, because they risk arousing emotional conflicts that she cannot cope with. Of course, no two cases of women suffering from this kind of emotional block are alike, and the reasons can be very complex.

Certainly, upbringing always plays a very big part in moulding our own attitudes towards sex, and our capacity to sustain a good fulfilling sexual relationship with a partner. But it's not **always the explicit 'do and don't' rules of parents** that matter as much as the implicit attitudes. However much a mother may talk in a relaxed way about sex, it's not much use if she herself is physically inhibited.

What *is* important is the mother's basic capacity for physical warmth, and the kind of physical relationship between the parents, because this is the image that the little girl incorporates into her own developing sense of femininity.

Of course, the early loss of a father or mother creates a loss of security which can affect relationships in adult life, perhaps creating difficulty in actual lovemaking. A woman may be afraid to 'let go' on the tide of rising passion from an instinctive fear of being let down – as she felt she was long ago by the loss of her parent.

The very early handling of the baby by her mother is also important. The nervous mother who holds her baby like a piece of fragile china **may, on a primitive non-verbal level, convey a sense of body insecurity. The warm, happily confident mother, holding her baby closely and securely, will implant in the child the sense of physical security which should grow into sexual confidence.**

Young people who have never had enough security and love as children, may grow up dreaming of a sexual relationship as the great event which will make up to them for all their earlier deprivations. It's more likely that reality will not match up to this idealized concept although, in time, they may hopefully learn to relax enough to find that intercourse can be a very deep and satisfying experience.

Is it possible to be frigid with one man and not with another?

For every woman (as for every man) there is a secret and very private image of what kind of lovemaking and lover makes them feel sexually aroused in a satisfactory way. The lover has to give them that very special something which makes them feel exquisitely feminine in a way which is pleasurable and good. Certainly there *are* partners who are right and wrong for any individual.

This may be a problem for people who marry very young; often they grow away from each other and their own private sexual needs may **diverge more and more. Other women who complain of frigidity turn out to have partners** who are simply ignorant about a woman's needs in intercourse, perhaps quite unable to caress them or even show tenderness. In such cases, frigidity can be a self-protective mechanism against the disappointment or frustrated desire the woman feels.

However, changing the man won't help solve a woman's difficulties if the main problem lies in her own inner emotional difficulties.

Can changes in your body turn you off sex?

A self-image of a good, healthy body gives a woman confidence in herself and her sexuality. If this image is interfered with in some way, she **may well start to lose this confidence which is so essential to her.**

Some women find they don't want or enjoy intercourse after having a baby. It's well known that post-natal blues is a phase that usually **passes, but some women have an underlying, deep fear that the actual birth of the baby has somehow taken away their capacity for sexual enjoyment for ever,** especially when there has been a long labour and perhaps painful stitching.

Changes in the menopause can also be very disturbing to a woman's self-image; hot flushes, cold sweats or unpredictable menstruation can all lead to a feeling that her body has taken over and she is no longer in control; vaginal dryness may mean that sex becomes painful, although it never has been before. Added to all this, the face in the mirror no longer seems to return quite the same reassuring image.

It seems that pleasure in one's own body is a very important component of a happy sex life. Certainly you should have no hesitation about consulting your doctor or a counsellor if any kind of physical change seems to lead to a loss of interest in sex.

Where can a woman go for help?

Books and magazines can be a comforting source of explanation and advice, if a woman happens to find an account of a similar problem to her own. On the other hand, books that are full of pronouncements on 'right and wrong' techniques might make her feel even more depressed. Generally, a woman is more likely to get help by talking to someone who can see the problem in the setting of her own personality and background. Her regular doctor may be able to help – if not he can recommend a specialist in this area. Also, a number of family planning clinics do have sessions for people with sexual difficulties.

Masturbation

Colin Ramsay

Is it true that men masturbate more than women?

Research suggests that it's more common in boys than girls – the ratio is 8:1. Physical differences make it much more likely that boys will masturbate. The penis is something which can't help but be noticed, especially as it hardens spontaneously. A boy soon finds that stroking it until it goes hard produces pleasant feelings. Female sexual organs are less obvious, however, so that girls may never discover the pleasure which they can get from self-stimulation.

Many women learn to masturbate as they grow older and may only get around to doing so in adult life. Men tend to masturbate a great deal in childhood and adolescence and then less and less as life goes on. In research, over 90 per cent of adult men say they have masturbated at sometime. The number of women who admit to masturbating is lower – about 60 per cent. However, since many people are shy about revealing their sexual behaviour – and some don't even know what masturbation is – these figures may be lower than is really the case.

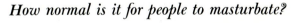

How normal is it for people to masturbate?

Masturbation simply means someone stimulating their own sex organs – it's a perfectly normal way of relieving sexual tension. From the earliest months, babies may learn to masturbate while exploring their bodies. They soon find that the sex organs are more sensitive and therefore much more fun to explore than the rest of their bodies, and touching them becomes a source of comfort and relaxation. Babies of both sexes may masturbate by rubbing their thighs together and pressing against something hard. Sometimes this reaches a climax with the baby 'thrusting' in a sexual way and crying, then relaxing, contented.

Men usually masturbate by stroking the penis by hand, while women stimulate the clitoris – either directly by hand or by pressing down on something hard.

Some women use a false penis to stimulate the vagina, or they may reach a climax just by rhythmically squeezing the thigh muscles.

Almost everybody masturbates at some time, and yet worry about masturbation is common. In fact it often causes more trouble than worries about sexual intercourse. The old idea that it's something dirty or harmful is certainly dying out, but many people still don't realize it is an absolutely normal stage in sexual development, which may continue to be a common part of people's lives.

Why is masturbation an important part of sexual development?

People who understand their own sexual functions through masturbation are more likely to have a fulfilling sex life. What they learn about themselves can play an important part in working out a good sexual relationship with a partner. The normal stages in sexual development start with masturbation then progress to petting with a partner. When two people know each other's bodies and needs, they can achieve the sexual closeness which most people hope for and need.

Once children develop sexual needs, masturbation may be the only outlet. Boys and men are highly likely to know about masturbation and they tend to discuss it with one another – even if it's only in a joking way. But many women who masturbate regularly never discuss it with anybody else, while some women don't even know what masturbation is. Women who masturbate in childhood, however, are far more likely to achieve orgasms during sexual intercourse than women who have never masturbated.

In this sense, masturbation could be seen as a kind of training for full sexual response, so it is an important part of sexual development.

Unfortunately, some parents still think that masturbation is sinful and must be stifled, and this often means that a child is smacked for touching his sex organs. Children who are punished and lectured about masturbation can certainly develop hang-ups about it which can spoil their adult sex lives. The taboos surrounding masturbation are so strong that the guarded way in which people talk about it – or usually avoid mentioning it at all – reinforces any sense of guilt caused by previous punishment or tickings off.

These kinds of attitudes can be one of the factors which inhibits normal sexual development but many sexual difficulties can be helped by therapy. Many of the remedies for certain sexual problems actually use masturbation as a starting point, as part of a treatment programme supervised by a special therapist. Talking about practising masturbation can help people to deal with the sense of guilt which has caused many of their problems.

Of course some of the problems associated with 'frigidity' may run very deep, and there are no 'mechanical' solutions, but it's also been found that therapy involving masturbation can help a frigid woman to build up a normal sex life. By first examining her own sexual organs, she is made familiar with her own sensations, and she can then progress to enjoying them with a partner. The doctor who introduced a mirror to women with sexual problems made a great breakthrough!

What is mutual masturbation?

It's usually called 'heavy petting' – in other words a couple touching and stimulating each other's sensitive parts without actually having intercourse.

Mutual masturbation allows two people to get close and to find out one another's needs before getting down to full intercourse. It helps a man to discover that a woman's 'equipment' is very different from his, and that it may take her much longer to become responsive than it does for him to get aroused. There are special nerve endings in the vagina and clitoris which only become sensitive when the blood supply to the area increases and the glands in the vulva produce the secretions to moisten the delicate mucous membranes. In the man, the same sort of nerve endings become sensitive when the penis is stiff and the end becomes hard and moist. His erection is obvious; the woman's equivalent is less so, but nonetheless real. Couples who go through this petting stage learn these extremely important facts, and lay firm foundations for a happy sex life together.

Children, too, may sometimes get involved in a kind of mutual masturbation – sexual games like 'mummies and daddies' and mutual sexual curiosity are far more common than most adults like to believe. Children are only damaged by these 'games' if they are forced into them, or if

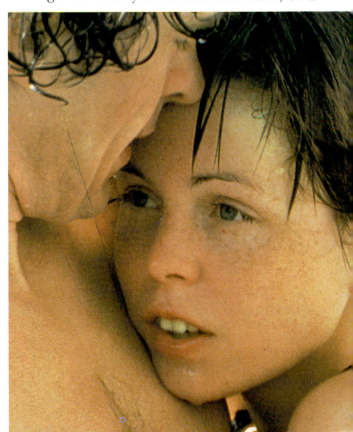

they are found out and punished, or are made to feel guilty about them.

The realization that it may be harmful to stop children from masturbating is one which is spreading slowly. If someone is prevented from exploring their natural sexual feelings, it may well create other hang-ups which can cause physical as well as emotional problems. A more relaxed and understanding upbringing can prevent many of these ever developing.

Is there something wrong if someone never masturbates?

Not really. Surveys show that at least a third of girls don't masturbate before they have sex, and about 5 per cent of men don't ever masturbate. Some of these people have sexual dreams or fantasies instead. Many people have simply never heard of (or thought of) it, and don't feel the need to stimulate themselves.

Some people, however, feel so guilty about masturbating when they 'find out' what it is, they stop doing it and suppress what are generally normal sexual feelings. It's hardly surprising that this happens – as a society we're still suffering from a hangover of the Victorian attitude that masturbation is an evil thing which could have terrible consequences.

Is masturbating a lot an 'unhealthy' sign?

Masturbation is only unhealthy when it leads to unhappiness. This kind of unhappiness is usually a result of feeling guilty. The problem usually begins in early life. A child who is unhappy because he is deprived of love or rigidly over-disciplined, or perhaps upset by parental quarrels, may find that masturbation is the only satisfaction he can get in life. He masturbates mainly because he needs reassurance, but this may anger the parents who then punish the child. An unhappy child who craves attention may think that even punishment is better than being ignored, so he continues to masturbate, undeterred. This sets up a vicious circle – the punishment meant to stop the masturbation just makes it more and more necessary.

As an adult he may continue to masturbate to relieve unhappiness. He feels guilty about it, becomes unhappy because of his guilt and so has to masturbate again and again – it all becomes rather obsessive.

This cycle can only be broken if he has a sympathetic partner who doesn't regard masturbation as sinful, but often it's only one half of a couple who sees masturbation as a normal part of their lives. Sometimes the other partner may feel rejected. 'He isn't interested in me, and I know he goes into the bathroom to masturbate. It's disgusting!' a woman might say, or 'I feel such a failure.' When quizzed as to why she regards a normal event as disgusting she'll admit to feeling ashamed of masturbation. If she can lose this inhibition and make it a mutual sexual activity, the barrier that has developed could be broken down.

For some individuals, masturbation *can* become an obsession. Brian's father died when he was three. He had a very religious and repressed mother who taught him that masturbation was extremely sinful and would lead to all sorts of terrible illnesses. She warned him that God would see and tell her if he either masturbated or discussed sex. Not surprisingly, Brian grew up horrified at his own sexual development and he never talked about it to anyone. He developed elaborate rituals to avoid masturbating, but sometimes he was driven to it and couldn't resist. Afterwards he would wash his hands again and again to try and clear his guilt.

He married a girl who shared his mother's narrow views about sex, had never masturbated and thought it was thoroughly sinful. She was shocked and unsympathetic when Brian owned up to masturbating occasionally, and was no help to him. Only after his attempted suicide did she realize that Brian's problems were hers too, and that if she wanted to save the relationship she would have to accept and try to understand his needs, and come to terms with them.

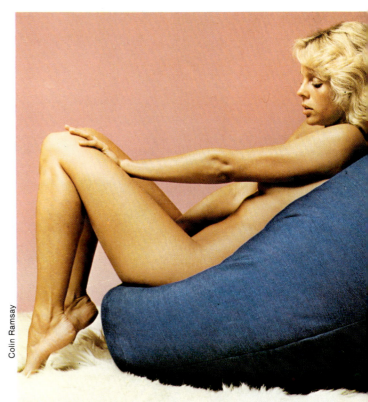

Colin Ramsay

Impotence

firm erection to have intercourse – but there are many different degrees of impotence, as well as a variety of causes. If failing to get an erection is an isolated, shortlived occurence, then it's nothing to worry about; this is quite normal and could be due to any number of things – too much to drink, strain and overwork, a temporary illness or worry.

When impotence is a more long term problem than this, it usually develops after a period of normal sexual function, although there are a small number of men who, right from adolescence, have never managed to produce an erection that's firm enough for intercourse.

Many women are fairly ignorant about male sexual problems; there's a tendency to think satisfaction is 'easy' for men, and it can be quite a surprise for a woman to get involved in a relationship where the man has some sexual difficulty. When a man has a problem getting an erection, his partner's attitude is crucial in trying to improve the situation. She can make things a lot worse by being demanding or derisory, while a sympathetic woman can contribute a great deal in helping a man to overcome his problem.

A man is 'impotent' if he can't get a sufficiently

What is wrong if a man can't get an erection?

Sometimes this is linked to an illness – about 10-15 per cent of impotent men have a physical basis for their sexual problem. If a man no longer awakes with an erection in the morning – as well as being impotent when he tries to make love – then it's likely that there is a physical cause. On the other hand, if he consistently wakes up with a firm erection and can masturbate normally, then the reasons are much more likely to be psychological, such as depression.

If a man suspects his impotence is linked to an illness, or perhaps to some drug he is taking

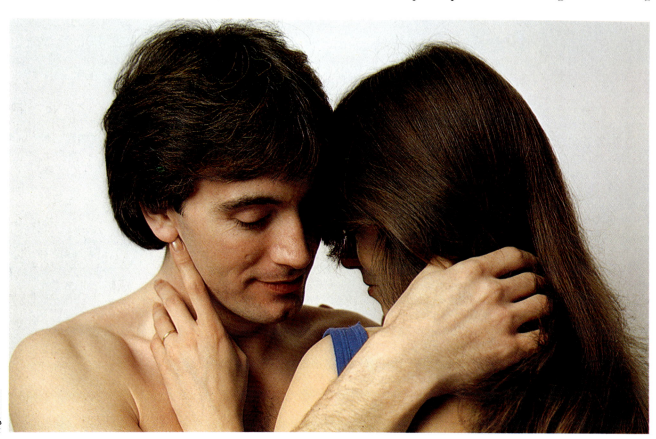

(those used to treat high blood pressure and some psychiatric problems have been known to affect sexual performance) then it's really a question he has to discuss with his doctor.

Sometimes there is a psychological factor involved as well; for example, quite a few men become impotent after prostate operations – not because this need cause any 'real' physical difficulty, but because they are ignorant and afraid about the effect it's going to have on their potency. Equally their wives may be unwilling to have sex after the operation, thinking that sex is now in some way forbidden. It seems that the men who are reassured about the operation and given all the facts are much less likely to develop problems after prostate surgery.

It's more common for the cause of impotence to be entirely psychological, related to a strong source of anxiety about sex — ignorance about 'what to do', fear of failure, a sense of guilt, or of being discovered and punished. This in turn may be related to the attitudes to sex that were impressed on a man in childhood, if he had a very negative, restrictive upbringing or his parents had the attitude that sex was something dirty and forbidden. Occasionally it may be that the man suffered a traumatic childhood experience, such as being sexually assaulted by an adult, or perhaps his first attempts at intercourse were disastrous.

Any kind of hostility, anger or resentment towards the woman he is trying to make love to may mean a man cannot respond sexually – sometimes this relates to a fear of making her pregnant or a fear of hurting her. It may be that she makes excessive demands on him; a man may feel so threatened if his sexual performance is criticized that the anxiety this sets up makes him impotent. Or it can reflect a general problem that affects the whole relationship – when sex has become a battleground for other conflicts.

Is it true that drinking a lot always makes a man impotent?

Not necessarily. The effect of alcohol varies to some extent with the physical and psychological make-up of the man concerned, the amount consumed and how frequently he drinks. Alcohol is a general brain depressant which has the effect of releasing a person's inhibitions to a greater or lesser extent, depending on how much of it has been consumed. The occasional evening of social drinking may reduce anxiety and tension in a usually inhibited man and cause a temporary increase in his sexual desire but, if a man gets really drunk, his sexual performance *is*

usually affected and becomes inadequate.

Prolonged bouts of heavy drinking frequently leads to a deterioration in a man's sexual response as well as the kind of loud-mouthed, bullying behaviour that is liable to disrupt his marriage overall. It is estimated that about half of all male alcoholics suffer from some sort of sexual disturbance – around four in ten become impotent.

Can a man be impotent with one woman but sexually all right with another?

Although it is possible for a man to develop impotence because he has become bored with his partner and no longer finds her attractive, this is not very common. On rare occasions, however, a man may be impotent with his wife but quite normal with his mistress. This may be because he 'splits' women into two categories – love objects and sex objects. He may fall in love with the pure, angelic, untouchable love object and find it impossible to have any kind of sexual relationship with this idealized woman. So he tends to confine his sexual activity to women for whom he has no respect or regard, embarking upon a sequence of meaningless, casual encounters.

Therapy with this kind of man involves exploring general sexual attitudes and relationships, trying to help him develop a more healthy approach to sex. Sex therapy could also be an essential part of his treatment, and ideally this should involve a woman for whom he feels positive affection.

How can a woman help her partner?

It rather depends on what kind of impotence the man is experiencing. Coping with a temporary problem within a basically good marriage is very different from taking on a relationship with a man who has always had a degree of sexual difficulty.

If some kind of short-term illness, worry or stress is at the root of the problem, then clearly it's not going to help if the man feels extra tension or pressure about his sexual performance. If both partners can talk freely about it, they may find it quite acceptable just to ignore sex for a while, though still enjoying the warmth and affection of their usual close physical contact. It's a balance between the woman making it clear she still wants him – when he's ready – but not making demands he cannot cope with for the moment.

On the man's side, he might spare a thought for the very natural feeling on the woman's part

81

What causes impotence?

For the majority of men, impotence is a short-lived state of affairs, brought on by factors including:

- fatigue
- certain prescribed drugs
- too much alcohol
- stress
- acute illness

But for some, the problem is longer term and will need professional assistance. It may be there's a physical cause that needs tackling (diabetes, emphysema or kidney failure *may* have this effect), but more often there's a psychological basis for the difficulty.

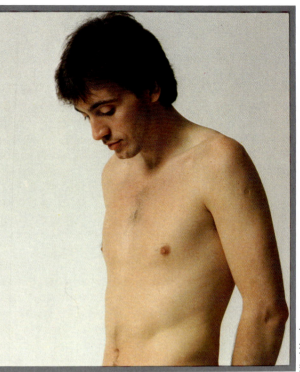

Nigel Heed

that 'he doesn't want me any more', and try to reassure his partner that he still very much needs her affection and support. And if oral or manual stimulation can give some sexual satisfaction, there is no reason to stop this kind of love play.

If the problem doesn't resolve itself, then it's certainly worth asking your doctor's advice. If the problem is a more long term one, then it's often essential for a wife to help by getting involved in whatever kind of counselling sessions or therapy are recommended by the specialist.

What kind of therapy is available?

If the impotence is a symptom of a general personality problem or neurotic illness, then individual psychotherapy may be the appropriate treatment. Anxiety-reducing drugs may also be used, and hormone preparations are sometimes helpful in the rare instances when hormone imbalance is causing the impotence. Sometimes, when the sexual problem comes second to some other source of tension in a relationship, then marriage counselling is the most useful first step.

The success of this treatment depends on both halves of the couple taking joint responsibility for their problem – and this is something the counsellor will help them to work towards. He will also encourage them to discuss with each other their sexual attitudes and fears, for recognizing them is the first step to overcoming them. The counsellor's suggestions and interpretations will help resolve any conflict.

One particular therapy technique, known as *sensate focus*, is commonly used to help overcome impotence. The counsellor will suggest a series of exercises for the couple to follow at home. These teach them to explore each other's bodies; to start with, touching the sexual organs and intercourse itself is banned. This removes any fear of failure or pressure to 'perform' from the man. So sexual stimulation is non-demanding and free from anxiety – the emphasis is on experiencing sensation, not achieving an orgasm.

Gradually, in this more relaxed atmosphere, the man will usually get spontaneous erections. The couple can then begin to stimulate each other's genital area. The man gains confidence as his erections come and go. The next stage is for the woman to lie on top of the man and to insert his penis into her vagina; she should thrust a few times but stop before the man becomes anxious and loses his erection. The man can reach an orgasm by manual stimulation, either from himself or his partner. Only once the man has sufficient confidence should the couple continue making love; and eventually they will progress to the man taking the so called 'dominant' position above the woman.

Is there a surgical cure for impotence?

During the last 10 to 15 years, a number of devices have been developed that can be implanted surgically in an impotent man to help him have intercourse. This treatment would usually only be used when his impotence was due to some irreversible physical cause, such as the effects of bowel or bladder surgery or a disease of the nerves that supply the sexual organs.

Either a fixed plastic rod or an inflatable device can be fitted. The disadvantage of the plastic rod is that it produces a permanent state of semi-erection, which may be embarrassing for the man. Infection is also a risk. The inflatable penile implant produces an erection only when the man wants it, and the penis looks entirely normal; both the patient and his partner seem to find this more acceptable.

Can a single man have therapy to treat impotence?

Many men without partners seek help for their sexual problems. Some have become so distressed and humiliated by their problem that they deliberately avoid socializing with women. Others become reluctant to start a relationship, knowing that before long their problems will be revealed and they will be subjected to further embarrassment.

These men pose a problem for therapists working in sex clinics, since sexual therapy nearly always involves treating the *couple*, improving their communications and encouraging them to collaborate in the kind of exercises described above. Some single women with sexual problems, such as those who have never experienced orgasm, can be helped with masturbatory exercises, but with men there are fewer treatment options.

Some clinics run special therapy sessions for males without partners. The group provides a setting where the men can discuss and share similar problems and experiences. Educational and erotic films are occasionally used, and the primary emphasis is on restoring the men's confidence. Some men can be helped by discussing the possible sources of their problem, by explaining the principles of sex therapy, and by reassuring them about the outcome should they find a suitable partner in the future.

When a single male with a sexual problem does meet a partner, he has to grapple with a number of problems. Should he disclose his problem and risk the consequences, or 'wait and see' hoping all will be well on the night? The second alternative is rarely successful and it's usually much better for him to discuss his difficulties before trying to have intercourse. If the relationship is reasonably stable and the woman is willing to attend a therapy clinic, there's every chance of a successful outcome. Your own doctor will be able to refer you to a suitable therapy clinic.

What should you do if your husband denies he has a problem?

This can create a considerable dilemma for a woman. If she believes that their relationship is being damaged by her partner's sexual problem she should try to discuss it with him; if he continues to deny that the problem exists then *she* becomes the person with the problem who has to decide on a policy of action. This really depends upon the degree of her commitment to the relationship, and in practice her options are limited.

If she wants the relationship to continue then she should seek advice from her doctor or a marriage guidance counsellor, who may be able to devise a method of getting the man to acknowledge his problem. One useful way is to adopt the 'what if' approach. This does not challenge a man who rigidly denies the problem, but merely asks him to consider the issue from a different viewpoint. For example, the man could be asked: 'What if your best friend developed a sexual problem and was unable to tell his wife about it?' 'What would you advise him and his wife to do?' 'If this were someone's problem, what do you think he should do?'

Of course, some women may choose to leave the man and seek sexual satisfaction elsewhere, but this decision obviously depends how committed she is to the relationship. It's worth emphasizing that once the man *has* been encouraged to seek treatment, the outlook for their sexual relationship is optimistic.

Should a man expect to become impotent when he's older?

Males reach the peak of their sexual drive and potency at 17 or 18; at this age erections may occur instantaneously. With increasing age a man requires more time and stimulation to achieve an erection. After the age of 50, orgasm gradually assumes less importance within the sexual experience and there is usually less of a physical need to ejaculate. It's quite usual for some men over 50 to be unable to have an erection for 12-24 hours after they have ejaculated, and a man over 60 will certainly have a slightly less firm erection as compared to someone younger.

For many men over this age, sexual activity can be satisfying without ejaculating at each attempt at intercourse, and there is no reason why the older man who has a happy relationship with his wife cannot enjoy satisfying love-play and intercourse well into old age.

The male orgasm

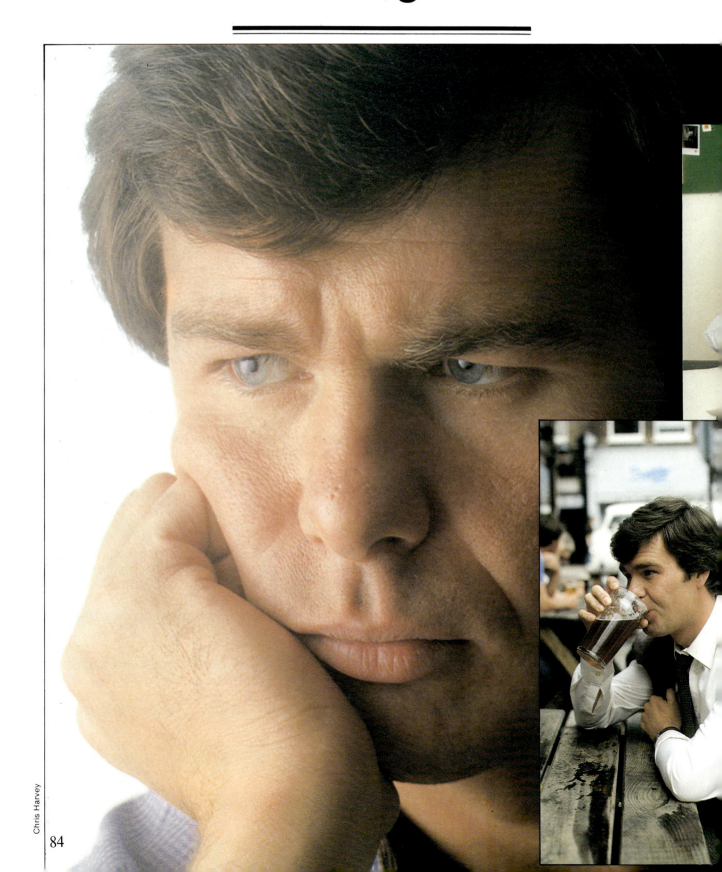

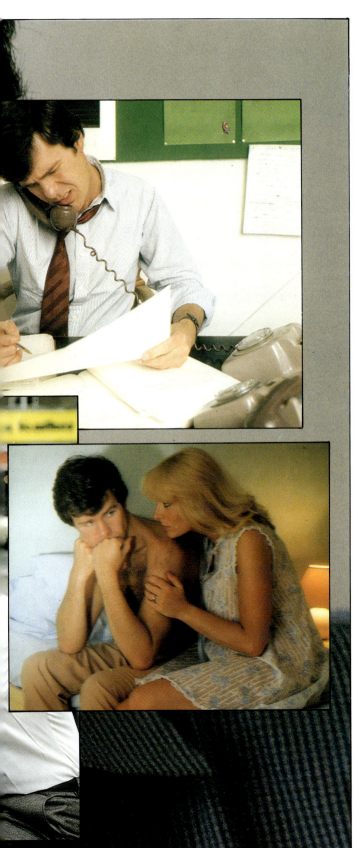

When a man finds he is unable to control his orgasm it can lead to a very unsatisfactory relationship for both partners. If he climaxes very quickly (premature ejaculation) it may well mean that the woman never reaches a high level of arousal or is unable to obtain orgasm when they are making love. Over a period of time she may become very frustrated and resentful and begin to doubt her own sexuality. And, even if she constantly reassures him, the man will often feel inadequate as a lover and guilty that he is letting his partner down.

How does a man normally control his orgasm?

Though male orgasm is a reflex action centred in the spinal cord, it can, like other reflexes, be partially brought under the conscious control of the brain. Most men learn to control their orgasm through a combination of practice and experience although it is possible to 'retrain' if things are going wrong.

The early experiences of orgasm are usually through masturbation and this is where many adolescents start to learn control. As a man becomes more aware of the sensations in his penis, he learns to delay an orgasm by stopping or slowing the rate of friction from his hand. Later on, he 'remembers' these experiences during sexual intercourse, where hopefully he adjusts and refines them to meet the changed circumstances of stimulation. However, it's not unusual for his early experiences to end in premature ejaculation.

Research has shown that when premature ejaculation occurs the man moves from a state of relatively low excitement to high orgasmic excitement with little intermediate build up. The penis erects rapidly and discharges at once without the usual relatively long period of erection. In time it is possible for a man to become more consciously aware of the sensations in his penis and learn to avoid the sort of excessive stimulation which can lead to premature orgasm. He should then be in a position to decide when he will 'come'.

Why do some men suffer from 'coming too soon'?

Though there are physical conditions and medical treatments which make it difficult to achieve orgasm, the commonest reason is psychological. And alcohol, etc, taken to alleviate anxiety and improve performance can actually make things worse, although one or two *small* drinks may help as a relaxant.

Anxiety is the major psychological cause of

premature ejaculation. For instance, a man may be able to control his orgasm with his wife but fail to perform adequately in an affair for fear of being found out. More general anxieties, such as worries about work, may also lead to a temporary bout of premature ejaculation.

Another very common anxiety has to do with fears about performing badly. Here, because the man worries so much about his 'poor' performance, he aggravates his condition even more and a vicious circle builds up – the more he worries the less control he has and vice versa. Clearly, if his partner is also unsympathetic the situation will deteriorate still further.

Anxieties may also originate from deep underlying causes related to his past experiences. If a man felt a lot of guilt about masturbating or making love when he was younger, he may have deliberately learned to come very quickly in order not to be discovered or to get it over as soon as possible, so as not to prolong his guilty feelings. His penis then becomes conditioned to ejaculate rapidly and once this pattern is established it may prove difficult to alter, so that the problem persists even in a relaxed atmosphere with a partner he loves.

Or a man who has learnt that it is dangerous to get close to another person because it is so hurtful to lose them may be afraid that in the closeness achieved during sexual intercourse (which is after all the most intimate of human activities) there is a danger of revealing his innermost feelings and giving his partner the power to hurt him. This anxiety about intimacy is alleviated by ejaculating quickly and reducing contact to the briefest possible interlude. It is common for such a man to find a partner who also has this fear of intimacy and unconsciously welcomes the failure as a solution to her own particular problem.

While most men who ask for sex therapy see themselves as having the 'problem' while their partner is completely 'blameless', sex therapists often find that the difficulty has arisen because of the general way the couple relates.

John referred himself for help with premature ejaculation. He was seen with his wife, Pam, who was very unsure whether she wanted help because she did not see the premature ejaculation as a problem. It emerged that she was very prudish about sex, had never really enjoyed it and saw it as primarily a way of making children. Her emotional ties were closer to her father and her children than to John. By preventing them from getting too close Pam 'used' the problem as a way of remaining faithful to the rest of her family. Also, a closer and more enjoyable sex life would, she felt, lead John to feel he was competing with her family for her affections. Somehow she believed that by reducing intimacy to a minimum she was sparing John from feeling rejected. In her discussions with John, she was mildly sarcastic, which increased John's difficulty.

Claire, on the other hand, referred herself for lack of interest in sex. It emerged that Peter, her husband, had always come, after a few seconds

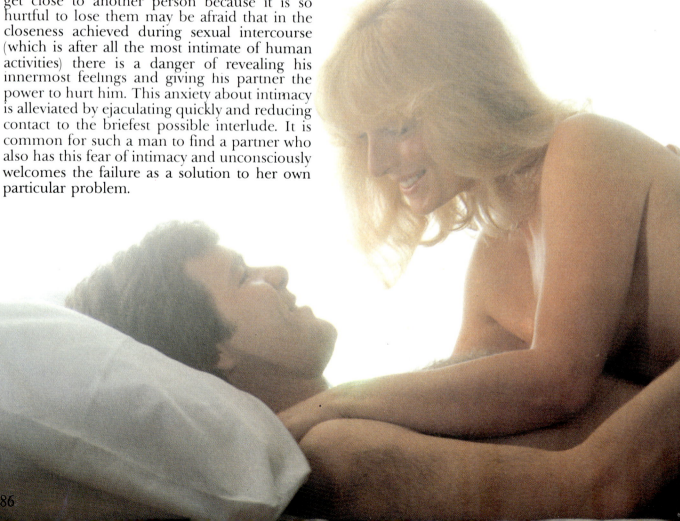

of entering her, and she had never been close to orgasm. Peter was very adamant that the problem was Claire's, largely because he was ignorant about sexual matters. However, it turned out that their sexuality mirrored other aspects of their relationship. They had never learned the 'give and take' philosophy of a happy relationship, both preferring to be on the receiving end of things. Both had come from homes where all discussions of sex had been avoided or carried on in hushed tones. Open discussions and the discovery that there is joy in giving helped them achieve a happy relationship.

What effects can this problem have on a relationship?

A man who suffers from premature ejaculation will often feel very inadequate, thinking himself as only 'half a man' and taking out his frustrations on his family, friends and work mates. At the same time his partner is probably feeling sexually frustrated and used, and she too may take it out on other people. She may also feel rejected and begin to doubt that she is sexually attractive.

The problem may create such tension that it indirectly causes some kind of emotional disturbance in the family. In some cases, a therapist may only become aware of sexual problems between a couple after he has been asked to help with a child who has trouble with delinquency or bedwetting.

Both partners may embark on affairs – the man to prove himself and the woman to cope with her sexual frustration and to reassure herself that she is sexually desirable.

How can a man overcome premature ejaculation?

Many men unsuccessfully attempt to treat themselves by distractions during intercourse – they think of non-sexual things or inflict pain on themselves by, for example, sticking their nails into their hands. The reason this won't work is because it takes the man's attention even further away from the sensations in his penis and so increases his lack of control.

It really is worth seeking professional help because premature ejaculation is the easiest sexual difficulty to treat, with some therapists reporting a success rate of up to 90 per cent. Overcoming premature ejaculation is a combination of learning to let go and learning that you have a right to enjoy sex.

What are the techniques used to treat it?

Most modern sex therapists prefer to see both partners, partly because treatment requires the co-operation of the female, but also in order to discover the underlying cause of the problem. They avoid blaming either of the partners, attempting to teach them to see the difficulty as a shared problem which hopefully can be resolved by changing not only the physical aspects of their sexuality but also the general problems in the relationship. After learning not to blame one another for the problem, the couple must be taught to accept and enjoy their own and each other's bodies and in this way to come to see sex as an act of love.

A therapist will teach the man control by suggesting exercises designed to increase the couple's awareness of each other's bodies. He will ask the woman to stimulate the penis manually and the man to concentrate on his own physical sensations rather than his partner's sexual needs. When the man feels an orgasm is close (the premonitory sensation) he must tell his partner to stop until these feelings have abated. The exercise is repeated four times, and only on the fourth occasion is the man allowed to ejaculate. After this, he can bring his wife to orgasm either manually or orally.

This technique is called the 'stop-start' method and is designed to teach the man to be aware of the sensations in his penis so that he can learn to consciously control them. When he has a reasonable degree of control by this method, the woman repeats the exercises with lubricated hands to simulate the secretions of the vagina.

When the man is able to exercise reasonable control in these circumstances he is asked to try the 'stop-start' technique as part of intercourse. He lies on his back and the woman straddles him and moves up and down on his penis. When he feels the premonitory sensation he asks her to stop until the sensation has passed. Again the exercise is repeated four times, at the end of which he is allowed to ejaculate. The woman is asked to be in this position because it is less stimulating for the man than when she is underneath. When they can do this with reasonable success, they can repeat the exercises in a side-to-side position and finally with the man on top.

Some sex therapists introduce a modification to this technique by asking the woman to firmly squeeze the ridge around the tip of the penis for about three seconds after the man has asked her to stop. This leads to the man losing the urge to ejaculate. There is also some loss of erection.

A similar sequence of stages is followed with this 'squeeze' technique as for the stop-start method. Here, however, the woman will have to remove the penis from her vagina during the later exercises to apply pressure to the tip.

Is it true that some men find it difficult to ejaculate at all?

This is a less common problem than premature ejaculation, but when it does occur it can have an equally disruptive influence on the man's self image and the relationship as a whole.

Most men will have had problems with delayed or absent ejaculation at one time or another, either because they were tired or had too much to drink. There is only a real problem if a man is frequently unable to reach orgasm or is only able to do so after very prolonged love play.

Men who suffer from delayed or absent ejaculation are, typically, able to maintain a firm erection for long periods and although the problem is often confined to intercourse it may also happen during solitary masturbation. In a small percentage of cases, the man may be unable to ejaculate with one partner but be successful with another.

Although the problem may be due to illness or medication (ask your doctor about this) it is more likely that the cause is psychological: the man is over-controlling his orgasmic reflex and is unable to 'let go'. In addition many retarded ejaculators

suffer from 'spectatoring' – they are too conscious of what they are doing during sexual intercourse and the more they observe themselves having sex, the less able they are to achieve orgasm.

There are many possible reasons why a man may find it difficult to 'let go'. He may have had a restrictive childhood when sex was equated with sin and masturbation, and was seen as something evil and shameful. Fear of making his partner pregnant or homosexual tendencies can also contribute to the problem.

It may be that the man was severely frightened while having sexual intercourse in the past – perhaps he was caught making love in his parents' house or in a car – or that he uses the affliction as a way of preventing himself from getting too close to his partner. Or he may have hostile feelings towards his partner and want to 'punish' her by not giving her his semen.

Joe, who was treated for retarded ejaculation, illustrates some aspects of these causes. While he had a great deal of sexual desire and could get and maintain an erection for over an hour, he had never ejaculated in a woman, although was quite capable of it during masturbation. He had been placed in a children's home at an early age and felt rejected by his mother. He had several bad experiences with bossy and sadistic female workers in the children's home who had punished him when he had 'wet dreams'. He had developed the idea that women did not deserve trust or love and subconsciously believed that they should be punished. He had never established a permanent relationship and his casual affairs tended to be with women who had an equally low opinion of men.

In order to stop over-controlling his orgasm a man must learn to relax and enjoy his sexuality and rid himself of his anxiety about coming in a woman. Therapists usually recommend a series of exercises which involve getting his partner to stimulate him and then allowing him to ejaculate by going into the next room and masturbating. On each successive occasion he is brought closer to the woman in order to ejaculate and eventually, if treatment is successful and he becomes confident in his ability to control his orgasm, he is able to come inside her.

Both partners need a great deal of patience and tolerance in carrying out the treatment. They must express their difficulties and even their anger with the therapist and with one another. These discussions are likely to embrace aspects of the relationship which appear to have nothing to do with sex. In doing this, they can achieve a greater degree of security and closeness which is, after all, what it is about.

CHAPTER 4

Pregnancy
and
Childbirth

Conception

At what time of the month is a woman most likely to get pregnant?

For a woman with a 28-day cycle, the most likely time to get pregnant is right in the middle of the month. Pregnancy can only happen when there is an egg in the Fallopian tube (see diagram) waiting to be fertilized by sperm.

Since the egg is usually produced 14 days before the next menstrual period, it is fairly easy to calculate the most fertile time. A woman with a 35-day cycle, for instance, would be most likely to get pregnant around day 21. Of course, if a woman has irregular periods, then counting back 14 days obviously won't work as a simple way of predicting the best date.

But there are other ways of working out when a woman is producing an egg. At this time, a hormone – called progesterone – is released, which causes the body temperature to rise. By taking your temperature every morning, you can see when a persistent rise in temperature takes place – indicating an egg has been released.

Some women notice a change in their vaginal secretions during ovulation – what's happening

When an egg is made

An egg is usually made 14 days before the start of a period. A persistent rise in body temperature takes place after ovulation. This chart shows the typical pattern, but actual temperatures fluctuate from one woman to another.

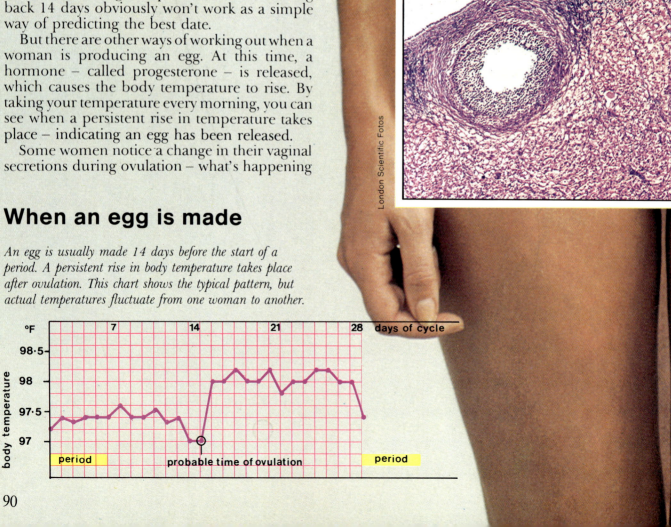

°F — days of cycle — 7 — 14 — 21 — 28

body temperature: 98·5, 98, 97·5, 97

period — probable time of ovulation — period

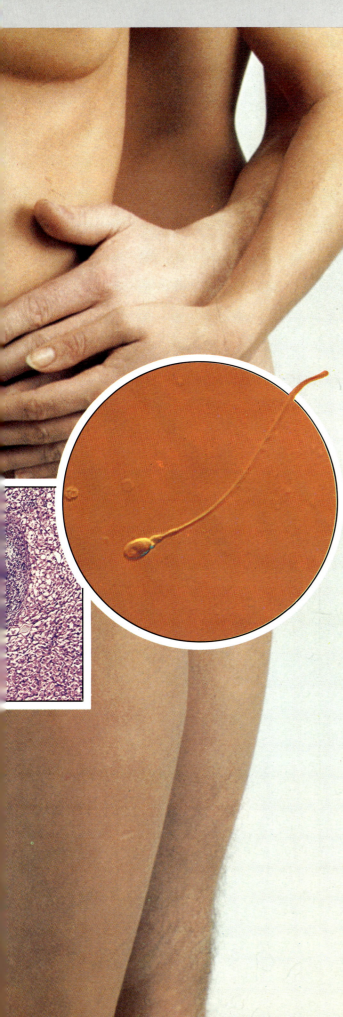

London Scientific Fotos

Mike Busselle

is that the mucus from the neck of the womb becomes very much thinner and less tacky than normal. Pain in the pit of the stomach is another sign of ovulation that some women experience. This is due to the release of a little fluid around the egg causing irritation of the lining of the stomach wall.

Once it has been released from the ovary, the egg lives only between 24 and 36 hours. If no sperm reaches the egg by then, it dies and is absorbed into the body's tissues.

How much sperm does a man usually produce?

Compared to a woman's egg production – usually limited to one every month – the quantities of sperm a man generates seem enormous. The actual amount produced varies according to demand. Anything between 60 and 200 million sperms may be ejaculated at any one time, although if he ejaculates, say, three or four times a day, the amount of sperm may diminish.

The sperm ejaculated during intercourse has been stored in the body for several weeks. The testicles store primitive sperm cells; as they mature, sperms are made and secreted from the testicle, passing into the system of tubes that lead up to the seminal vesicles – a pair of sacs behind the prostate gland. Here the sperms are stored and continue to mature for some weeks.

When a man ejaculates, most of the fluid actually comes from the prostate gland; as this fluid passes down the pipe to the penis, just before ejaculation, a small jet of sperm is squirted into it from each of the seminal vesicles. The amount of fluid ejaculated varies from about half a teaspoonful to a tablespoonful.

Provided the sperm count is above 20 million sperms per cubic centimetre, the man is probably perfectly fertile. Below this level, the chances of an active sperm reaching the far end of a woman's Fallopian tube become rather less.

How easy is it to get pregnant?

Outside the 24 to 36 hours period when the egg is present, the chances of getting pregnant are nil. Since sperm lives only 24 hours, intercourse taking place more than a day or so outside the time of ovulation will not result in pregnancy. This is the basis of the so-called 'safe period' or 'rhythm' method of contraception; but of course this does rely on a woman being able to calculate precisely her times of ovulation – which is not always a straightforward matter.

The vast number of sperm released during intercourse are necessary to give a reasonable chance of fertilizing an egg. The sperms move in all directions once they are deposited in the upper end of the vagina, and they have a long way to travel to reach the egg.

The diagram on this page shows the route: through the neck of the womb, through the cervical canal, then on to the moisture lining the womb, and along the Fallopian tube to meet the egg at the outer end. Relative to body size, this is equivalent to a man running from London to Oxford in just over an hour!

This gives some idea of the vast mobility required for the successful sperm to get to the far end of the Fallopian tube. Of the many millions of sperm deposited in the vagina during intercourse, probably only 50 or so will actually make the long and hazardous journey to reach the egg.

As far as we know, there is no chemical kind of attraction or other force that guides the sperm to the egg – until the sperm is very close. So the journey is partly a matter of chance.

Of the sperms which reach the egg, it is only a single sperm which penetrates the outer layers that causes fertilization. Once the sperm head has passed into the egg, the outer layers change to form an impenetrable block to stop any other sperm entering. The *nucleus* of the sperm is the part which contains the genetic material from the father; once this has fused with the egg, the new embryo is provided with all the vital genetic 'blue prints' from the mother and father in equal amounts.

Is it true that you can get pregnant without having intercourse?

Though getting pregnant is a chancy business, it can be achieved without the penis actually penetrating the vagina. Sperm deposited around the lips of the vagina by merely placing the penis between a woman's legs, may travel upwards through the cervix and on into the uterus and Fallopian tube.

The chances of this happening are rare, and of course conception is much less likely than if the sperm is deposited close to the cervix. But there are many instances of pregnancies in girls who are virgins who have had 'intercourse' between the thighs.

How sperm is made and stored

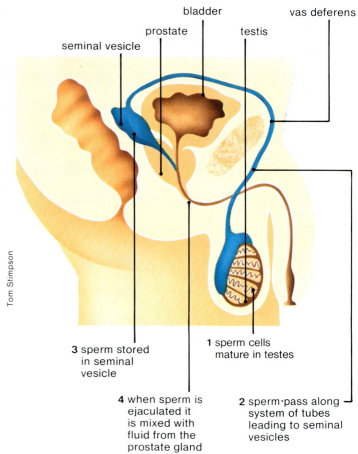

seminal vesicle · prostate · bladder · testis · vas deferens

3 sperm stored in seminal vesicle

4 when sperm is ejaculated it is mixed with fluid from the prostate gland

1 sperm cells mature in testes

2 sperm pass along system of tubes leading to seminal vesicles

Tom Stimpson

Are there any techniques which increase the chances of getting pregnant?

There are very few ways in which you can influence nature in this. Of course, as already explained, intercourse has to take place at the time of ovulation to result in pregnancy, but there are also some variations in technique which may slightly improve the chances of the sperm reaching the egg.

If a woman is particularly keen on getting pregnant, she might try to stay lying on her back after intercourse, and falling asleep in that position. This should minimize the amount of semen which passes down the vagina and escapes, and the pool of semen in the vagina will bathe the cervix for much longer than usual, thus slightly increasing the chances of sperm travelling up through the cervical canal. But it's doubtful just how big a difference this makes and, in any case, most people move in their sleep to adopt whatever position their body prefers.

Some people say that the quantity of sperm ejaculated during intercourse can be increased

How the egg is fertilized

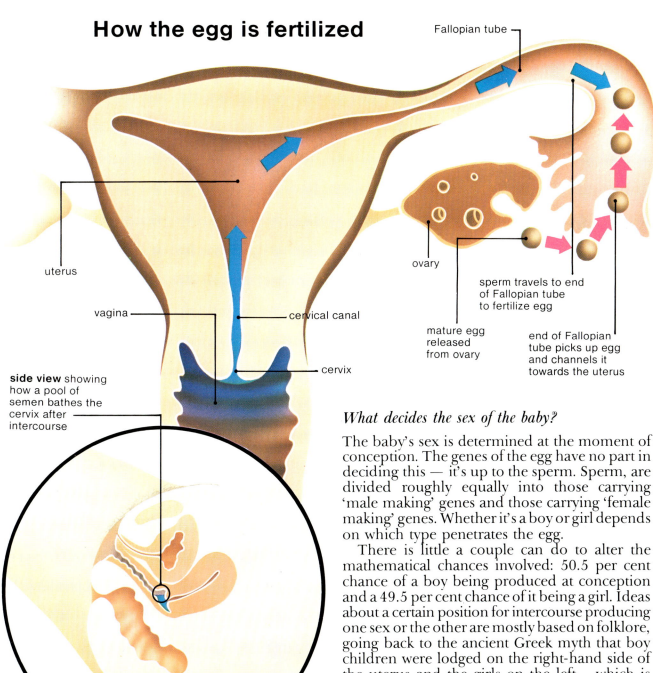

Fallopian tube

uterus

vagina

cervical canal

side view showing how a pool of semen bathes the cervix after intercourse

cervix

ovary

mature egg released from ovary

sperm travels to end of Fallopian tube to fertilize egg

end of Fallopian tube picks up egg and channels it towards the uterus

after a few days abstinence. For a man with a normal sperm count this actually makes no great difference. With a low sperm count, this 'saving up' of sperm for two or three days helps a bit, but longer than that makes no difference.

Some women produce a particularly thick mucus from the neck of the womb which sperm find difficult to penetrate. Medical treatment may help thin this to make fertilization easier.

What decides the sex of the baby?

The baby's sex is determined at the moment of conception. The genes of the egg have no part in deciding this — it's up to the sperm. Sperm, are divided roughly equally into those carrying 'male making' genes and those carrying 'female making' genes. Whether it's a boy or girl depends on which type penetrates the egg.

There is little a couple can do to alter the mathematical chances involved: 50.5 per cent chance of a boy being produced at conception and a 49.5 per cent chance of it being a girl. Ideas about a certain position for intercourse producing one sex or the other are mostly based on folklore, going back to the ancient Greek myth that boy children were lodged on the right-hand side of the uterus and the girls on the left – which is simply not true.

Research work is being done on how the acidity of the vagina may affect the odds; it is believed that male-making sperm are more active in a slightly acid vagina while female-making sperm are more active in a slightly alkaline environment.

In the past some people used to be recommended a douche using vinegar or sodium bicarbonate. These were a terrible nuisance and used to put many people off intercourse completely. Newer techniques include the use of gels – which are more elegant than douches and are formulated to alter slightly the acidity of the vagina. Research into this is still in progress.

How are twins conceived?

There are two sorts of twins – identical and non-identical. Identical twins are made from one egg fertilized by one sperm. When the fertilized egg divides to form two cells, normally these stick together, and go on to reproduce, making 4, 8, 16, 32 cells and so on. In some rare cases, however, at the two cell stage the clump divides completely and instead of going on to form a four cell unit, makes a *pair* of two cell *individuals*. So two absolutely identical clumps of cells are made. Each of these goes on to develop into a separate individual with a common genetic background – the result is identical twins.

Non-identical twins are the result of a woman making more than one egg during the menstrual cycle. If the two eggs are fertilized by two separate sperms they will develop into two separate individuals with *different* genetic backgrounds. They may also be of different sex, and bear no more resemblance to each other than any other brother or sister – they simply share the same womb at the same time. Identical twins, however, not only look like each other, they often resemble each other mentally and psychologically – even if they are separated and brought up in different families.

How twins are made

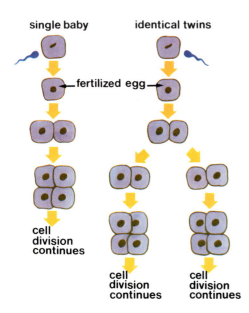

Identical *twins develop when a fertilized egg splits at the two-cell stage into a further two groups of two cells; each of these then goes on to develop into a baby.*
Non-identical *twins follow two 'single baby' patterns – two **separate** eggs are fertilized and develop in the womb together.*

What is the best age to get pregnant?

Nature probably intended women to conceive very soon after puberty. In primitive societies, a girl would have intercourse fairly soon after reaching sexual maturity and would probably soon get pregnant. From then onwards she was likely to be pregnant or breastfeeding for the next 10 or 15 years, bearing between eight and twelve babies, many of whom would die. This is of course far removed from the experience of women in modern Western societies. Few women now marry until their early 20s and having children is often postponed until the early 30s in order to pursue a career or job.

Statistically, the safest age for women in Britain to have children is between the ages of 20 and 29. Providing a woman is in reasonable health, there is no reason, however, why she should not wait until her 30s before starting a family.

The groups at greatest risk are the very young – those under 20 – and women over 40. Among the younger group, the risk is not their age, but the fact that many of them don't accept proper medical care.

Women in their late 30s may also face problems, but of a different sort. A child conceived by a woman of this age will be a teenager when the mother is in her late 50s. This in itself may produce a certain amount of family strain. Nowadays, any woman has to consider all these kinds of emotional and social factors – and not just purely medical ones.

How soon after having a baby should you get pregnant again?

When a mother is breastfeeding her baby, she will not usually produce any eggs. (But this is *not* a reliable means of birth control.) Once breast-feeding stops, egg production is likely to resume six to ten weeks later. If planning another pregnancy, the ideal interval between each one depends very much on the background of the mother, her age, the size of her existing family and what domestic help she has.

For most women there is no serious medical risk in a series of pregnancies in quick succession. Problems when they do occur tend to come later, when the mother has to cope with satisfying the demands of two babies. As a general rule, it makes life easier if a woman does not have to carry two children at once; leaving an interval of between 20 to 24 months before the birth of the next baby means the previous child will be toddling or walking. A lot depends on circumstances, however, and an older woman may want to have another child sooner than this.

The developing baby

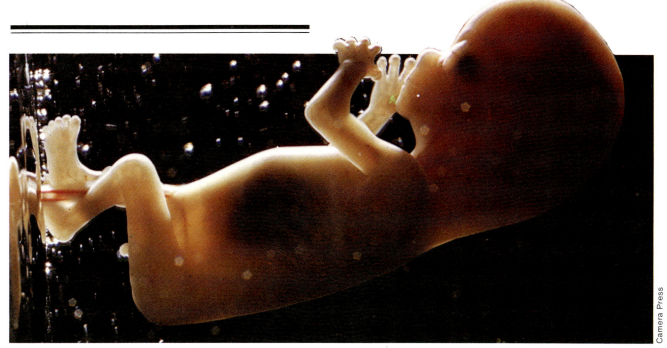

Long before a woman is aware she is pregnant, the fertilized egg she is carrying has already started to grow very rapidly. When a sperm fertilizes an egg it creates one complete cell — a tiny unit which contains all the genetic material to develop into a fully formed human being. The cell keeps dividing until in seven days it has grown into a clump of several hundred cells. Each of these continues to carry the complete genetic code which will determine the development of the baby – this is vital, for if the code is incomplete some kind of imperfection or abnormality will appear later on.

As the fertilized egg divides it passes down the Fallopian tube towards the womb. At the same time, the lining of the womb prepares to receive the egg: it grows thicker, nutrients are laid down in the cells and changes take place in the glands, making them ready to produce the amniotic fluid which will surround the foetus in the womb. It takes about 4-6 days for the fertilized egg to reach the womb, where it sticks to the wall and buries itself into the lining. At this stage, there will be a miscarriage if the egg fails to get a firm anchorage.

The term embryo is used to describe the fertilized, developing egg, up to the point when all the organs are formed. A foetus is considered to be a fully formed minute human being. So an embryo becomes a foetus after about 10 weeks.

How does food and oxygen reach the foetus?

An essential exchange station lies between the unborn child and its mother, known as the *placenta*. This vital link starts to develop once the egg is embedded in the lining of the womb. Cells from the outer edge of the embryo form a mass of finger-like projections which contain minute blood vessels. These invade the mother's tissues and develop into the placenta – it's rather like a thick plate or disc clamped onto the inside of the womb. By the time the baby is full term this is about 9 inches in diameter and an inch thick.

The 'fingers' in the placenta are bathed in a pool of the mother's blood; the placenta is linked directly to the foetus by large blood vessels which run along the umbilical cord. So, when nutrients and oxygen from the mother's blood pass into the blood vessels of the placenta, they are

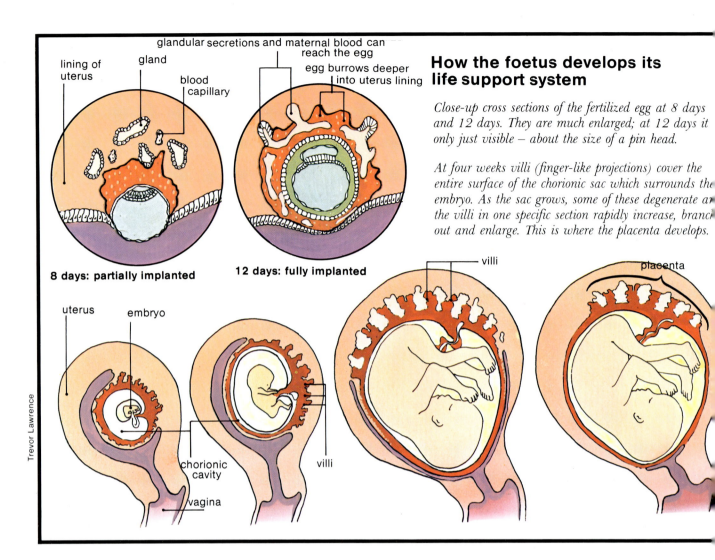

How the foetus develops its life support system

lining of uterus

gland

glandular secretions and maternal blood can reach the egg

blood capillary

egg burrows deeper into uterus lining

Close-up cross sections of the fertilized egg at 8 days and 12 days. They are much enlarged; at 12 days it only just visible – about the size of a pin head.

At four weeks villi (finger-like projections) cover the entire surface of the chorionic sac which surrounds the embryo. As the sac grows, some of these degenerate and the villi in one specific section rapidly increase, branch out and enlarge. This is where the placenta develops.

8 days: partially implanted

12 days: fully implanted

villi

placenta

uterus

embryo

chorionic cavity

villi

vagina

Trevor Lawrence

---

channelled through to the foetus. Waste products from the foetus can pass back into the mother's circulation in a similar way. The placenta is expelled shortly after the baby is born – hence the popular name 'afterbirth'.

Why is the foetus surrounded by fluid?

The foetus grows inside a sac (a bag of membrane) which is filled with amniotic fluid. The fluid has several functions; if the mother falls or bangs her abdomen against something, it will absorb some of the shock and so protect the foetus. It also helps to maintain an even temperature around the foetus, and provides a comfortable, sterile environment where the foetus can move its limbs freely. By the end of pregnancy the amount of fluid varies between 1 and 4 pints.

How quickly does the foetus develop?

The foetus grows very rapidly indeed – if a child were to continue growing at the same rate after birth as before, it would be 75 feet tall and weigh

several tons by the age of 19 years!

Different parts of the foetus grow at different rates. Most of the blood which contains oxygen is pumped to the head area of the foetus, so the brain and head grow most quickly. In the early stages of pregnancy the foetus appears to be almost all head and, even at birth, a baby's head still looks disproportionately large for the size of its body.

The limbs are of little use inside the womb so they have a relatively poor blood supply – at birth they are rather puny in relation to the rest of the body. It's not until the baby starts to toddle that the legs become stronger and grow longer than the rest of the body.

When can you feel the first 'kicks'?

Usually a mother first feels her baby move during the 18th to 20th week of pregnancy. However, the foetus has been moving much earlier than this – a doctor using an ultrasound machine can detect movements at about 8 to 10 weeks. Pregnant women should write down

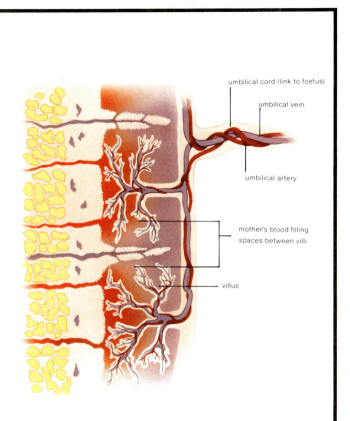

The detail of the placenta shows how it acts as an exchange station between the mother and foetus.

weeks, 8 weeks, or 12 weeks after the first day of the last normal period. If a pregnant woman notices any loss of blood, however slight – even brown staining from old blood – at these times she should stay in bed and contact her doctor. Most miscarriages which occur in the early stages are caused by the embryo being abnormal.

What's the normal size for a full-term baby?

The average length is about 20 inches (50cms) and boys are often a little longer than girls. The average weight of a full-term normal child is 7-7½ pounds (3-3.5 kilograms), with boys usually weighing a little more than girls. But a baby who is under this weight at birth is not necessarily abnormal or premature. Taller mothers may expect to have slightly longer babies.

Why does a premature baby look so wrinkly?

A newborn child has a layer of fat beneath its skin which makes it look quite rounded. In the first weeks of pregnancy an external layer of fatty material protects the baby from loss of temperature, but proper fat is not laid down until the last six weeks of pregnancy. A premature baby has not had time to lay down much fat and so will have wrinkled skin and look rather wizened.

How soon is it possible to tell the sex of a baby?

If you could actually see the foetus around 12 weeks it would already be clear whether it's going to be a boy or girl. Testing this from the 'outside' is not quite so straightforward. The only reliable method of checking the sex while the baby is in the womb is to examine the chromosomes in the baby's cells – these are shed from the baby's skin into the surrounding fluid. The test involves passing a needle through the stomach wall into the womb to draw out fluid and to collect some of the cells. They are then processed and examined under a microscope.

This is only done after about the 16th week of pregnancy, since there would be too few cells before this time. There is a risk of causing a miscarriage, so it's only done for medical reasons, not just to satisfy the curiosity of impatient parents! A doctor might want to know the sex of an unborn child if he suspected it was carrying a sex-determined disease, such as haemophilia.

Later in pregnancy (30 weeks) an ultrasound scan of the foetus may show up a scrotum on the 'picture'. However, this is difficult to achieve as it depends on the ultrasound beam travelling in the exact plane between the baby's legs. For this

when they first feel the baby move, as this may be useful later in deciding exactly what date the baby is due.

When does the baby's heart start beating?

In the early stages of development there is simply a 'tube' which will eventually develop into the baby's heart. But research has shown that there are pulsations in the tube as early as 22 days after conception – that's about 5 weeks from the first day of the last normal menstrual period. These pulsations can be detected at about 14 weeks using a hand-held ultrasound machine, and a bigger hospital ultrasound instrument might pick them up a week or two earlier. The human ear can usually hear the baby's heart beat, through a special stethoscope, at about 20 weeks of pregnancy.

When is the greatest risk of miscarriage?

The embryo is most likely to be dislodged at the time when a period would be expected — at 4 reason it is not commonly used as a method of determining sex.

Another way of testing may be to detect the very small amounts of a male hormone which pass into the mother's body fluids (blood or saliva) if she is carrying a boy. If these hormones could be detected with certainty they might give an indication of a male child, but work on this test is still at an early stage and is by no means conclusive.

It is often thought that male and female babies have a different heart rate at the foetal stage, but most doctors will not suggest it as a guide to indicating the sex.

How much do we know about life in the womb?

There are various techniques nowadays which can help to give an idea of how the foetus grows and responds inside the mother's body. Some of the techniques, such as ultrasound – which builds up an echo picture of the growing foetus – were developed primarily to monitor the baby's health. Likewise a fetoscope – a special telescope – can be inserted under anaesthetic through the mother's stomach wall and into the uterus; this can give information about any visible problems, such as a limb deformity.

Recent research has produced a lot of information about how the unborn baby moves, sees, hears. For example, in the early weeks after conception, the baby is sufficiently well formed to bend his fingers around an object, and in response to a touch on the sole of his foot he curls his toes. It seems that the level of the baby's activity – kicking and squirming – increases when the mother is under emotional stress. With prolonged stress, there is an increase in movement up to 10 times the normal level.

Quite early on in pregnancy, the eyes of the foetus move when it changes position or goes to sleep and in late pregnancy, when some light can penetrate into the womb from outside, the baby's activity increases in response to a bright light.

After about 20 weeks it seems that the ears are working, as the foetus responds to a wide variety of sounds, including loud outside noises such as a door slamming. Of course, the foetus is surrounded by noise in the womb, such as the rhythmic sound of blood circulation, and of air passing through the mother's intestine. A mother's natural tendency to hold a new born baby on the left side, where he can hear her heartbeat, may have a calming effect because it is providing the same reassuring rhythm which he has been used to inside the womb.

How the foetus grows

0 – 6 weeks
☐ The embryo is beginning to form a 'body' shape with a head and tail
☐ The brain and spinal column start to form, along with the limb buds (tiny bumps from which the limbs will grow)
☐ The heart starts beating

6 – 12 weeks
☐ The head is tucked down onto the chest and is very large in proportion to the rest of the body
☐ The tail has almost disappeared and the limbs have grown to become arms and legs with recognizable hands and feet. The curves of the shoulders, elbows, hips and knees appear. The brain and spinal column are near completion and the spine makes its first small movements
☐ All the internal organs are there; the heart is circulating blood cells around the body but the lungs are still solid
☐ Traces of the mouth, nostrils and eyes are visible but the skin that will become the eyelids still covers the eyes. The internal parts of the ears are forming but no external ear shows

12 – 16 weeks
☐ The head is still bent forward but is now more rounded. Webbed fingers and toes can be made out and the ankles and wrists are clear. All the limbs are growing, developing muscles and starting to move
☐ The skin over the eyes has become eyelids but they remain shut. The nose and mouth are more fully developed and the ears begin to grow
☐ Most of the vital organs are starting to function; the heart is completely formed and is pumping blood through the foetus and the umbilical cord. The ovaries or testicles begin to grow

16 – 20 weeks
☐ The limbs are now properly formed with moving joints. The webbing between the fingers and toes disappears and the nails appear
☐ The external sexual organs start growing, so the sex of the foetus is now evident
☐ The head, still looks over large, but is well rounded; the neck is now grown so the head can move. It starts to look familiar with proper ears, nose and eyes and the beginnings of eyebrows and eyelashes. A membrane still covers the pupils
☐ Soft hairs, called 'lanuga' begin to appear all over the body
☐ All the internal organs are complete with only the lungs, kidneys and intestines continuing to grow
☐ The baby can drink some of the fluid around him and starts to pass urine
☐ The skin is transparent so the body is bright red from the blood vessels beneath the skin

20 – 24 weeks
☐ Hair begins to grow on the head, baby teeth form and the nails harden. Nipples appear and the eyebrows and eyelashes are fully grown
☐ The muscles gain in size and strength and the mother can feel her baby moving

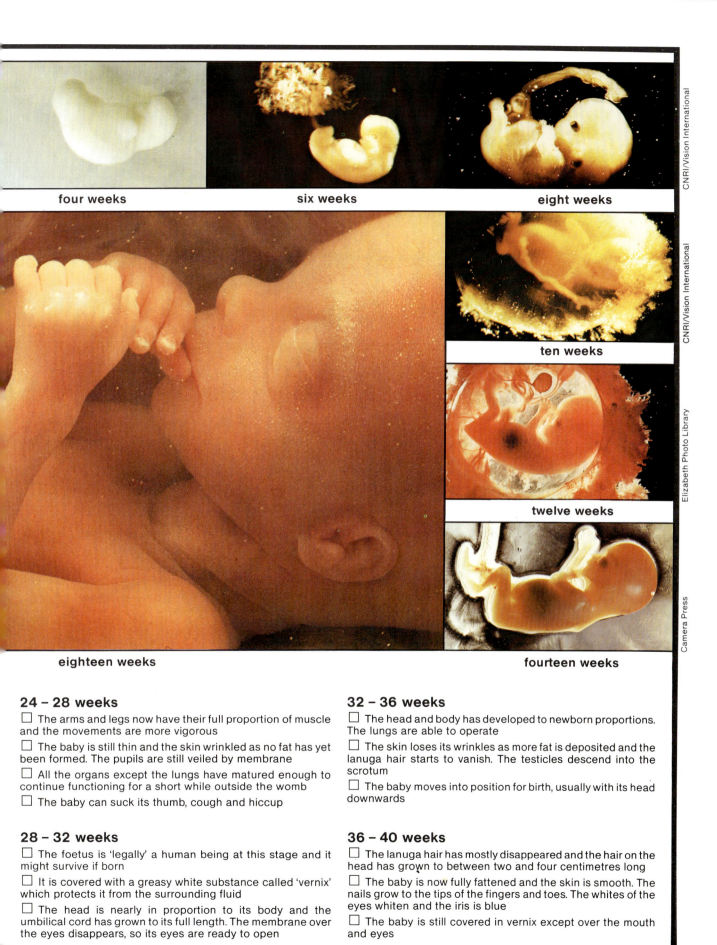

four weeks

six weeks

eight weeks

ten weeks

twelve weeks

eighteen weeks

fourteen weeks

CNRI/Vision International

CNRI/Vision International

Elizabeth Photo Library

Camera Press

24 – 28 weeks

☐ The arms and legs now have their full proportion of muscle and the movements are more vigorous

☐ The baby is still thin and the skin wrinkled as no fat has yet been formed. The pupils are still veiled by membrane

☐ All the organs except the lungs have matured enough to continue functioning for a short while outside the womb

☐ The baby can suck its thumb, cough and hiccup

28 – 32 weeks

☐ The foetus is 'legally' a human being at this stage and it might survive if born

☐ It is covered with a greasy white substance called 'vernix' which protects it from the surrounding fluid

☐ The head is nearly in proportion to its body and the umbilical cord has grown to its full length. The membrane over the eyes disappears, so its eyes are ready to open

32 – 36 weeks

☐ The head and body has developed to newborn proportions. The lungs are able to operate

☐ The skin loses its wrinkles as more fat is deposited and the lanuga hair starts to vanish. The testicles descend into the scrotum

☐ The baby moves into position for birth, usually with its head downwards

36 – 40 weeks

☐ The lanuga hair has mostly disappeared and the hair on the head has grown to between two and four centimetres long

☐ The baby is now fully fattened and the skin is smooth. The nails grow to the tips of the fingers and toes. The whites of the eyes whiten and the iris is blue

☐ The baby is still covered in vernix except over the mouth and eyes

How your body changes

Once a baby has been conceived, the mother's body starts to go through some dramatic changes – all aimed at producing the best possible conditions for the embryo to grow. These changes are controlled by a number of powerful hormone signals.

When the fertilized egg implants in the lining of the womb, the usual pattern of hormone control that produces the menstrual cycle is disrupted. Normally, the level of the hormone *progesterone* would gradually fall off in the last two weeks of the cycle; however, part of the fertilized egg starts to produce a hormone (*human chorionic gonadotrophin HCG*) which stimulates the ovary to continue excreting a high level of progesterone. This actually stops you ovulating again, now that the pregnancy has begun.

Progesterone levels are very high in early pregnancy, but the other major hormone involved, *oestrogen*, doesn't rise so quickly. A certain base level continues to be excreted by the ovaries, but it rises more significantly later on, around the 12th to 14th week. At this stage, the developing placenta and embryo act together in taking over the production of both progesterone and oestrogen.

Is it true an increase in breast size is one of the first signs of pregnancy?

Yes – it's noticeable very early on. A woman may sometimes experience a feeling of fullness in the breasts even before she realizes she is pregnant. The size of the breasts increases with amazing speed, and by the 6th week of pregnancy (two weeks after your missed period) they will be very noticeably enlarged. The hormone *prolactin*, produced by the pituitary, causes the milk-producing glands in the breasts to get bigger, and this continues gradually throughout the pregnancy.

How the hormones work in pregnancy

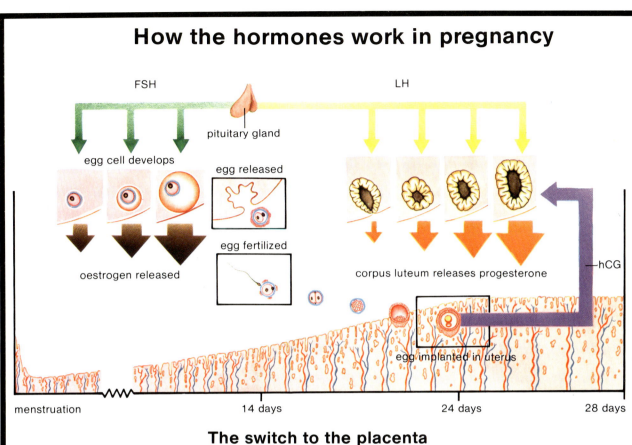

FSH

LH

pituitary gland

egg cell develops

egg released

egg fertilized

oestrogen released

corpus luteum releases progesterone

hCG

egg implanted in uterus

menstruation

14 days

24 days

28 days

The switch to the placenta

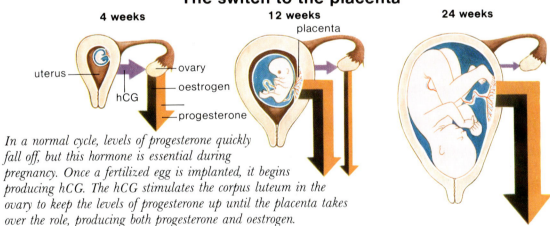

4 weeks

12 weeks

24 weeks

placenta

uterus

hCG

ovary

oestrogen

progesterone

In a normal cycle, levels of progesterone quickly fall off, but this hormone is essential during pregnancy. Once a fertilized egg is implanted, it begins producing hCG. The hCG stimulates the corpus luteum in the ovary to keep the levels of progesterone up until the placenta takes over the role, producing both progesterone and oestrogen.

Hormone levels in normal pregnancy

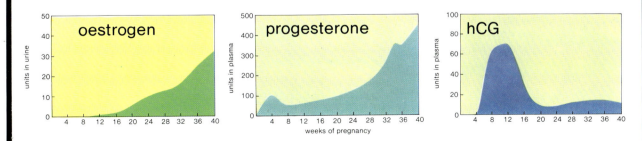

oestrogen — units in urine

progesterone — units in plasma — weeks of pregnancy

hCG — units in plasma

The levels of oestrogen and progesterone continue to rise steadily throughout pregnancy, but the hCG levels will

drop as dramatically as they rose, once the hormone is no longer necessary to stimulate the corpus luteum.

Dee McClean

Bernard Fallon

Most other changes in the breasts become noticeable at about the same time. Because the skin is stretched you may find they are unusually tender at this stage and an increased flow of blood through the breasts makes them tingle and throb. Don't be surprised if you see lots of little surface veins appearing; this is also due to the increased blood supply.

The nipples will usually become more prominent and, in a first pregnancy, little white bumps will appear on the *areola* – the pinky-brown area round the nipple. Some women again experience tender breasts in the last few weeks, combined with a leaking fluid from the nipple. This fluid is called 'colostrum' and is a normal and healthy sign.

What causes morning sickness?

The precise reasons are not known, but it's probably due to one of the hormonal changes. There is a rapid rise in the production of various hormones in early pregnancy, but the high level of the hormone gonadotrophin is much reduced by the third or fourth month – and this is when most women start to feel *less* sick. So it seems there could be a link between this hormone and the sickness.

The sickness may be partly 'psychological'; this is not to say that anyone who is being sick is not looking forward to having her baby – simply that some of the natural anxiety a woman feels at this time shows itself through sickness.

Sickness affects about two-thirds of pregnant women, in the early months. For quite a few expectant mothers it's nothing more than a feeling of nausea when they wake up in the morning. Others may go on feeling sick at

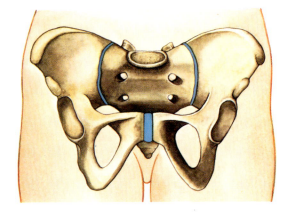

The joints 'soften' during pregnancy, meaning that the gaps between the bones of the pelvis open slightly. This will be important during childbirth, because the passage through which the baby must pass can expand that bit more.

intervals throughout the day and some women actually vomit. Eating a dry biscuit or cracker before you get up in the morning does seem to help a lot of women – no one knows exactly why.

Although being sick is inconvenient and unpleasant there is no cause for alarm. Occasional vomiting cannot harm the baby or cause a miscarriage, as some women fear.

Why do many women feel so tired, and dizzy, during the first three months?

Most women are totally unprepared for the tiredness that results from all the increased hormonal activity. The baby is still relatively tiny by the end of the first three months, and the tiredness seems out of all proportion to the actual 'weight' they are carrying. But in fact there are many other body changes going on in this time – besides what's happening in the womb itself – all of which can contribute to a general feeling of fatigue.

One important change is in the pattern of blood supply. The pelvic area, containing the womb, demands more blood to ensure rich supplies of oxygen and nutrients for the developing embryo. If this results in a decrease in blood supply to the mother's brain, it may make her feel faint. However, the sense of dizziness usually passes by mid-pregnancy, when the body has adjusted to the new pattern of blood supply.

There's another major change which can contribute to general tiredness. The progesterone levels cause a softening of the ligaments that support the joints; this has a slightly weakening effect on the major muscles, so many activities can feel like much more of an effort than usual. The whole point of this 'loosening' is to allow the pelvis to expand to accommodate the baby, and make it sufficiently wide for the labour and delivery (see diagram).

When can you start to feel the womb getting bigger?

The womb in its normal state is slightly smaller than your clenched fist; by stretching of the inside cells it will gradually enlarge to hold a seven-pound baby plus placenta at full term. It enlarges quite slowly until the twelfth week, when it is usually about the size of a grapefruit. At this stage it becomes too large to remain hidden in your pelvis and it can be felt through the abdominal wall.

Just when others will notice you are pregnant depends on the strength of your tummy muscles. If they have been kept strong by regular exercise,

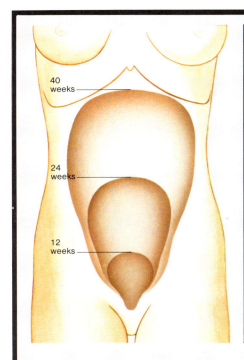

Landmarks in pregnancy

1 – 12 weeks	13 – 27 weeks	28 – 40 weeks
breasts enlarge and may be tender; surface veins become visible	nipples and areola darken	colostrum may leak spontaneously from breasts in last few weeks
morning sickness	'frequency' and morning sickness may disappear	'frequency' may return
frequent need to empty bladder	pregnancy starts to 'show'	tiredness almost inevitable
feeling of extreme tiredness	linea nigra may appear	difficulty in sleeping due to size of tummy and leg cramps
possibility of dizziness and fainting		possibility of varicose veins
sense of taste and smell may alter		'butterfly mask' may appear

40 weeks

24 weeks

12 weeks

Dee McClean

At 12 weeks there are few external signs of pregnancy; not until the 16th does the abdomen start to enlarge. Note that the uterus may drop in the 40th week, when the baby's head goes into the pelvis.

the muscles may act like a very good corset and hide the growing womb until about the 20th week. Also, if it's your first child, your muscles may hide the growing child for longer. If they've been stretched by previous pregnancies you may be noticeably pregnant as early as the 14th week.

However it's an interesting point that your external size at full term doesn't necessarily have much bearing on the size of your baby; both the amount of fluid surrounding the foetus and the strength of the tummy muscles may affect the overall size you reach.

How much weight are you likely to gain?

Most women put on between 24-28lbs during pregnancy and this is considered quite normal. As the baby usually only accounts for 6-9lbs of this, you may wonder how the rest is distributed.

The breasts and womb increase in size and therefore add to the weight of the baby itself; together with the amniotic fluid (which surrounds the baby) and the placenta, this comes to a total of around 15lbs. The natural increase in the volume of the mother's blood accounts for some increase too, but the rest is due to increased body fat and fluid retention.

The increased level of oestrogen encourages fluid retention in the tissues, which may show as a slight puffiness in the ankles, fingers or face.

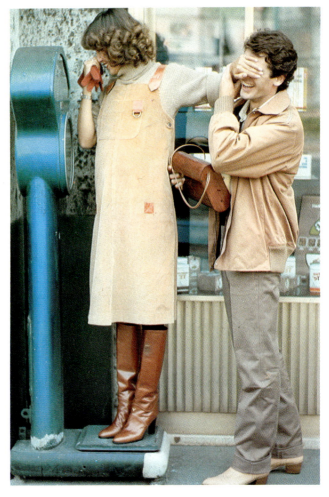

Most pregnant mothers retain some extra fluid in this way; it's only a cause for concern if it rises too dramatically.

You may start putting on more body fat – usually as a result of eating too much. Although a healthy, balanced diet is more important than ever, it's a common misconception that you have to start 'eating for two'. This is not necessary, and if you start eating a lot more than you used to, any excess calories will normally go into store, not into the baby!

It's difficult to lay down hard and fast rules about weight gain as it varies so much from woman to woman but in a normal pregnancy it might average out in the way shown in the graph on this page. Overall a weight gain of between 26-28lbs is usually advised. After this you can expect your weight to remain fairly constant until the baby is born.

Why do some women get varicose veins in pregnancy?

The surface veins on the legs are responsible for draining blood up towards the heart, and the main channel through which the blood has to pass runs up through the pelvis. In late pregnancy, when the growing womb pressed on these veins in the pelvic area, it has the effect of 'damming' the blood back into the legs, causing the skin veins to become swollen. In addition, the hormones produced in early pregnancy have the effect of making the veins a little saggy. Many women who get mild varicose veins during pregnancy find they improve afterwards, although in some cases they do become a permanent problem. The same sort of trouble can affect the veins at the bottom of the rectum, which is why piles are also common in pregnancy.

Is it normal for moles and freckles to get darker during pregnancy?

Yes. One of the pregnancy hormones tends to make skin cells containing dark pigments enlarge and any birthmarks, freckles, moles or scars will become darker after about the 14th week of pregnancy. Some women – more usually the fair-haired, thin-skinned type – develop a dark-coloured area over the cheeks on either side of the nose, sometimes rather like a butterfly shape.

At about the same time you may notice a dark line – the *linea nigra* – developing on the middle of your tummy, from the navel downwards. This usually fades when pregnancy is over, though occasionally a trace of it may remain. The nipples and areola also become much darker after the 14th week but this is a change which is permanent in most women.

Apart from changes in pigmentation, many women notice their skin looks in exceptionally good condition during pregnancy, and some acne sufferers find their skin troubles clear up – though the effect is not necessarily permanent.

Is it common for a woman's sense of smell and taste to alter?

Yes. This happens to nearly all women and is often another very early sign that you may be pregnant. It's thought that the reason why many women suddenly complain of a 'metallic' taste in the mouth, and start to 'go off' things they've always liked, is due to an alteration in the blood supply to the lining of the nose and tongue. Both the sense of taste and smell seem to change, and many women can't bear coffee, alcohol, cigarette smoke, or spicy foods.

It's not unusual to develop a special craving for certain foods – like shellfish, pickles, or doughnuts. Some women develop a really bizarre appetite, craving for something that's not normally thought of as food.

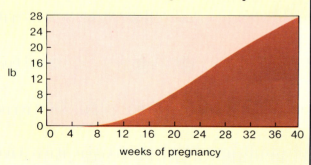

Where the weight goes

	Optional	Total
breasts 2lb (plus or minus 1lb)		
baby 7lb (plus or minus 2lb)		
placenta 1lb (plus or minus ¼lb)		
amniotic fluid 1lb (plus up to 1 lb)	fat and fluid 8lb (plus or minus 4lb)	24lb (plus or minus 10lb)
uterus 2lb (plus or minus ½lb)		
blood volume 3lb (plus or minus 1½lb)		

*The figures in brackets indicate the possible variation.

Tony Stone Associates

What you can expect to put on

lb / weeks of pregnancy

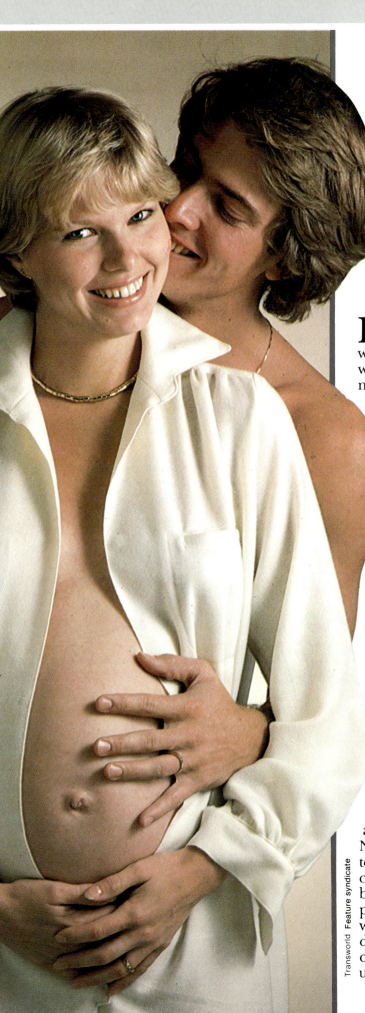

Common ante-natal anxieties

For most women, pregnancy is a time of anticipation and curiosity, but even for those who have been longing for a child, it is not without its anxieties and sometimes even resentment. Many women still have gaps in their understanding of pregnancy and childbirth which makes them more vulnerable to the horror stories and old wives' tales which they are almost certain to encounter. The more, then, that a woman can learn about the whole process she is undergoing, the more confidently she can face the prospect of birth and motherhood.

Why do some women grow to resent being pregnant – even if the baby was planned?

Although it sounds a contradiction, it is possible for a woman to want a baby very much and at the same time dislike the actual process of bearing a child. While some women will look and feel marvellous during pregnancy, this is not always so. The first three months is sometimes an uncomfortable time, with nausea in 50 per cent of woman and actual sickness in 30 per cent. Tiredness and a lack of normal energy are commonly experienced.

Apart from feeling resentful about this constant state of feeling unwell, many women interpret such typical discomforts as signs that they are going to have a terrible labour or an abnormal child. But of course this is not so. Nausea, vomiting and many of the other symptoms of early pregnancy are produced by increased amounts of hormones which help the baby to grow. An excess of these hormones can produce what seem to be endless symptoms, which can be daunting for the mother-to-be, but does not mean that the entire pregnancy will carry on in this manner, nor that the child will be unhealthy or adversely affected in some way.

Transworld Feature syndicate

In addition, as her pregnancy progresses, a woman may come to resent losing her figure, believing that she has also lost her sexual attractiveness. She may worry that she will never regain her normal curves, and lose 'the bulge'. And, of course, the growing size is a constant reminder of the enormous responsibilities to come.

If a woman has been very active, she may find the physical and mental slow-down, which generally happens in pregnancy, especially frustrating. Some women become very absent-minded – and very angry about this! The gradual curtailment of activities such as certain sports, smoking and drinking may upset others. Women who have to give up their work – 'a job which I loved, gave me great satisfaction, and helped me earn my own money' – can find the break harder than they anticipated; the loss of independence and the new financial worries make them feel less than welcoming about the expected baby.

A certain loss of self-confidence is involved in all of these experiences, and so adds to the sense of vulnerability already felt by some pregnant women. Many complain that people – even friends – treat them merely as 'baby-makers' and not as individuals. All they ever talk about is, 'When are you due?' 'What sex do you want?' 'Have you thought of names?'

Similarly, it's not unusual to find many women who intensely dislike the interference in their lives which seems to descend on them from all sides as soon as they're pregnant. In-laws and relations, neighbours and even passers-by will offer advice, often unwanted and ill-informed, on anything from how to change a nappy, to the best school for the child!

When the time comes for a woman to have her baby, she has to rely on the professional 'experts' such as doctors, nurses, clinics and even books. And while these experts are necessary and generally very helpful, they can inadvertently make some women feel as though they are no longer in charge of their own bodies and that the whole business has become unnecessarily clinical and complicated, which adds to their resentment.

What effect might a pregnancy have on a couple's relationship?

Relationships cannot fail to be affected by a pregnancy, and some adjustment will have to be made every time there is a new addition to the family. Naturally, if a man has difficulty in expressing his feelings about the event, his wife may jump to the wrong conclusions. For instance, if a woman already feels sensitive about her size and shape, she may interpret any passing interest in the female shape as confirmation that he no longer finds *her* attractive. A man may simply be taking it for granted that he loves his wife, not realizing that she may need a lot of extra reassurance at this time.

Certainly, too, a couple's sex-life will alter somewhat when a woman is pregnant, and it's most important that the pair are able to discuss what this means to each of them. Many women, for example, show an increased interest in sex during the middle five months of pregnancy (due, probably, to hormonal changes) just at the time when some men may be starting to worry that intercourse may hurt either their partner or the growing baby! Talking openly can prevent

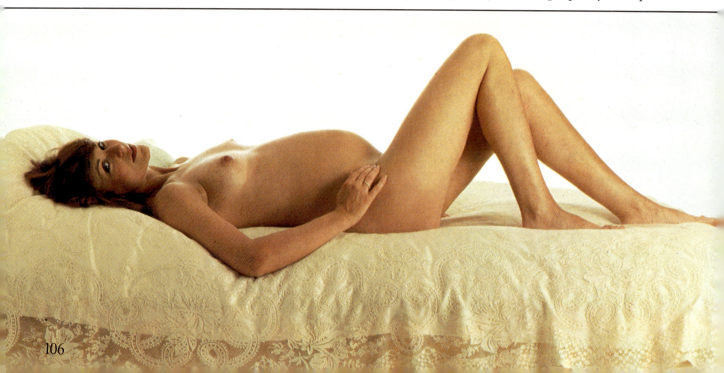

unnecessary emotional problems arising from such conflicting needs and worries. Research has shown that in a normal pregnancy there is no need to fear that intercourse is a risk to the baby or mother except during the last month, when it is wiser to avoid it. Those in danger of miscarrying or having a premature delivery must follow their doctor's advice. Throughout pregnancy love-making positions will need to alter (to avoid deep penetration which in any event can become uncomfortable), but that may just help to make things more interesting!

Why do some men seem changed or moody at the prospect of becoming fathers?

Apprehension can have a lot to do with the way in which a prospective father reacts to pregnancy. It's easy to forget that he may have to face just as many new situations and changes as the prospective mother, and so undergo his own emotional upheavals. Since society, especially in the past, decreed that childbearing was a woman's business only, men tended to play very much of a background role. Now, however, they are generally encouraged to participate in antenatal training programmes, to be present at the birth and, in most hospitals, can visit their wives and infants freely during most hours of the day.

While these changes have helped greatly to reduce the anxieties men may have towards childbirth, and can help a couple establish a special bond with one another, would-be fathers may still have difficulty in coming to terms with their feelings. Some secretly remain very worried about the well-being of their wives and babies. Others simply dread having to be present at the birth for fear that they will make fools of themselves or break down in some way. Such reactions are very normal – and should be shared with the woman, who more than likely understands them best, as they are not unlike her own anxieties and apprehensions.

It is in fact very common to find that a man feels excluded when his wife is pregnant. He may feel that she is so absorbed in what is happening to her that he is left out in the cold, or he may be a little jealous of all the extra attention she is receiving. If it's a first child, he may be very concerned about the changes to their relationship that are bound to occur. Will his wife reject him in favour of the baby? Will they (or she) become so tied down with responsibilities to the child that their social life disappears? And, above all, will he be able to provide the emotional support needed by the child, and be a good father? If his wife is giving up work financial worries, too,

can make a man depressed or apprehensive about becoming a parent. In all these instances his reaction may be to draw even further away from the experience, by 'burying' himself in work, for example.

If a man has been at the centre of his wife's attentions, the coming of a baby can bring out all sorts of insecurities in him. And what is even worse is that he may be afraid or ashamed to talk about them – after all, being a man he is not supposed to have such emotions! Once again, a woman who can be sensitive to and patient with her partner's altering attitudes and moods may be the greatest help to him. Getting him to talk with friends who have gone through some of the same things themselves can also be reassuring. Doctors, midwives and health visitors are all very aware of the anxieties prospective fathers may have. They may be especially helpful in letting a man know that he is certainly not the only one to have such feelings and that his wife and baby will be given the best of care by experienced medical and nursing teams. Above all they can make him aware of how much his support means to his wife and of how rewarding the shared experience of having a baby can be.

Why do some parents become so anxious about which sex their baby may be?

Very often the cause of such an obsession lies far deeper than the parents realize, and has its roots in psychological and cultural considerations. Because of this, such anxieties are often not easy to overcome, or even to recognize.

Some people, men more frequently than women, will desperately want a son as their first child, in order to inherit the family name, title, business or wealth, and to act as 'head of the house' in the father's absence. Men, too, will sometimes feel that it is 'inferior' to have daughters, or, conversely, they may be afraid that sons will challenge their authority, and so want only girls who, they feel, will be more docile.

In other cases people may want a child of their own sex to 're-live' their own lives – to have the advantages and experiences they themselves wanted but never had. The 'ballet mother' or 'rugby father' are just two, almost cliché, examples. Then again, some people who are very insecure about their sexuality may believe that they can 'prove' themselves by producing a child of their own sex: a woman who seriously doubts her feminine appeal may believe that by giving birth to a daughter she will be demonstrating her womanliness to the world.

In contrast, if a woman has had a difficult

relationship with a parent, she may feel threatened at the thought of having a child of that sex for fear of repeating a painful pattern all over again – she may, for example, fear having a daughter because her own mother was very critical and over-possessive with her.

Finally, many women still feel frightened of disappointing their husbands, or even losing their love, if they don't produce the child of the sex he desires. This is ironic, as it is the father's chromosomes which primarily determine the sex of the child, not the mother's.

Is it usual to feel worried about the baby being normal?

Yes. Almost without exception women worry at some time during a pregnancy that they may be carrying an abnormal child, or that the baby may be harmed during birth, although in Western countries having a baby is generally considered to be safer than going on a long car journey.

Naturally, there are certain general precautions which all women can take to avoid any special risk of harm to the growing child – eating a sensible, balanced diet, taking regular, moderate exercise, cutting out smoking, drinking strictly in moderation and taking no drugs, unless specifically prescribed by the doctor.

In some cases a woman may have a rather primitive superstitious fear – that as a 'punishment' for some slight wrongdoing in her past, her baby may be abnormal. However, a woman who continues to worry about having a handicapped baby, in spite of reassurances to the contrary from doctors, may really be afraid of something slightly different – that she won't be a 'good' mother maybe, or will 'fail' to go through labour and birth easily and successfully.

The so-called 'maternal instinct' is something which large numbers of women claim not to have – especially in a first pregnancy. And, in fact, it is not any one identifiable emotion. With no previous experience of handling babies or caring for young children, it's not surprising that many women feel quite devastated at the thought of being *totally* responsible for another human being. It's easy for self-doubts and fears to project themselves on to the unknown baby growing inside the womb – and to make yourself believe that because you don't seem to be coping with pregnancy well enough, the baby won't be 100 per cent healthy.

Any woman who is isolated from friends or family during her pregnancy may be more prone to such worries, and it is especially important for her to be able to talk with others and share these anxieties. Antenatal classes, run by almost all hospitals and various private groups, generally provide an excellent opportunity for having chats with other prospective mothers – where you are sure to find your own fears echoed – as well as with trained nursing and maternity staff who will almost certainly be able to reassure you.

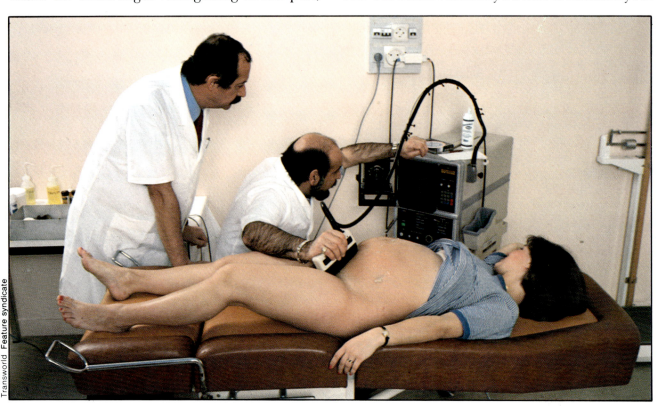

Is it normal to be frightened about the pain involved in the birth?

Probably the most common antenatal fears are those concerned with the actual birth – and these are perfectly understandable. For many women, having a baby is still the only occasion on which they will have to experience pain. A woman having her first baby will naturally wonder, 'What is it really like? Will I be able to cope? Will I lose control or make a fool of myself?' Even those who have previously had children may feel somewhat apprehensive if they have unpleasant memories of earlier births.

Unfortunately, no one can tell a woman precisely what will happen, as each birth proceeds differently and, more importantly, each person will react to the experience differently; a sensation of mild discomfort to one may be felt as extreme pain by another. Simply having to go into hospital may frighten some women greatly.

Natural childbirth methods are based on the principle that not knowing what to expect makes a woman more tense than need be during labour, and so increases the experience of pain. It follows that learning all you can about labour – about what causes contractions, how they will alter at different stages of labour and what you can be doing to relax – will be the best way of confronting fears about giving birth.

By all means go to the special classes held for expectant mothers (and fathers). If going into hospital worries you, then don't simply avoid thinking about it; make a point of going along to the labour ward and ask about the policies and techniques practised there. If there is anything you don't understand or don't particularly want for yourself, then discuss it with the staff and your doctor beforehand. Labour is not something which happens just to one part of you – it is a very intense, concentrated effort involving your whole body, mind and emotions. It can be an extremely rewarding and even pleasurable experience if you prepare for it, and deal with any queries regarding techniques or medical help (drugs or methods of delivery) *before* you are actually in the thick of it.

Above all, remember that giving birth is *not* a performance which you will pass or fail; your own capabilities are not being tested. Do not be ashamed to ask for any help you feel you need – and that includes asking your husband for his presence and support at the birth, if possible.

Most hospitals are quite willing for fathers to help out during labour, recognizing that pain and discomfort are greatly eased when shared with someone you know and love. Remember,

too, that the pain of labour is unlike that of most injuries or accidents – it is the pain of creating. Knowing that there is a purpose to it can help you to cope with it positively. And many women find that once labour is over any pain is soon forgotten.

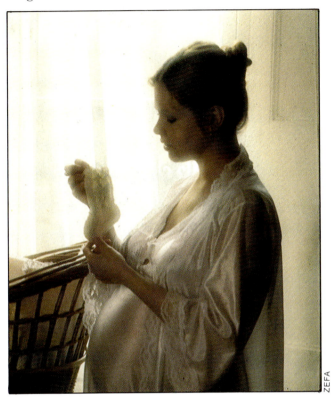

ZEFA

What should a woman do if she feels seriously trapped by being pregnant?

A woman who comes to feel utterly 'trapped' by her pregnancy will need to seek help and advice. The first person to turn to for sympathy and support is her partner, but the depth of her anxiety may require expert help.

Various difficulties are often brought to light by an understanding counsellor. Is the woman in a stable relationship? Is the baby wanted? Is the woman's career being interrupted at a crucial point? Has the woman several children already? These are all examples of concerns which often underlie feelings of being trapped.

Having said all this, however, it is often the woman in an apparently happy situation who suffers from this feeling. Motherhood can be made to seem horrifying if you think you have to give up all the other facets of your life. Don't drop friends or leave work, and close all doors behind you when you enter the final stages of pregnancy. For your own peace of mind, work out a plan whereby you can continue doing at least some of the things you find most satisfying.

Health care in pregnancy

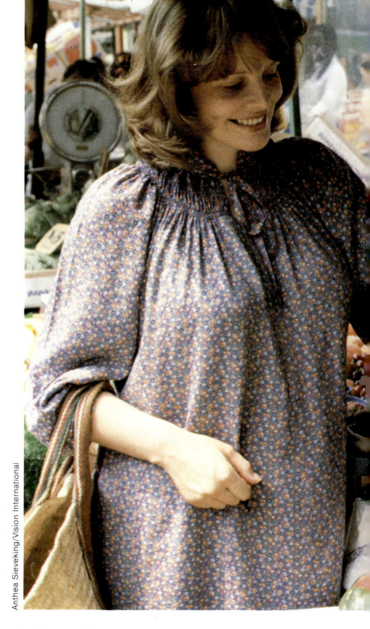

Anthea Sieveking/Vision International

Are extra vitamins and minerals necessary?

It's true that vitamins and minerals are essential for a baby's health and well-being, but doctors say that most of them are present in quite sufficient amounts in an ordinary mixed diet. As long as you eat a protein meal containing a good portion of meat or fish once a day, you'll be getting adequate supplies, but take care not to increase your carbohydrate intake. This won't be of any benefit and will just add extra unwanted calories. Above all, don't be tempted into 'eating for two'!

The only two substances which most pregnant women need supplements of are iron, and folic acid, the vitamin required for growth. However, in many countries these two supplements are usually prescribed for pregnant women and there's little risk of a deficiency occurring. So, unless a pregnant woman is short of a particular vitamin or mineral for some reason, there's no point taking supplements of any substances other than those mentioned.

Although you don't normally need synthetic calcium supplements, you do need to increase your calcium intake slightly to ensure that your diet contains sufficient to keep your teeth and bones strong and healthy, and help the baby's bones to grow. Even though bones appear to be fairly static, they are in fact continually dissolving and being renewed. Normally these counter activities are carefully balanced out so that your bones and teeth remain strong, but certain hormone changes in pregnancy tend to increase the dissolving action and slow up the laying down process. This alteration allows the baby to take what it needs but it may leave the mother a little deficient. The calcium imbalance could make your bones slightly brittle and can cause leg cramps at night. However, you can help overcome both problems by making sure that your daily diet contains some milk and cheese —

both are rich sources of calcium.

It's also particularly important to eat plenty of roughage. You can get this from high-fibre foods like whole-grain cereals, wholemeal bread, fruit and vegetables. And if you're not particularly fond of cabbage, spinach, and other high-fibre vegetables, then bran is a very useful alternative, either the coarse health-food variety or the more refined manufactured breakfast cereal type. If you drink enough fluid (minimum of 2 pints a day) and eat sufficient fibre you'll minimize the risk of suffering from constipation.

Why is smoking harmful during pregnancy?

Smoking is harmful at all times, but it can have a particularly detrimental effect on the foetus.

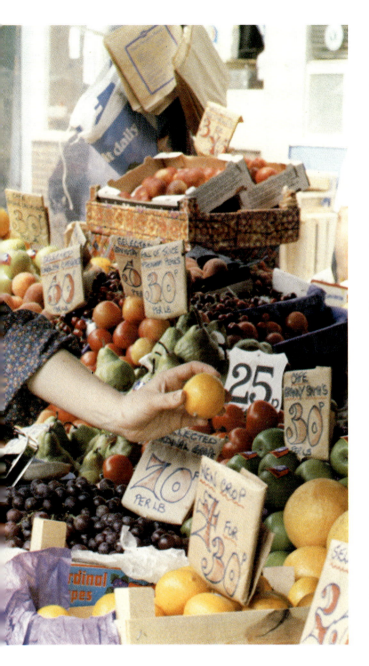

mature than one to a non-smoker. There is a further risk in that if the woman should develop toxaemia (when blood pressure rises, protein leaks into the urine and the limbs become swollen and puffy) it tends to be very much more severe than in a non-smoker, and is more likely to cause the death of the unborn child. As well as these hazards, it seems that the baby born to the smoking mother shows a marked retardation of reading ability and educational capacity later.

You can see from this how important it is for a pregnant woman to cut out smoking for the sake of her unborn child, even if she is prepared to take a risk with her own health.

Why is sleeping often a problem late in pregnancy?

Discomfort in bed and trouble staying asleep are usually due to the increase in size of the uterus. It may be hard to find a comfortable position to sleep in, especially if you normally sleep on your back or your tummy. In addition, the sheer size of your stomach tends to interfere as you turn over. We all turn many times during a night's sleep so when you're pregnant it can mean that you wake up in order to turn over. This soon becomes very irritating and can build up into a habit of waking in the night. If this proves really difficult to cope with, consult your doctor and he may prescribe some treatment to help.

What causes stretch marks and what can be done to prevent them?

The basic cause of stretch marks is the pulling of skin above its own limit of elasticity. A certain amount of elastic fibres are present in your skin and when they're stretched fairly suddenly, as in pregnancy, and tighten above their elastic limit, the fibres in the deeper layers start to tear and red irregular marks show on the skin's surface.

The reason that stretch marks are worse in some women than others is simply due to the fact that elasticity of the skin varies from person to person. Although there's not much you can do to increase your skin's elasticity, some women find it helpful to massage their skin daily as this seems to postpone the appearance of stretch marks.

There's no evidence that the specially formulated creams which claim to prevent stretch marks are of any use in themselves, and doctors say that if there is any benefit from these it's most likely due to the massaging action of the fingers during application, rather than the properties of the cream.

Making sure you don't become unduly over-

The nicotine and carbon monoxide in cigarette smoke are the substances which do the damage. Nicotine may cause the blood vessels of the placenta to narrow bringing about a reduction of placental blood supply, and therefore of oxygen and nutrients, from mother to child. Carbon monoxide can enter the baby's circulation, and, because the baby's blood pigment has a strong affinity for carbon monoxide, the poison becomes even more concentrated. These and other harmful chemicals absorbed from the smoke, combined with the reduction of placental blood supply and the generally poorer appetite of mothers who smoke, affect the nutrition and growth of the developing baby.

It's a fact that the child born to a cigarette-smoking mother will be born lighter and less

Stretch marks

Whether or not you get stretch marks, or how badly, depends on the proportion of elastic fibres to non-elastic fibres your skin contains. The more elastic fibres, the less likely you are to get stretch marks.

elastic fibres   non-elastic fibres

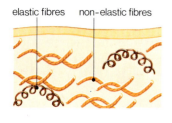

The fibres which give the skin its elastic quality are found in the epidermis.

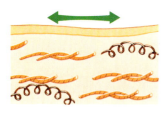

When stretched in moderation, the epidermis can usually take the strain; the elastic fibres pull out and the non-elastic fibres straighten.

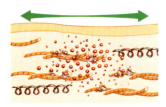

But if the stretching is prolonged or is too extreme, the non-elastic fibres tear and a little bleeding occurs.

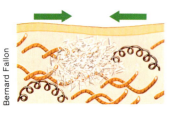

Afterwards, the epidermis will return to its old size, but the area of bleeding is replaced by white scar tissue which shows through the skin as a pale area.

Bernard Fallon

weight won't actually prevent stretch marks appearing on your tummy since in this area they're mainly due to the expanding uterus. But it may well help you to avoid them on your bottom and thighs. However, changes in hormone levels during pregnancy can affect the fluid content of these areas and this may cause stretch marks to occur here, even in the best weight-regulated women.

Unfortunately, once they have formed the damage has been done to underlying skin tissues. Even though the marks will pale when pregnancy is over, as white fibrous tissue takes the place of the acute red reaction, they may never go away completely. Sunbathing and acquiring a tan sometimes help to disguise them, and if you feel they are really obtrusive there are various body makeups available which may help.

Should you try to avoid all medicines during pregnancy?

Wherever possible it's best not to take medicines and drugs while you're pregnant. However, it's a fact that very few medicines actually produce abnormalities in human beings, and any that can are only available on prescription. All doctors know about them and would not willingly prescribe them for a woman they *know* is pregnant. If you have to consult a doctor for illness, and you think you might be pregnant, it's vital to tell him

While you're pregnant is it best to cut down on exercise and sport?

If you're used to doing a certain amount of physical exercise or sport such as tennis, cycling, swimming or walking there's no reason why you shouldn't continue, providing pregnancy progresses normally. However, you must take care not to overtire or overstrain yourself: always stop when you become tired and never allow yourself to become exhausted. Doctors believe that the two best and safest exercises to keep you fit while pregnant are walking and swimming (provided deep underwater diving is avoided).

It's not a good idea to take on any *new* form of exercise and sport and, if you're not used to it, avoid vigorous exercise. Pregnancy itself imposes quite a lot of extra work on your body, both physical and metabolic, and anything extra that you're not accustomed to will cause unnecessary strain. Indeed, for most women who have a home to look after, or a job to do, or other children to take care of, the duties involved will provide quite enough exercise during pregnancy. (Information on special ante-natal exercises – which you can learn at a class and practise at home – is covered in a separate chapter).

In fact, adequate rest is much more important than physical exertion when you're pregnant. Obviously the amount of rest you need varies enormously from one woman to another, but ideally it's wise, in the second half of pregnancy at least, to rest on the bed for two hours every afternoon. If you can't manage this try to make sure that you get as much rest as possible at night: avoid late nights and do lie-in.

When you think of the extra weight you're carrying around it's not really surprising that you need lots of rest. If your total weight gain is say, 25lbs, then towards the end of pregnancy it's much the same as carrying a 25lb suitcase all day. If this were so you'd certainly need to put it down occasionally!

so, however slight the possibility. That way there's no danger of him prescribing drugs which could damage the baby.

For instance, a certain type of commonly used antibiotic, harmless in normal circumstances, may seriously affect the growing foetus. Potentially damaging drugs are especially harmful in the first three months of pregnancy. It's during this time that abnormalities are produced and that you should be particularly careful about taking any new medicine. It's especially important not to go to the bathroom cabinet and take some medicine prescribed for another person at this or any time during pregnancy.

Most of the common over-the-counter pain killers, containing aspirin and codeine, are safe as long as taken in reasonable doses. For example, a couple of aspirins for the occasional headache won't do you any harm, but the same dose taken regularly every four to six hours for two or three days is not recommended. It's also perfectly all right to take heartburn and indigestion preparations in reasonable doses. On the whole, it's safe

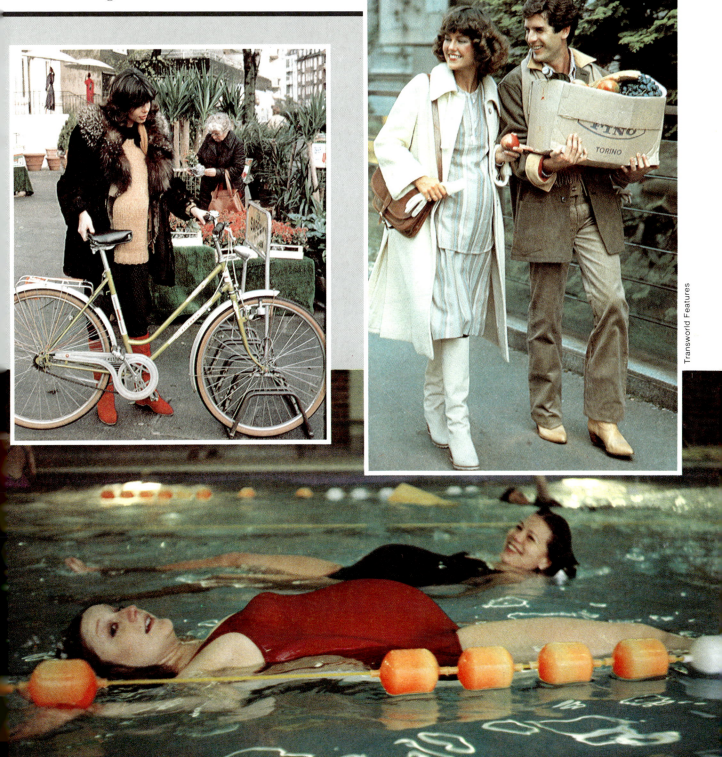

to take sleeping tablets during pregnancy, and if you're having great difficulty getting a good night's rest your doctor may prescribe them. However, it's obviously much better if you can manage without them.

Despite some controversy over anti-nausea pills, the latest scientific evidence has shown those available to be safe. Indeed, in cases of severe morning sickness doctors say their use is necessary and fully justified. Not only do they help relieve the intense discomfort but they may prevent damage to the baby – due to metabolic alterations in the short term, or, if the vomiting goes on for more than three months, to deficiencies in the mother's diet.

Over all, the decision to take a specific drug during pregnancy involves your doctor balancing out its benefits against the disadvantages of any possible side effects. For example if a woman is being treated for a long standing condition that started well before pregnancy, it's likely that the advantages of continuing the treatment will outweigh any disadvantages.

Is there any need to avoid intercourse during pregnancy?

For most couples there is no reason why a normal sex life should not be continued throughout pregnancy, since sexual intercourse does not disturb a normally implanted growing baby. However, if a woman has any bleeding from the vagina, in early pregnancy, indicating a threat to miscarry, intercourse should be stopped until her doctor advises that it's all right to start again.

Towards the end of pregnancy, the size of the baby may make intercourse mechanically more difficult but this can usually be overcome by a change of position. In the last few days, some people believe that intercourse actually promotes the onset of labour. There's little evidence to prove this, but there is no reason why intercourse should be stopped. It does not increase the risk of infection in delivery, so it's entirely up to the couple whether or not they want to make love.

Should you worry about severe backache? Why does it happen and can it be avoided?

Backache is very common throughout pregnancy. It's mainly due to the fact that most women change their posture and it throws extra strain on the bottom part of the spinal column and surrounding muscles. Trying to compensate for the weight of the uterus as it grows upwards and forwards, you tend to lean backwards as you walk, pushing out your stomach and arching your

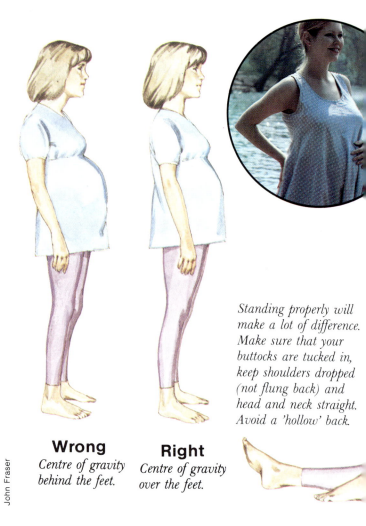

Wrong
Centre of gravity behind the feet.

Right
Centre of gravity over the feet.

Standing properly will make a lot of difference. Make sure that your buttocks are tucked in, keep shoulders dropped (not flung back) and head and neck straight. Avoid a 'hollow' back.

John Fraser

back. As pregnancy advances this stance becomes even more exaggerated. If you're a bit overtired or especially if the balance of muscles in the pelvis is upset, backache is the inevitable result.

Correct posture is essential to help relieve or better still, prevent this kind of backache since, by redistributing the weight, it puts less unnatural strain on the muscles and ligaments of the back. You should aim to stand with your back straight and your shoulders loose and relaxed rather than braced and flung back, holding your tummy and bottom 'in', so that your centre of gravity is immediately over your feet. Practise this by pressing the whole length of your spine against a flat wall and trying to maintain that posture. Towards the end of pregnancy you may well find that it's almost impossible not to arch your back a little, and that the only points touching the wall are your shoulders and bottom! The strain on the surrounding structures can cause backache and discomfort. And if there is any tendency to weakness here, it will be made worse in early pregnancy.

The only cure for backache of this sort is extra rest. If you're already taking rest make sure that

How to avoid backache

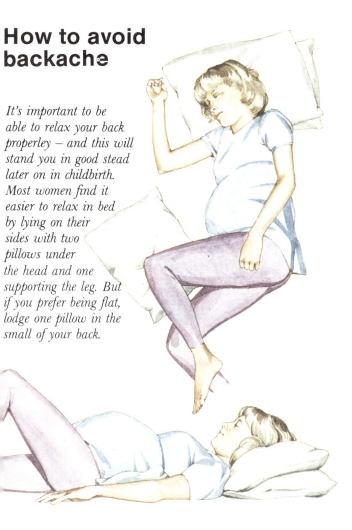

It's important to be able to relax your back properley – and this will stand you in good stead later on in childbirth. Most women find it easier to relax in bed by lying on their sides with two pillows under the head and one supporting the leg. But if you prefer being flat, lodge one pillow in the small of your back.

you take more, particularly lying down, and don't let yourself get overtired. Local heat either in the form of a hot water bottle or linament may help a little, and if the discomfort is severe it may be necessary to take pain relievers.

How can you avoid swollen feet?

Swollen ankles and feet are common in the latter half of pregnancy, especially in the afternoon during warm weather. While it's obviously not practical if you're working, doctors say that best cure is to sit down and put your feet up for an hour or two, or better still, lie down with your feet resting on a pillow.

Since your feet are carrying the brunt of the increased weight, shoes that give adequate support are essential. Avoid very high heels at any time since the last thing you want to do is to tip the pelvis further forward. Going bare foot round the house won't do any harm but try not to alternate between high heels during the day and no shoes at all in the evening. Ideally all shoes, whether walking shoes or slippers, should have a similar height of heel throughout pregnancy.

Should you stop drinking alcohol during pregnancy?

Alcohol is as much a drug as anything taken in pill or tablet form, but because it's socially acceptable it's easy to forget that its use should be restricted during pregnancy.

Alcohol almost certainly has a damaging effect on the unborn child, although the exact extent of the damage is still to be finally assessed. There's a growing body of research on it and some experts claim to have demonstrated a definite relationship between a mother who drinks heavily daily, and what's called foetal alcohol syndrome. It seems that in severe cases, for instance where the mother is an alcoholic, the baby is born both jittery and shaky, and is in fact experiencing withdrawal symptoms in the form of DTs. In addition, the baby is likely to be born with some degree of mental backwardness, to be small in size, and may even suffer from spinal or lung abnormalities.

If you're a regular drinker and you discover that you're pregnant you must cut down drastically, and long sessions with alcohol at a party are definitely to be avoided. In fact doctors say that it's best to drink as little alcohol as possible during pregnancy, and certainly to try and avoid spirits. Many doctors now recommend that you limit your drinking say, to a *maximum* of a couple of glasses of wine (or the equivalent) with a meal twice a week.

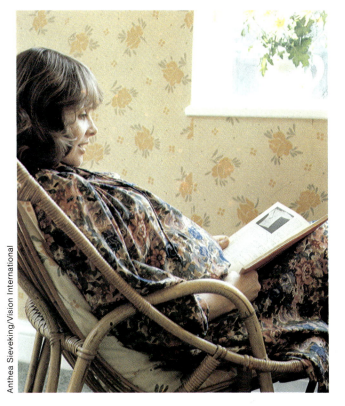

Approaches to childbirth

aving babies is no longer the hazardous business it used to be a century ago. Many women weren't then afforded the luxury of a choice between a home or hospital delivery. The baby would be delivered in a bedroom by the midwife. Without electricity or running water and without modern drugs and instruments the birth would probably have been painful for the mother and almost certainly hazardous to both mother and child.

There have been dramatic changes since then. Labour can be painless and the baby can be delivered on a chosen date. If he is born sick, he will no longer have to fight alone for his life, there are now machines to help him. All this, and more, is now available. But, as technology marches on, some parents and doctors have started to question whether a return to more 'natural' methods of childbirth would be better both for the mother's physical health and her emotional well being.

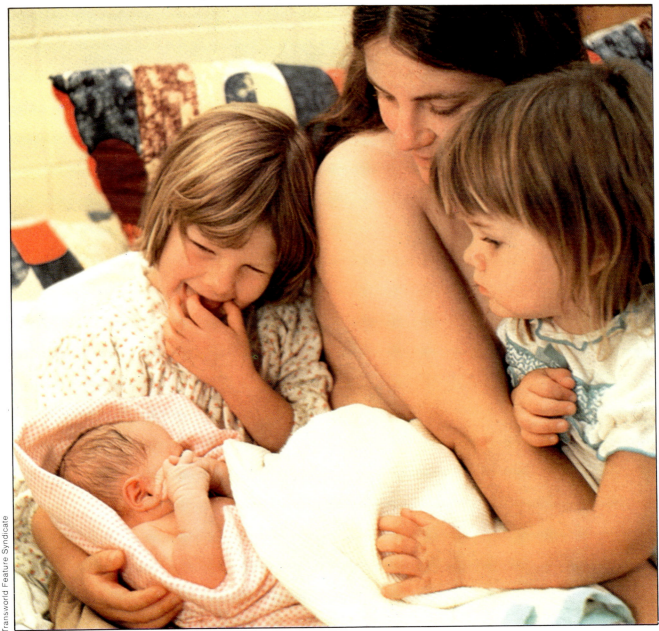

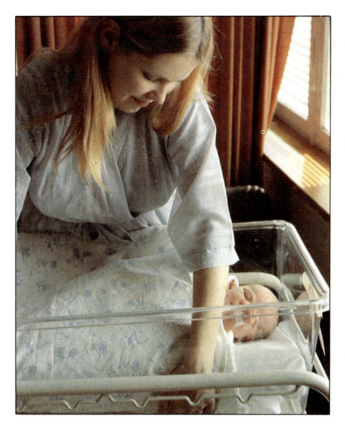

Why is there so much pressure on women to have their babies in hospital?

In an ideal world, happy healthy babies would be born every time and giving birth would always be an uncomplicated business requiring only mid-wife, mother and a baby who's ready to be born. In most cases this *is* all that's needed and the baby who's born in hospital is lucky in that he doesn't need the incubator, the intensive care unit or any of the specialized medical attention which is to hand. But, until a baby has actually been born, there's no way of knowing whether or not such facilities will be needed.

In the early stages of a woman's pregnancy a number of tests may be used to try and establish her baby's shape, position and whether he appears to be healthy. All the indicators may show mother and baby to be in good shape. Indeed, the first stages of labour may go without a hitch but then something unpredictable and un-expected may happen. The baby may show signs of *foetal distress*; his heart-beat may be irregular or show signs of slowing down. The mother may start to haemorrhage after she's given birth. Such things don't often happen, but when they do specialized medical attention and equipment will be needed and this is something which only a hospital can adequately provide.

If a similar situation were to occur during a home birth, the chances of both mother or baby

surviving are going to be reduced. This is not to doubt the expertise of your doctor and the midwife who's attending you. It's just that it's not possible for transfusion or resuscitation equip-ment to be installed for a home birth. And, although most areas are serviced by an obstetric flying squad which can be called up if complica-tions do occur, the time before its arrival may mean vital seconds are lost.

Most babies who are born at home are delivered safely; out of every 1,000 births in England and Wales, for example, only five die. The perinatal mortality rate – the number of babies who die during birth or within the first week of life – is low because only the healthiest mothers, having the best antenatal care, are advised to have their babies at home. Some 5 per cent of expectant mothers in England and Wales feel the advantages of a home birth outweigh the slight risks and opt to have their babies at home. Just over 1 per cent of women in America do so, and the figure is even lower in Sweden and Australia.

However, if you do decide you'd like to have a home delivery, it won't only be your feelings that count. The baby's physical well-being will also have to be assessed, something which your doctor will be able to establish.

Why is hospital delivery vital for a first baby?

Some women come under a high risk category which makes hospital delivery vital *just in case* there are complications. Into this category come women who are over 35, those suffering from diabetes, high blood pressure or other illnesses and the woman who's expecting her first child.

In the animal world the perinatal mortality rate among first-born sheep, cows and dogs is so high that farmers tend to regard the first preg-nancy merely as a warm up to the second, usually successful one. Of course perinatal mortality isn't anything like as high amongst first-born humans, though the contrast between first and subsequent births is still present. There are 23 deaths per 1,000 births for first babies compared to 16 per 1,000 for second babies. Birth simply gets easier the second or third time round. For a start you know what's going on and are familiar with the routine so breathing and relaxing properly should be easier. More importantly, the birth canal will also be slightly different from the one your first baby encountered. With the first it'll be muscular and rigid and will consequently hinder the baby's descent. With subsequent babies it will be slightly more flexible, making labour easier.

Planning a home delivery?

Good lighting is important so the midwife can see what she's doing. It doesn't need to be overhead; a strong sidelight will be adequate.

Heating is very important. The room should be warm with no draughts – babies chill easily.

The midwife will need to scrub her hands so make sure there's a nailbrush, soap and hand towel for her to use; alternatively ensure these items are in the bathroom.

At least three pillows to support the mother's back.

Change of sheets for bed and clean towels.

Accouchement sheet, often provided by local hospital. This protects the mattress from getting soiled.

Baby bath or a clean plastic bowl in which to wash baby.

Soft clean blanket to receive baby in.

Electric kettle to boil water. Sterilized water will be needed to wash mother's vaginal area, as well as for cleaning baby once he's been born.

Bedpan or chamber pot – only really necessary if the toilet is downstairs and difficult for the mother to get to.

Newspapers or plastic bags in which to put afterbirth

Paul Williams

Do most women feel a home birth is a happier experience?

Most women feel that birth is a happy experience wherever it takes place, providing the end result is a healthy baby. You may feel happier at home because you're in your own bed – perhaps the same one in which the child was conceived – and the familiar surroundings can greatly add to feelings of security. There's a privacy at home which no large hospital could ever hope to match. If you have other children you won't have to be separated from them. There are practical advantages, too, such as not having to travel.

Generally, women who opt for a home birth do so because they feel it'll be a more emotionally satisfying experience. But, although it can be argued that medical staff are obviously going to be more concerned with the physical well-being of mother and child rather than with providing emotional support, more and more hospitals are making their maternity wings brighter and more attractive places to be in.

Approaches to childbirth are changing, too. No longer is it routine for babies to be whisked away as soon as they are born, to be returned to their mothers only when feeding time arrives.

Increasingly, a cot is kept by the mother's bed so she can feed and touch her baby when they both want this. Fathers are encouraged to be present during the birth – one hospital even makes it routine to position an armchair behind the father just in case he's overcome by the proceedings! In another hospital, immediately after the delivery, the medical staff leave the room, leaving mother, father and baby together so they can enjoy the first hour or so of a new life quietly together as a family.

Of course, hospitals are going to differ in their approach – one may welcome anything innovative, another may regard *all* variations on the usual routine as a nuisance. Before you're due to go into hospital, find out how far the staff are willing to go in accommodating your wishes. Talk things over with the obstetrician who'll be attending you.

What is natural childbirth? Does it mean a pain-free birth?

Natural childbirth simply means a labour which doesn't require any medical intervention – no anaesthetics, induction, episiotomy, no forceps and no Caesarean – just you and the baby working together to push the baby out. It's based on the idea that if a woman knows exactly what's happening to her body during the different stages of labour, she is likely to experience less anxiety and pain, and can control – even enjoy – the birth.

Natural childbirth relies considerably on how you breathe and when you push, techniques which you will need to be taught in antenatal classes. But other factors, too, which no amount of preparation will be able to influence, are also important — how the baby's head is positioned, for example. Ideally it should be head first and facing your back. The size of the baby is significant – if he's too big, he may be impossible to push out without medical assistance. Ideally, also, labour should start between the 37th and 42nd week from the first day of the last menstrual period. If the baby is born much later or earlier there may be complications making medical assistance vital.

Women who give birth without medical intervention regard it as a more emotionally satisfying experience. Quite naturally, they feel a stronger sense of achievement when it's their uterus which has done all the work.

The advocates of natural childbirth say that labour doesn't need to be painful, or certainly not painful in the way you'd recognize the sensation of a smashed rib, say, or a badly crushed finger. They believe that the right attitude, correct breathing, knowing when to relax and when to push, and being aware of what's going on can all help to create pain relief without the need for drugs or injections.

However, natural childbirth can't guarantee a pain-free labour. Some women are more sensitive to the pain of birth than others – everyone has a different pain threshold and, even if you've completely mastered all your breathing and relaxing techniques, this is no guarantee that the birth will be painless. In fact, the only way to *guarantee* such a thing would be to have an *epidural*, an injection which numbs the body from the waist down but leaves you fully conscious. Lots of women do, in fact, opt for some pain relief.

The idea that natural childbirth must be painless stems, in part, from the notion that women in primitive societies are capable of having babies without fuss, bother and pain. It's argued that because these women haven't been culturally conditioned into expecting childbirth to be painful, it isn't. Because, too, they have children with more frequency and from an earlier age, the experience becomes a familiar one which is gone through without fear. Anxiety and tension do tend to make pain feel worse than it actually is.

But it's difficult to generalize. Just because women in a primitive society don't have access to epidurals, it doesn't mean to say they wouldn't ask for them if they could. They do, in fact, use herbs and plants as pain relieving agents during labour which suggests that it's not the entirely painless procedure it's made out to be. It's perhaps also significant that the number of babies who die during, or immediately after, birth in such places is extremely high, as is the number of women who die in childbirth through lack of proper medical facilities.

Is it true that with natural childbirth there's no need for induction or episiotomy?

No, not necessarily. You may start your labour *intending* to use natural childbirth methods but it may become clear to you and the medical staff who are looking after you that you're going to need assistance in delivering the child. Alternatively, you may yourself decide that you'd like pain relief after all, it's not always possible to predict such things in advance.

Anthea Sieveking/Vision International

When nature needs a helping hand

There are several ways in which an obstetrician may help a woman to deliver her baby more quickly. While every woman has a right to say whether or not she wants this type of assistance it's important to bear in mind that a labour lasting longer than 12 hours can be bad for mother and baby. Understanding the advantages and disadvantages of the medical procedures and in which way each is designed to help in the delivery, as well as *talking things over with your obstetrician*, will help you to decide just how much medical assistance you want.

Medical term	How it's done	Effects
Amniotomy	Rupturing the membranes by passing small surgical instrument through cervix	A painless procedure. Labour usually starts within a few hours and no other assistance may be needed. State of amniotic fluid (and therefore health of baby) can be assessed
Oxytocin drip	Drip set up through vein in the arm containing a drug which stimulates the uterus	Contractions will be stronger and more effective but may therefore be more painful. Drip will mean mother can't move very far from her bed
Prostaglandin pessaries	Inserted into the vagina	Causes cervix to dilate and may also start contractions. Pessaries don't restrict the mother's movements, but aren't yet available in all hospitals
Episiotomy	Surgical cut made in vagina – local anaesthetic will be administered	Makes prolapse in later life less likely. But stitches may be painful while they are healing, and the scar may be sore during love-making at first
Forceps delivery	Episiotomy has to be given first of all. Forceps gently hold the baby's head allowing the obstetrician to ease it through birth canal	With a forceps delivery a mother may feel her involvement in the birth is less because she can't push the baby out herself
Venthouse delivery	Suction cap placed on baby's head so that the baby is helped through birth canal	The suction cap has the virtue of allowing the mother to help by pushing down

There are several reasons why doctors may need to interfere to speed up or bring on a labour, and generally they are in the interests of both mother and baby. The monitoring which goes on during labour means that any abnormal patterns can be detected early and corrected. For example, very few women are able to put up with 12 hours of contractions and backache with a baby facing the 'wrong way' without wanting some form of pain relief. In the same way, three days of weak, ineffective or irregular contractions can be dangerous to both mother and baby. She will be exhausted, and probably unable to put in a final effort to push the baby out. The baby itself may also become distressed, suffering through a depletion of oxygen. Many obstetricians feel that any labour which continues for longer than 12 hours is going to be bad for both mother and child; others consider even 12 hours as being too long.

In cases like this an obstetrician may decide to speed up the labour by giving the mother an *oxytocin drip.* This, like the hormone produced by your own brain, has the effect of increasing the strength and frequency of the contractions and thereby causes the *cervix* (the neck of the womb) to dilate, allowing the baby's head to pass through.

If your baby is overdue it is probably in your best interests to start the delivery with some medical assistance. With late babies there's a danger that the *placenta*, which supplies the baby with its nutrients, may be ageing and unable to perform its function so well. Many obstetricians believe that any pregnancy that continues for longer than two weeks after the estimated delivery date ought to be helped on its way. If the membranes – the sack of fluid which surrounds the baby – haven't ruptured, this can be done by making a small incision with an instrument. This may be the only assistance that a mother needs and she may then be able to complete the delivery herself.

An *episiotomy* is a surgical incision made in the vaginal muscle so that the baby can pass out of the vaginal opening more easily. Without an episiotomy the baby's head pushes on the mother's vagina, until the pelvic floor muscles relax sufficiently to allow it to pass through. With a baby showing signs of foetal distress when speed of delivery is crucial, this simple cut will generally be made. Some obstetricians believe this should be routine for all women having their first baby because, by cutting the birth opening, the stress is removed from the vaginal muscles and this will make prolapse in later life less likely.

Are episiotomies really for the best?

There's a considerable controversy going on at the moment over whether these, and other methods of speeding delivery, should be carried out or whether it's best just to leave the whole process to 'nature'. Some people argue that since technology has entered into the delivery room many mothers have been robbed of the chance to experience the full emotional and physical impact of giving birth. They argue that the baby doesn't arrive when it 'wants' to arrive, but comes when the doctor decrees. Episiotomies are given, they say, when instead it would be better to either wait for the vaginal muscles to fully relax, or to allow the baby to push its way out naturally. This way the baby determines the size of the tear and whether there's to be one.

There are equally valid arguments from the other side. While it may be untrue to say that doctors *always* know best, nature is likely to be even more fallible. For this reason, many parents feel more confident when they know that the very best technological equipment is going to be used to bring their new baby safely into the world. Lots of women want some pain relief during labour. Analgesics, such as *pethidine*, numb the muscles but leave the mother awake and able to continue to contribute to the delivery of her child. Epidurals are also popular, although, because the mother feels nothing below her waist, there is a slightly increased risk that she will be unable to push the baby out herself and a forceps delivery may be necessary.

As for the controversial use of episiotomies, before they were as common as they are today, the birth opening was left to stretch for hours to avoid a tear or allowed to tear randomly. Consequently muscle was devitalized, nerves destroyed and prolapse was more common. Technological developments such as machines which monitor the progress of mother and baby now allow a baby's journey down the birth canal to be charted continuously. The size of the cervix, the frequency of contractions, the mother's blood pressure and the foetal heart rate are all recorded so that the pattern of labour can be observed and compared to the 'average' labour. By using such monitors, doctors can see problems early and correct them.

If the obstetrician decides that your baby needs to be induced then there will probably be a good reason for it and it's unlikely to be something that's done for the convenience of the medical staff. However, it's important to remember, too, that you always have a right to know what's going on and, generally, your obstetrician should be willing to tell you.

Are women ever given anaesthetics without being consulted?

Yes, this may occasionally happen, but generally with good reason. Sometimes the birth process can proceed very quickly. Occasionally there may not be time to ask a woman if she wants an anaesthetic nor even time to explain what's happening. If the mother has suddenly become unconscious due to a haemorrhage, say, the medical staff who are attending her will have to act very rapidly to deal with the emergency and, in some circumstances, to save her life.

The important thing to remember about giving birth is that it's often full of surprises – generally nice ones; finding out whether the baby's a boy or a girl; whether it has dark or fair hair and seeing whether it bears any resemblance to other members of the family. You may even be surprised to find that, although you may have expected your labour to be a long, drawn out and painful one, it's quite the opposite. Keep an open mind about things. Don't resolve in advance to refuse pain killers; rather wait and see how things turn out. After all, labour shouldn't be an endurance test. No woman should ever be made to feel guilty about the fact that she wants pain relief during childbirth.

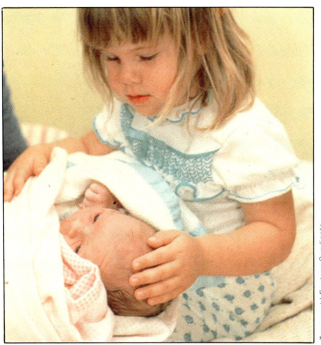

Transworld Feature Syndicate

Labour and childbirth

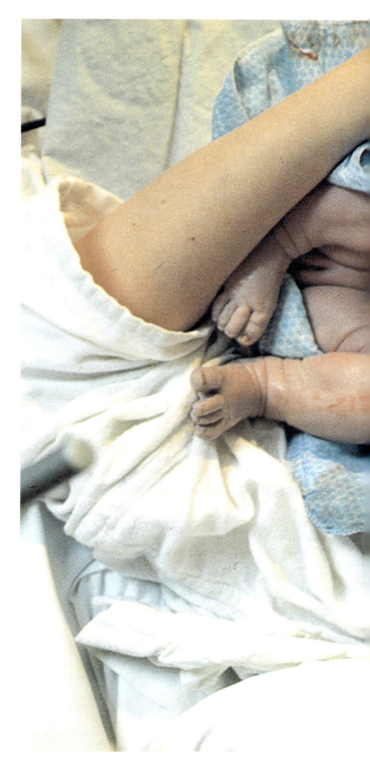

What are the signs that labour has started?

Many women are worried that they won't recognize labour when it begins, but there are three clear cut ways it can happen:
- **Contractions:** during the later stages of pregnancy the uterine muscle contracts every so often. These contractions are felt only in the front and are not true labour contractions (see about false labour, later).

True labour contractions start as a low backache, moving round to the front of the stomach. They come in regular bouts, occurring every half hour to begin with but rapidly progressing to once every 15 to 20 minutes (in the delivery stage they come about every two minutes).

With a first baby it is wise to wait until they are coming regularly, every 15 minutes or so, before going to hospital. With a subsequent baby, you may find it harder to decide on the right moment to leave home. With the responsibility of a larger family, you'll want to make sure your other children are all right before you go. However, things happen much faster in a second labour, so if you want to be sure of getting to hospital on time, leave as soon as the contractions are coming every 20 minutes or so.
- **A 'show' of blood** or bloodstained mucus is another sure sign that labour has started. It's usually only a slight bleeding but it's unmistakable. As soon as you notice it you should go to hospital straight away.
- **Breaking the waters:** in the womb the baby is bathed in fluid and covered by a membranous sac. This sac has to be ruptured before the baby can be born. When this happens clear fluid gushes out of the vagina and is an obvious indication that labour has started.

This is a very unusual way for a woman having her first baby to start labour as the neck of the womb is closed and the membranes are well supported – but it can happen. It is more usual in subsequent pregnancies, as the neck may be a little more open, and the sac unsupported.

How can you be sure that you are not going to have a false labour?

It is sometimes difficult to be certain whether labour pains are the real thing. In the last weeks of pregnancy, the uterus contracts, limbering up to prepare for delivery. This is perfectly normal but, like any other muscular action, if it goes on too long it may be painful. These contractions are different from actual labour contractions

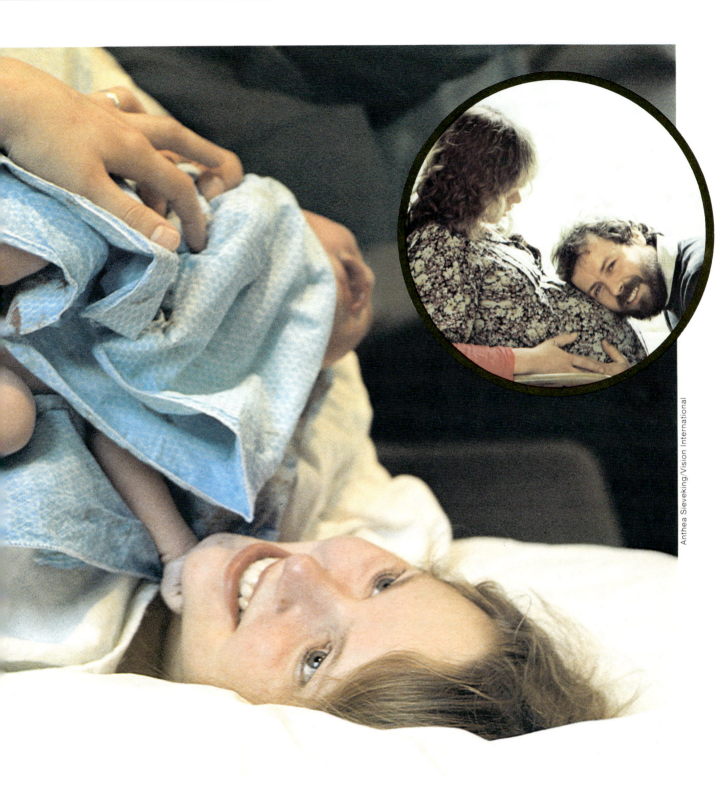

Anthea Sieveking/Vision International

which are caused by the opening of the cervix and the descent of the foetus through the pelvis. However, these false labour contractions can be mistaken for real labour.

Don't hesitate to contact the midwife or hospital if you are uncertain; they never mind 'false alarms'. It is far better to play safe than for the baby to be born *en route* to the hospital. False labours are more common in first pregnancies, though they can occur in later ones – particularly

if a woman has been induced before and has no idea how labour starts.

Is the beginning of labour always painful?

No. It is more of a dull ache, felt at first in the lower back and moving around to the front. This 'stomach' ache is often mistaken for colic and a woman may suspect she has eaten too much raw fruit. The clue lies in the ache beginning at the

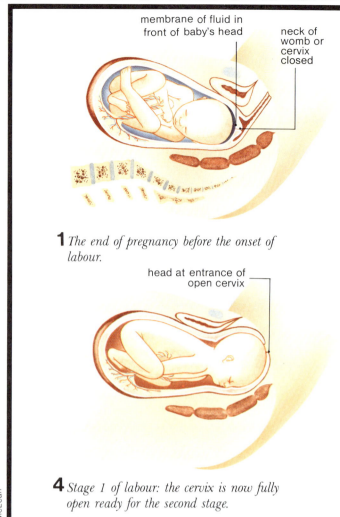

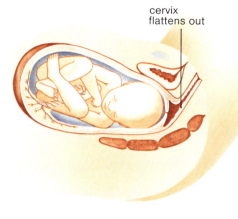

1 *The end of pregnancy before the onset of labour.*

2 *Late pregnancy or early labour: the head begins to descend.*

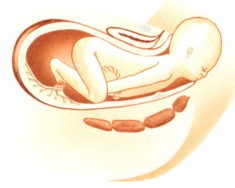

4 *Stage 1 of labour: the cervix is now fully open ready for the second stage.*

5 *Stage 2 of labour: the baby begins to emerge. Once the head and shoulders are born the rest is an easy matter.*

Dee McLean

back and moving round to the front. Gut colic rarely manifests itself in this fashion. In the case of a contraction, by placing your hand on your stomach you can feel the uterus harden as its muscle tightens.

Do some women not notice labour has begun?

This is very rare. Occasionally, a woman who has had several children and happens to be a little plump may not notice the difference between the contractions of late pregnancy and actual labour pains. Either the former have been a little more painful than usual or the latter less intense. As a result, the woman stays at home unaware that she is in labour and either arrives in hospital very late or even has the baby outside the hospital. However, this is most unusual and almost unknown in someone new to motherhood.

What are the normal procedures once you reach hospital?

A midwife will greet you when you arrive. She will usually check the antenatal notes that are prepared at the clinic in previous weeks. It's a good idea to take the communication card with you if you have it, just in case the notes are not readily available. The midwife will quickly examine your stomach to make sure that labour is proceeding well and that delivery is not imminent. She will ask a few simple questions and probably check your blood pressure.

Some hospitals have now stopped giving the traditional enema at the onset of labour. Its original purpose was to encourage uterine contractions and guard against the embarrassment and possible infection of the bowels emptying during the birth. But it is now thought that the use of an enema doesn't make the delivery any cleaner, nor does it bring on uterine contractions. If a woman's bowel is full she may be given a suppository, but that is all that needs to be done.

Similarly the regulation close shave of all the pubic hair is no longer usual. Some hospitals still shave round the back of the vagina and between the legs. This is done to provide a clean area so that when the baby is being born the skin around the birth canal can be properly cleaned with antiseptic. Also, if an *episiotomy* (see later) is

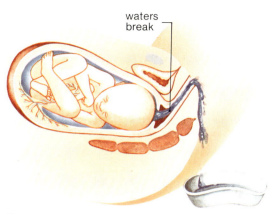

3 *Stage 1 of labour: the membranes have ruptured and the cervix begins to open.*

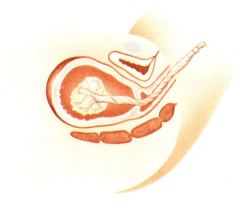

6 *Stage 3 of labour: giving birth to the placenta.*

needed or a tear occurs, this can be sewn up more tidily if there is no pubic hair in the way. Other hospitals only require a woman to clip the hair between her legs with a pair of small hair scissors in the last few days of pregnancy. This is quite enough preparation for a normal delivery.

Some hospitals still give a bath on admission. After this, if the membranes have still not broken, you may be encouraged to sit up or even walk around as you wish. Once the 'waters' have ruptured, you will be asked to stay close to bed and offered pain relief as and when you need it.

What are the stages of labour?

Labour is divided into three stages. The first begins with the start of regular contractions and the gradual opening of the neck of the womb (dilation of the cervix) until it is fully open and wide enough to take the baby's head.

In the second stage, the baby is pushed through the open cervix, normally head first, down the vagina and out into the world.

The third stage of labour is the placental stage which ends when the placenta, membranes and cord are completely delivered.

The different stages of labour vary in length. The first is by far the longest and, for the woman, the most tedious. In a first pregnancy it can last as long as 18 hours, though usually it is around eight to 10 hours. The second stage generally takes about an hour, though again, with a first baby, it may be longer – up to two hours. The third stage is very quick, lasting for a few minutes only. It is speeded up by giving the mother an injection when her baby is delivered (i.e. at the end of stage two), thus accelerating the arrival of the placenta and reducing blood loss.

How do I know when I am in the second stage of labour?

The second stage starts when the neck of the womb is fully dilated. Some women anticipate this with a feeling of fullness in the pelvis. There is a sensation of wanting to open the bowel and a little blood may pass from the vagina. A vaginal examination should clinch the matter.

How can I be sure that I will push efficiently?

You will need practice here. Most hospitals run antenatal classes which teach the art of pushing. Other classes are run by local authorities, and many private organizations, such as the National Childbirth Trust in Britain, have their own instructors.

When a contraction of the uterus is on the way, you will sense a tightening in the abdomen. You should first of all take a few quick breaths in and out, then a large breath in and hold it. For 10 to 15 seconds keep your pushing steady, down into the bottom of the pelvis, and hold your breath. Next, let the breath out and take in another large chestful of air to give a second push, again for 10 to 15 seconds. With control you should manage four or five pushes per contraction, each of which will ease the baby's progress down the vaginal passage. Relax as much as possible in the minute or two between contractions, so as to be ready to tackle the next one when it comes.

Most women find the second stage of labour a relief after the more passive first stage. They feel comforted and reassured from taking an active part in delivering their own baby.

Is it true that some women are reluctant to push?

Some women do have difficulty in pushing. Often this is due either to fear of pain or lack of training during pregnancy. This is a pity, as pushing is a primitive, instinctive response to the feeling of something filling the pelvis. They can be helped, however, by a good doctor or midwife.

What is the best method of pain relief in labour?

Doctors will prescribe safe, pain-relieving drugs that will not affect the baby. In the first stage of labour, the best of these is *pethidine*, injected into the muscle of the buttock. It takes about 20 minutes to start working and the effect usually lasts two or three hours. If labour is lengthy, more than one injection will be needed and the mother should warn those around her when the effect is wearing off so that she can be given a second one in time.

Another method of relieving pain is by the *epidural* anaesthetic, which numbs the nerves as they flow from the uterus towards the spine. This calls for a skilled anaesthetist to be present. It is an effective method and popular with many women as it leaves the mother fully conscious to take an active part in the birth process.

Top: listening to the child's heart beat. Right: still in the first stages of labour. Far right: the head appears. Below right: the new born baby with umbilical cord still attached. Below: giving an epidural.

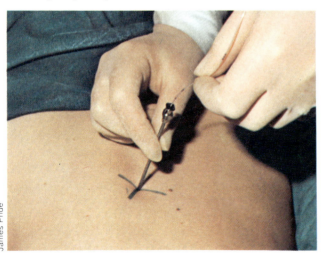

James Pride

In the second stage of labour pethidine injections should not be administered as they can affect a new born baby's breathing. An epidural would be difficult to insert for the first time at this stage, and so most hospitals recommend nitrous oxide and oxygen. This gives pain relief very quickly as it is inhaled and absorbed through the lungs. Women wishing to use nitrous oxide need to be shown how to use the face mask during pregnancy so that they know how to control the gas when the time comes.

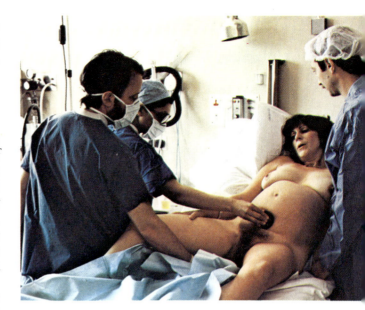

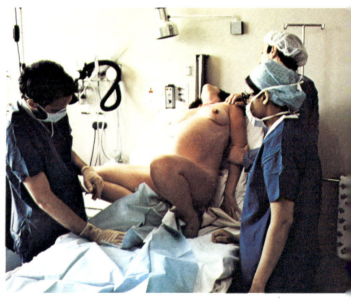

What happens at the moment of delivery of my baby?

The baby's head moves down the vagina, gradually stretching the opening ahead of it. With each contraction and bout of pushing, more of the surface of the head becomes visible. Between contractions it may retreat a little, but soon re-emerges when the next one occurs. Eventually, the head reaches the point of no return, and passes through the entrance.

There is no need for any more pushing. From now on, the midwife takes over delivery. The hardest part of labour is over, and the shoulders and body slip through easily. You can see your baby being born if your head and shoulders are raised up on pillows.

It is vital to follow the midwife's instructions at this stage, to avoid pushing too hard once the

Anthea Sieveking/Vision International

baby's head has passed the entrance. This would damage the tissues of the lower end of the vagina. The best way not to push is to pant quickly in and out when the midwife asks you.

What is an episiotomy and when is it necessary?

Often during delivery the baby's head over-stretches the tissues and they tear. To try to prevent a tear, an episiotomy may be carried out; this is a small surgical cut which is made under local anaesthetic to relieve tension at the bottom of the vagina.

This mini-operation is usually hardly felt, and all doctors and midwives have been trained to perform it. Afterwards, the area will be stitched up carefully to bring tissues together and allow

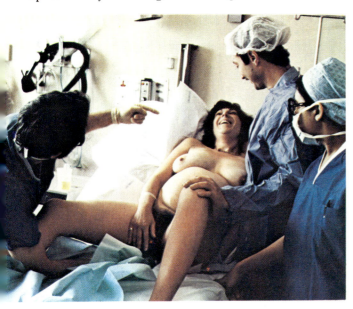

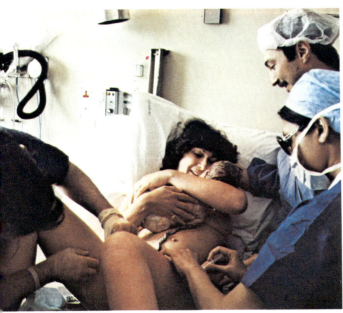

them to heal neatly.

It is up to the person doing the delivery to decide whether or not an episiotomy is necessary. If it is your first baby, you are more likely to need the operation than if you have already had one or more children.

What happens to baby when it has been born?

Being born is one of the greatest shocks in life. Inside the uterus the baby has been living in a gravity-free, dark, warm, quiet environment. Suddenly he is pushed into the outside world where the force of gravity is influencing him. He has to breathe – through lungs which have never been used before – to get his oxygen, while light, touch and a cool temperature are all new sensations for him.

He starts to breathe by sucking in a big breath. But before this happens the midwife removes any excess fluid from his nose and mouth with a very small suction tube. Most babies take their first breath within 30 seconds of birth, and 96 per cent of them do so in three minutes. Once breathing is established it is essential to keep the baby warm. The midwife will wrap the baby in a prewarmed blanket, as a damp child can lose heat very readily even in an apparently warm room. Most rooms are not more than 75°F and a baby has been used to an internal body temperature of 98°F. The midwife examines the baby soon after it is born, to make sure there are no external abnormalities.

How is the placenta delivered?

Once the baby is born and breathing well, the midwife awaits the arrival of the placenta. She feels for the next contraction which often comes within five minutes of birth. When this happens she can usually guide the placenta out of the uterus by pulling at the cord in a controlled fashion. The placenta is soft and causes no pain, being much smaller than the baby. Usually an injection has been given during the birth, to help the uterus contract and expel the placenta, so reducing blood loss. Any stitching needed is usually left until after the placenta has emerged.

Are second babies easier to have than first?

Usually, yes. The labour tends to be shorter and the woman is more mentally prepared for what is going to happen. She has been through the experience before and knows the ropes. Most women, as a result, find it easier to have their second and third babies.

Post-natal depression

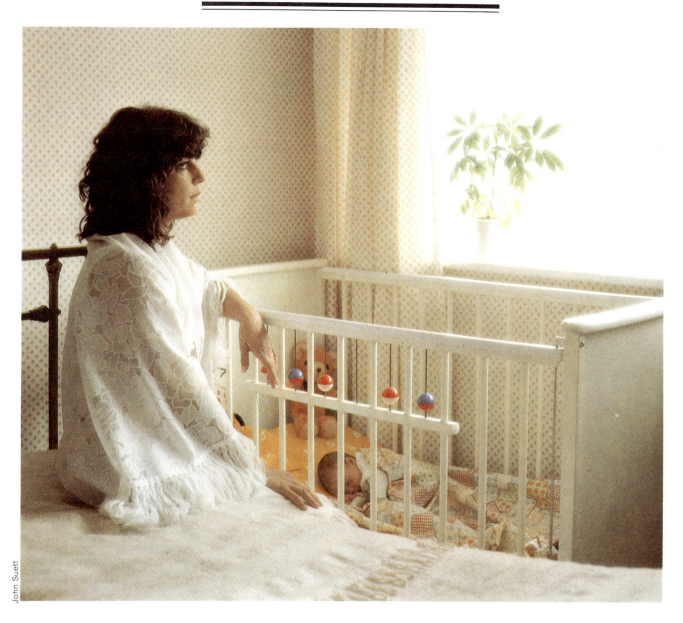

John Suett

Do many women get depressed after the birth of a baby?

Yes, in the early days after having a baby mild depression is so common that it is regarded as normal. It happens after at least 50 per cent of births and usually shows up during the third or fourth day. It doesn't last very long – normally a day or two, or sometimes just a few hours — and it is rarely troublesome. This brief low is often called *'baby blues'*.

At the other end of the scale one or two mothers in every thousand suffer from depression so severe and intense that it causes derangement, loss of contact with reality and the risk of suicide. Such deep depression as this is called *psychotic depression.*

The condition in between these two extremes is called *post-natal depression* which follows about one in 10 births. It is not as mild nor as common as baby blues. It happens more often than psychotic depression, however, and it's considerably less severe.

It's certainly not a normal event any more than

catching 'flu could be considered normal. But it's not so rare that it's very abnormal either; any woman can get it. Post-natal depression is one of the most common and unpleasant complications of the *puerperium* – the period of six weeks or so after having a baby when the body is supposed to be getting itself back to normal.

It's perhaps rather artificial to try to draw a clear-cut distinction between 'the blues' and post-natal depression. Most women have their babies in hospital these days and they can easily feel under a certain amount of strain in trying to establish some sort of routine for the new baby. This strain could be expressed as anxiety, spells of despondency and a few tears.

It's not clear whether this readjustment period is normal or something in between 'blues' and post-natal depression – but it's not usually something to worry too much about. However, a woman who is still troubled by despondency between six and eight weeks after the birth and who is not usually so depressed, is suffering from post-natal depression.

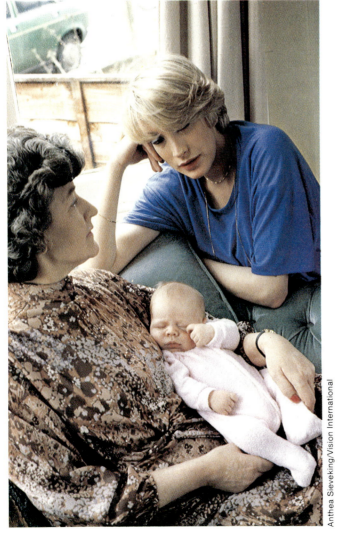

What are the typical signs?

Not unexpectedly, the main symptoms of a woman with post-natal depression are that she feels low and depressed. The new mother is unhappy, fed up and demoralized. She is sad, tearful and feels guilty. The mood can vary every day, but often gets worse as the day goes on.

Usually the mother cannot explain her misery, especially at such a traditionally happy time. When other mothers in her social circle have appeared to cope happily with motherhood she blames herself for her self-pity and inability to 'pull herself together'. To be in such a state is an unusual, perhaps unique, experience for her. She is often irritable, particularly with her partner as well as with any other children she has, and this makes her feel all the more guilty.

She is anxious to the point of panic and feels that she cannot cope. She worries unduly if the baby doesn't take all its feeds, doesn't bring up its wind, keeps crying or even if it sleeps too soundly. These are common, and natural anxieties for many new mothers, but they utterly and painfully pre-occupy the mother who is depressed.

Fatigue nearly always goes hand in hand with the depression. It adds to the awful feeling of not coping. By the end of the day a depressed mother is completely exhausted and longs to go to bed. But when she gets there she cannot sleep, tossing and turning instead. Eventually, when she does drop off, sleep is fitful and disturbed by alarming dreams which generally involve the baby. By this time, because she is so weary, she may think that there is something physically wrong with her. She may well visit her doctor for iron or a tonic to treat imagined anaemia or a hormone change.

Depression usually causes a loss of appetite and therefore of weight, but sometimes it has just the opposite effect. Eating for comfort and consolation leads to weight gain which does nothing at all for an already poor self-image.

A number of depressed women go off sex too. This denies them an important source of pleasure, closeness and self-esteem. It may also estrange the baby's father who is already perplexed.

Baby blues cause tearfulness, despondency, anxiety and difficulty in coping too, but the symptoms are short-lived and never severe. Psychotic depression goes much further than post-natal depression and is so severe that the mother feels both she and the baby are beyond hope. She feels unfit to live and is preoccupied with desperate ideas of removing herself and the baby from her wretched world. Tragically she sometimes acts in accordance with such dismal thoughts.

Anthea Sieveking/Vision International

How long does it usually last?

Rather surprisingly there have not been many follow-up studies of post-natal depression, so there is no accurate answer to this question.

To be recognized for what it is, the depression has to last at least a month. After that the mood usually runs its course in a matter of weeks, but it can sometimes last for months or even for longer than a year.

Baby blues are over within a day or two. Psychotic depression is less likely to go unrecognized and untreated than post-natal depression. Though it's a more severe disorder this means, ironically, that psychotic depression stands a better chance of being curtailed quickly.

What causes post-natal depression?

There are several possible causes, none of which apparently apply in all cases. A stillbirth, early death or severe handicap of the baby are events which anyone would find depressing. Generally, however, there isn't such an obvious cause for post-natal depression.

Some sufferers have gone through similar bouts of depression which have no connection with childbirth. They may well be the type who experience depression anyway when under stress. This is very much so in cases of psychotic depression where there is often a personal and family history of severe depression. However a lot of women who suffer from post-natal depression never get depressed at other times, not even after other births.

On occasions there seems to be a reason why the birth of one particular child should bring about depression. A woman who had coped well with her first daughter became very anxious and low after the birth of her second. She explained that as a second daughter herself she had felt that her older sister was their mother's favourite. She was afraid that history might repeat itself.

There is little evidence to connect post-natal depression with complications in pregnancy, difficult childbirth, hospital confinement or the use of anaesthetics which may prevent the mother and baby being together after delivery. (This separation can delay the attachment or 'bonding' process.)

Although hormone theories are popular, none are proven. For example, there is a huge build-up of oestrogen and progesterone during pregnancy, followed by a sudden fall after delivery. It has been suggested that this change in hormone levels contributes to baby blues. But this doesn't explain post-natal depression which develops more slowly and lasts a lot longer. No hormone therapy has proved to be effective in the treatment of post-natal depression.

Why do some women suffer from it when others don't?

Doctors don't know. The few clues they have fall a long way short of giving a complete picture.

It has been suggested that personality contributes to post-natal depression. For example the obsessional, compliant woman who is brought up always to do what she's told and not as she feels may be more at risk. Her instincts have been thwarted for so long that they don't tell her how to deal with an uncontrolled, demanding newborn baby. It's difficult for her to identify and cope with her offspring. An immature woman who may see her baby as a rival is also said to be at risk. But there is no really solid evidence to relate this type of depression to personality.

Current theories include suppressed anger and a learned state of helplessness as factors which provoke depression. Following these lines, situations which give rise to anger that cannot be aired, or which promote feelings of incompetence or helplessness, may lead to depression.

The loss of a woman's mother at a tender age through death or divorce has been associated with increased risk of post-natal depression. A spate of bad luck during the year before the birth of the baby, and the absence of a supportive partner or friend are also contributing factors.

What's the best kind of approach to take with a depressed mother?

In the first place it's an enormous relief for a depressed mother to be told that she is suffering from post-natal depression. It's a well recognized disorder which is unpleasant while it lasts but likely to get better nonetheless.

She is not a spoilt brat, wallowing in self-pity, ungrateful or unmotherly. She is not physically ill, she is not a freak, nor is she going mad. It is her sheer bad luck to be afflicted this way.

It is good for her to talk about how she feels. She will appreciate the chance to cry on someone's shoulder without being interrupted too quickly, scolded or being 'jollied along'.

The health visitor, the family doctor and occasionally a psychiatrist should be involved. Sometimes an anti-depressive drug helps a lot. The husband or partner and other members of the family (the grandmothers for example) should be brought into the picture so that they can understand what's going on, and help out.

CHAPTER 5

Tests
and
Operations

Pregnancy testing

Up until the 1930s the diagnosis of pregnancy was based on a combination of physical signs and symptoms such as missed periods, early morning sickness, breast tenderness and possibly a gain in weight. During the last 50 years however, scientists have developed objective tests which can detect biochemical changes in the body associated with pregnancy. In addition, the development of techniques such as ultrasound scanning now enables the embryo to be *seen* in the uterus without fear of damage.

Quite simply, if you consider that it is during the first few weeks of pregnancy that all the major organs of the body and the brain itself are being formed, you can understand why it's important for a woman to know she's pregnant as soon as possible.

Apart from the general value of pregnancy testing, special tests can confirm the presence of an ectopic pregnancy (one that develops in a Fallopian tube instead of the uterus). It is vitally important that this condition is detected as early as possible, as it is extremely dangerous to the woman concerned. The accurate early diagnosis of pregnancy also helps the woman with an unwanted pregnancy to take the option of having it terminated simply and effectively.

Is it true that animals are used for pregnancy testing?

Not any longer. This used to be the case until the early 1960s. Until this time a test called a *bioassay* was commonly used to determine whether HCG was present in the mother's blood or urine. Bioassays depended upon the measurement of the response of the ovaries or testes of an experimental animal (mice, rats, rabbits, frogs or toads) to an injection of HCG. These tests were not only relatively insensitive, they were also costly and time consuming, taking anything from five hours to five days to perform. Furthermore, there was the added disadvantage that large numbers of animals were required to carry them out. With these limitations, plus the fact that simple, quick and more accurate tests are now available, there is very little reason for bioassays to be performed nowadays.

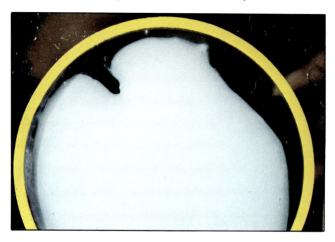

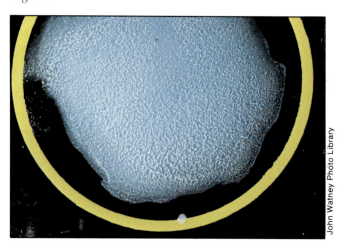

The results of a slide test are easily visible to the naked eye. The top picture shows a positive result and the bottom is negative.

John Watney Photo Library

What is the most common pregnancy test?

Tests called *immunoassays* superseded bioassays during the mid-1960s, and they remain the most commonly used test of pregnancy. There are two different types – an *agglutination immunoassay*, and a *radioimmunoassay*. Immunoassay is a term used to describe any test which involves the use of *antibodies* to the substance being tested, and does not refer only to a pregnancy test.

Antibodies to HCG (anti-HCG) are produced

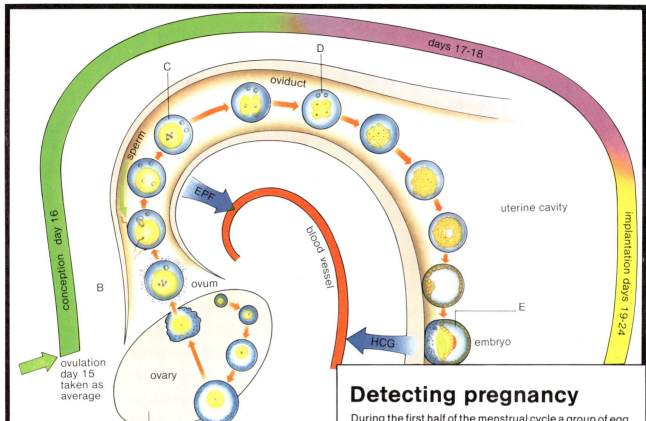

Labels on diagram: days 17-18, oviduct, D, C, sperm, EPF, blood vessel, uterine cavity, implantation days 19-24, E, embryo, HCG, B, ovum, conception day 16, ovulation day 15 taken as average, ovary, follicle, A

by injecting an experimental animal (rabbit, sheep or goat) with HCG extracted from the blood or urine of pregnant women. Because the animal has been injected with a foreign substance its natural defence system immediately begins to fight against it by producing antibodies which are released into the bloodstream. These are then extracted (causing no harm to the animal) and used to monitor the presence of HCG in samples of blood or urine from a woman who suspects she may be pregnant.

The most common type of immunoassay is the agglutination immunoassay. This can be further divided into *tube* or *slide tests*, but the principles of both are the same. They are both quick and simple, and results can be read with the naked eye.

With the slide test a drop of anti-HCG is put on to a glass slide, and a small drop of the mother's urine is mixed with it. If the sample contains HCG it will neutralize the effect of the antibodies as the two are mixed together. If there is no HCG present to neutralize the antibodies they will remain active in the solution on the slide. In order to make the results of the test easily readable, a few drops of a milky substance made of rubber latex particles coated with HCG are added to the mixture after a one-minute interval.

Detecting pregnancy

During the first half of the menstrual cycle a group of egg follicles start to develop in the ovary (A). Any time between days 12 to 21 (the first day of the menstrual period is considered to be day 1 of the menstrual cycle) one of them, the *leading follicle*, will reach a size where it breaks and releases the egg into the oviduct (B). Taking day 15 as the average day on which this happens, *conception* – fertilization of an egg by a sperm – will probably take place the day after ovulation, in this case on day 16 (C). It is unlikely to happen any later as an egg has a limited life span – usually less than 24 hours.

When a sperm fertilizes an egg it creates one complete cell. This keeps on dividing, and the number of cells increases rapidly during the following two days, 17 and 18 (D). *Implantation* (E), the embedding of the developing embryo into the lining of the uterus, can occur from days 19 to 24 in this instance. It is at this stage that pregnancy is considered to be established.

It is now possible to detect pregnancy very early on indeed, in fact immediately conception has occurred. This is because a protein substance not normally present in the mother's body, known as the *early pregnancy factor* (EPF) begins to be produced at this time. Although tests, called *rosette inhibition tests*, are available in certain countries to detect and measure the presence of EPF, they are usually only carried out on women whose pregnancies are being monitored in hospital, possibly because of trouble in previous pregnancies. In normal circumstances, of course, a woman would not even begin to suspect she was pregnant until some time after this earliest stage of pregnancy – probably not until after the first period is missed.

So, although in theory it is possible to detect pregnancy any time after the moment of conception, it is in fact easier and far more common to test for a substance called human chorionic gonadotrophin (HCG). This hormone is produced in increasingly large quantities by the implanted embryo. HCG can be identified in the mother's blood and urine, and its presence is a good indication that the woman has conceived.

If the antibodies are still present they will automatically be drawn to the HCG coating on the latex particles, and the two will clump together to form 'curds' in the milky substance. The binding reaction takes place within three minutes and indicates that the woman is *not* pregnant. However, if all the antibodies have been neutralized by HCG in the urine there will be no clumping together (see diagram), indicating a positive result.

In the tube test, red blood cells from sheep are coated with HCG and used instead of latex particles. Apart from this, the test is performed along similar lines. After mixing a small sample of urine with a known amount of anti-HCG, the HCG coated red blood cells are added. Unlike the slide test, results are not immediately detectable and the tube has to be left in a rack for two hours.

If a dark ring forms at the bottom of the tube, the woman is pregnant. The HCG in the urine sample has neutralized the anti-HCG and the HCG coated red blood cells sink to the bottom of the tube, forming a distinct ring as shown on the previous page. However, if the woman is *not* pregnant no HCG is present in the urine, the HCG coated red blood cells will clump together with the antibodies and remain suspended in the solution so no ring forms.

What other tests are available?

The other type of immunoassay, the *radioimmunoassay*, can also be used to test for pregnancy. Although based on the same principle as the agglutination immunoassay, it is more expensive and more complicated. A radioimmunoassay takes about four hours to perform and, unlike the agglutination immunoassay, which can be performed in an outpatients' clinic, it has to be done in a laboratory with specialized equipment.

It is, however, an extremely sensitive test capable of detecting the very low levels of HCG produced in early pregnancy. Two factors make this test extremely precise. One involves the use of antibodies found only in a fractional part of HCG. A molecule of HCG can be split into two parts – the *alpha unit*, whose chemical structure is identical to some other hormones, particularly the luteinising hormone (LH) produced prior to, and just after, ovulation; and the *beta unit*, which is structurally unique. When antibodies to the whole HCG molecule are used, an early radioimmunoassay pregnancy test may also detect LH and so provide inaccurate results. If antibodies specific to the beta sub-unit are used, the test immediately becomes more precise since it is only measuring for the presence of HCG.

The other factor that makes a radioimmunoassay an extremely sensitive test is the use of HCG which has been 'tagged' with radioactive iodine, in place of HCG coated latex particles or red blood cells.

The test itself consists of incubating a sample of serum or urine with a pre-determined amount of antibody to the beta sub-unit. The radioactive HCG is then added, and a gamma ray counter is used to measure how much radioactive HCG has been bound to the antibodies. If the woman is *not* pregnant all the unneutralized antibodies will have adhered to the radioactive HCG and the reading on the gamma ray counter will be high. If she *is* pregnant however, much less radioactive HCG will bind itself to the antibodies, and the reading on the gamma ray counter will be low. Radioimmunoassays are particularly valuable in detecting an ectopic pregnancy. If a doctor suspects that this may be the case he will arrange for a radioimmunoassay to be carried out, in order to test for the extremely low levels of HCG produced by this type of pregnancy.

A test called a *radioreceptor assay* may also be used to detect pregnancy. It involves the use of what are known as *receptor proteins* to attract the HCG instead of antibodies. The test only takes about an hour to perform, but because the method also measures LH it can only be used after the time of the missed menstrual period when this hormone will no longer be present.

How accurate are pregnancy tests?

Pregnancy tests are not 100 per cent reliable, but if they are performed correctly and at the recommended time, they should be at least 95 times out of every 100.

Because the amount of HCG produced at any one stage of pregnancy varies considerably from woman to woman, the least sensitive tests – the agglutination immunoassays – cannot be performed with 95 per cent accuracy until six weeks after the LMP (the first day of the last menstrual period). This time span allows for a positive result even in the case of a woman producing fairly low levels of HCG.

As you can see from the diagram, the results of a radioimmunoassay may be accurately determined by four and a half weeks after conception.

Very occasionally a test may give a false positive result, indicating a pregnancy when one is not present. However, this occurs very rarely. False negatives – no indication of pregnancy when one is in fact established – are more common and may occur because the pregnancy has been dated incorrectly. For instance, if the woman conceived later than was originally estimated, HCG levels may not have been high enough at the time of the test to give a positive result. If a woman is in any doubt the test should be repeated one week later.

The most recent development in the detection of pregnancy has been the use of *ultrasonography*. With an ultrasound scan – which has the great merit of taking less than five minutes to perform – it is now possible to see the developing embryo in the uterus as early as six weeks after LMP.

This ultrasound scan reveals a developing embryo.

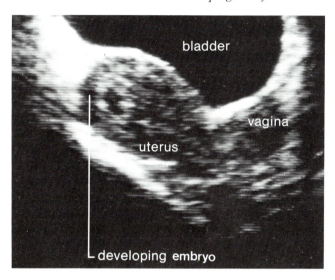

Are there any new advances in pregnancy testing?

Yes. New tests are being developed which concentrate on detecting chemical changes in easily accessible body fluids like saliva and urine.

Scientists in this field are trying to move away from any tests involving the use of blood samples (simply because they are more difficult to obtain), and attempts are also being made to develop tests that avoid the use of radioactive chemicals. And further, there is a move towards producing anti-HCG in cultures rather than extracting them from the blood of animals.

It has been found that several different protein substances, not normally present in a woman's body, are produced when she is pregnant. Work is being done to develop tests that detect the presence of these substances. Tests are also being developed to detect a particular enzyme known to be present in the saliva of pregnant women.

A further recent discovery has been that pregnancy alters the body's production of white blood cells. It could be that the detection of this alteration in *lymphocyte* function will form the basis for a future pregnancy test, but this line of research is in its early stages at present.

In addition, the sensitivity of ultrasound detection is continually being improved. It is already possible to 'see' ovulation and, as mentioned earlier on, the developing embryo can be seen in the womb by the sixth week of pregnancy. A leading specialist in the field claims that soon, the stages between ovulation and the six-week-old embryo may also be detected visually. In fact it is thought likely that the ultrasound scan will probably be the main form of pregnancy testing in the not too distant future.

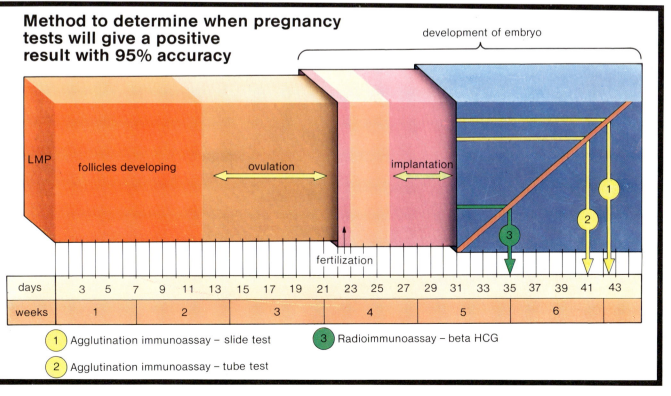

Method to determine when pregnancy tests will give a positive result with 95% accuracy

development of embryo

LMP — follicles developing — ovulation — implantation — fertilization

days	3	5	7	9	11	13	15	17	19	21	23	25	27	29	31	33	35	37	39	41	43
weeks	1		2			3			4			5			6						

1 Agglutination immunoassay – slide test   3 Radioimmunoassay – beta HCG

2 Agglutination immunoassay – tube test

Bernard Fallon

Hundreds of thousands of women each year give birth to healthy babies after a trouble-free pregnancy. Nature has provided an ideal environment in the womb.

Unfortunately, complications do occur, but with an ever-increasing battery of tests at their disposal, doctors can identify problems early and, if necessary, intervene to help both mother and baby. But for this checking process to be effective, it must be regular and must start early in pregnancy. Each appointment for an ante-natal check-up may be crucial to the health of the developing baby.

What are the normal screening tests done during pregnancy?

A programme of physical examinations and medical tests help doctors to identify any potential problems early in pregnancy. Some of the procedures are 'one-offs', others become a regular part of each ante-natal visit, so that doctors can monitor the progress of both mother and baby.

This 'screening' starts at the first ante-natal visit, which should take place within 12 weeks of conception, and continues until the birth of the baby. Apart from regular physical check-ups – internal and abdominal examinations and weighing – certain medical tests also become part of the routine. Urine samples and blood pressure readings are taken at every visit while cervical smears or blood tests may only be needed once or twice throughout the pregnancy. Ultrasound screening is also a normal check in some centres. The chart on this page tells you exactly what these medical tests are for.

After the first ante-natal visit, mothers are usually asked to come back every four weeks. At the 28th week, the gap between visits closes to two weeks, and then to one at the 36th week up until the baby is born. Sometimes the findings of these routine check-ups will indicate that further tests may be necessary.

Why do doctors sometimes recommend special screening tests?

At the first ante-natal visit, doctors will review the expectant mother's medical background and the progress of any earlier pregnancy. Any illness, perhaps running in the family, may affect the unborn child.

Women suffering from diabetes, high blood pressure, kidney or heart disease, and even alcoholism or drug addiction are all considered

Ante-natal tests

to be "high risk". They will automatically be given tests to check on their baby's size and growth. Indeed, whenever a doctor suspects that a baby is not thriving properly he will recommend that these tests be given. Small babies with a low weight are more likely to be born prematurely and to risk physical or mental handicap. Doctor's will also run tests if they suspect that a mother is carrying more than one baby, or if she has a previous history of miscarriage or stillbirth. Older women and very young women particularly those who are single or living in very deprived circumstances, will also be candidates, since they are more likely to encounter complications.

Older women run a greater risk of having a mongol baby too (Down's syndrome) – one of the better known of the 'genetic' problems. A complication of this kind, which results in malformation, is one of the things parents fear most and a major reason for running special tests. There are a number of disorders which can cause abnormality in babies, some of which do run in families. Fortunately, it's possible to detect them while the child is in the womb, and if necessary to terminate the pregnancy.

Hormone levels in the mother's blood and urine can sometimes give doctors guidance on the progress of 'high risk' babies, and some abnormalities may be detected during routine ante-natal tests. For instance, signs of spina bifida, which can cause major malformations, can be seen in blood tests. But pre-birth screening has been revolutionized over the past 10 years by two new techniques – ultrasonic screening and amniocentesis (the fluid test). Women with a high risk factor or a family history of inherited disease can now be screened by these methods as a matter of course.

What does an ultrasound test show?

Ultrasound gives doctors a 'window' on the womb, providing information that often cannot be gathered in any other way. It is now commonly used in the routine examination of pregnant women, even when there is no suspicion of any abnormality, just to confirm dates.

The technique uses a series of high frequency

Pre-birth medical tests

TEST	PURPOSE
Urine	Detection of toxaemia, 'pregnancy diabetes' and kidney infection.
Blood	Detection of anaemia, German measles and presence of 'neural tube' disorders such as spina bifida. Blood group is checked to see if it is compatible with baby's ('rhesus' babies) or in case a blood transfusion is needed.
Blood pressure	High blood pressure may indicate toxaemia.
Ultrasound	Helps determine baby's birth size. Confirms multiple births. Allows examination of the placenta. Checks for baby's heartbeat; internal bleeding; expected date of delivery and foetal disorders.
Cervical smears	Detects early signs of cervical cancer or infections such as 'thrush'.
Fluid test (Amniocentesis)	Detection of a wide range of disorders and defects including mongolism, spina bifida and 'neural tube' disorders. Also guide to baby's maturity and rate of growth.

sound waves – inaudible to the human ear – which 'bounce' back from the foetal tissue according to its density and depth. These sound waves build up to form an impression of the baby – his first 'photograph' in fact. Unlike X-rays which are only used as a last resort, it also has the advantage of being harmless.

The mother lies on a couch and her stomach is given a smearing of olive oil to give the scanner 'head' a good 'contact'. The scanner moves backwards and forwards and up and down and the mother can often see the baby's outline appearing on the 'screen' – an exciting moment.

Ultrasound screening can be valuable in preventing handicaps in babies. Premature births, for example, can be avoided, since screening allows doctors to assess the exact age of the foetus and so time delivery. Diabetic babies, can also be closely watched, and signs of bleeding from behind the placenta can warn doctors that the baby is in danger of oxygen starvation – one of the major causes of either handicap or death.

One of the most important functions is in aiding amniocentesis (the fluid test) in detecting malformation. In skilled hands, an ultrasonic scanner can actually reveal the damage caused by 'open' spina bifida.

Regular checks will follow the baby's progress. A sudden fall in the growth rate could mean that the mother needs to rest, or that the placenta is failing to deliver enough oxygen and that the baby must be delivered. A misplaced placenta can confirm the need for a Caesarian delivery.

The baby's weight can also be assessed with the aid of the ultrasonic scanner, and this can ensure that the best facilities and care are available to very small babies. Similarly, twin and multiple births can be diagnosed as early as seven weeks, so that both parents and doctors can be forewarned and preparations made. A baby's heartbeat, too, can be detected long before any stethoscope would be able to pick it up.

The ultrasound test

The image that appears on the screen during an ultrasound screening test is built up from sound waves; it's not easy to make out unless you are an expert. This one shows a foetus at about 17 weeks old.

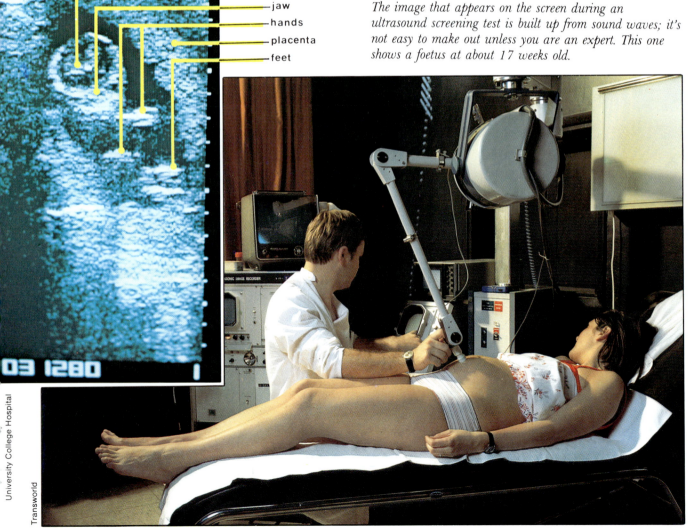

head
jaw
hands
placenta
feet

03 1280

What is the fluid test?

Basically, this involves taking a sample of the amniotic fluid which surrounds the baby.

The sample is drawn off by inserting a fine, hollow needle through the mother's abdomen into the womb. This is neither as frightening nor as strange as it sounds. The woman lies comfortably on her back, while the doctor checks the position of the baby so that he knows precisely where the needle should go. A small amount of local anaesthetic is rubbed over the skin, so that as the needle goes in there is no pain, only a slightly strange feeling.

The fluid does not 'leak' out of the womb – the tissue in the wall simply closes over the 'puncture' as the needle is withdrawn.

The fluid contains cells shed from the baby's skin, and from these doctors can detect signs of any inherited defects. It also contains traces of a substance called alphafetoprotein (AFP). High levels indicate the presence of 'neurological' disorders such as spina bifida.

It is crucial that the tests are carried out at the correct time – usually between the 16th to 18th week of pregnancy – when results should be much clearer. But the one disadvantage of this timing is that, should an abortion follow, it will take place later in pregnancy than is normal.

Many doctors would like to see the screening of blood, followed by a fluid test if necessary, introduced all over the country to detect spina bifida. Three or four out of every 1000 pregnancies result in 'neural tube' disorders of this kind, and screening is estimated to detect three in every four affected infants. Already, a large number of doctors recommend that all pregnant women aged about 40 or over should be tested for mongolism, if they wish, since the risks rise steeply at this time. No mother is obliged to have these tests, and if your doctor recommends that you have them you can always discuss it with him if you have any doubts.

Is it true that fluid tests can predict the sex of a baby?

Yes. When the fluid is tested for inherited disorders, it can also reveal the sex of the child, but the test is not available to those who simply want to know whether their baby is a boy or a girl. This is not because it would take the mystery out of pregnancy – and many parents enjoy this guessing game – but because it could be open to abuse. Already some parents have begun to demand abortion as of right if the child is of the 'wrong' sex.

What new screening tests are in the pipeline?

The most up-to-date equipment, which is not yet commonly available is a 'real time' scanner which can also pick up the baby's movements as they take place. Such movements can be detected in a foetus that is only eight weeks old.

Blood can be seen coursing through the veins and the heart beating. In late pregnancy the scanner can show the baby 'breathing' or making some form of respiratory movement. This has enormous benefits in checking the baby's well being, and some researchers believe that in the future this scanner may make it possible to operate on the baby in the womb; in the case of heart defects for example.

The newest techniques also permit the exact diagnosis of some disorders for which a blood sample from the foetus is needed. A fetoscope can extract a sample from the placenta and this can be tested for haemophilia or muscular dystrophy. The fetoscope has a tiny built-in light and may even help to explore the baby for defects such as a cleft palate.

Is there a test that can detect the exact date when the baby will be delivered?

No. Babies do not follow such a strict timetable that they all require exactly 40 weeks in the womb. Some may need a little more, some a little less. Although ultrasound is the most reliable guide to estimating the age of the foetus we have, it is not infallible, and doctors and midwives are warned not to rely on it too heavily.

Are the new tests safe?

As with all medical procedures, risk must be balanced against the advantages. As far as we know the high frequency sound waves of the ultrasound scan do not damage the foetus, and there has been considerable research to support this belief.

Amniocentesis carries a slight risk – perhaps a two per cent chance of miscarriage. But in the centres with the best experienced and most highly skilled operators, the risk is even less. Nevertheless, because of the slight chance of harming the child, doctors do not always encourage the test. If a woman over 40 is carrying a much-wanted first baby, after years of infertility, the doctors may advise against amniocentesis, though mongolism may be a risk. Younger women, who have much lower chances of having mongol children are not normally tested either. And in any case, you are not obliged to have them.

Infertility in women

How long should you 'try' for a baby, before consulting a doctor?

Some couples are lucky and conceive a child at the first attempt; others may have to wait longer– for years perhaps rather than months. Conception is a very complicated business, and if a woman is to conceive, a number of 'conditions' must be satisfied:

● she must have healthy, active ovaries regularly producing fully ripe eggs – so she must have normal periods.

● there must be a clear passageway for the egg to travel down and the sperm to travel up – via the vagina, through the cervix to the womb and along the Fallopian tubes to the ovaries.

● there must be a normally developed womb, complete with prepared lining, ready to receive the fertilized egg and nourish it.

● last, but not least, there must be healthy sperm deposited high enough in the vagina to make their way through the cervix to meet and fertilize the egg.

Not only must all the reproductive organs be in working order, but the hormone messengers which control them must also be operating properly. And that's not all; even if all these physical requirements are met, timing is crucial. If the sperm don't arrive within the 24 hours before an egg is released or up to 10 hours afterwards then there is no chance of pregnancy.

Given this, it's quite surprising that, on average, 90 per cent of married couples conceive a child within one year of deciding to start a family.

If after one year of trying you still haven't conceived, it's well worth while consulting your doctor. It's estimated that about 40 per cent of 'infertile' couples do eventually have children.

But there is a lot you can do to encourage pregnancy before you need involve your doctor (see previous chapter on *Conception*).

What are the most important causes of infertility in women?

Of the many causes of infertility, some are more important than others, either because they are more common, or because they interfere quite seriously with the chance of having a baby.

Any blockage of the reproductive gland will, of course, restrict the passage of egg and sperm. In such cases, surgery is often the only answer. One of the commonest and best known of this type of problem is a blockage in the Fallopian tubes.

This is usually due to an inflammation following an infection somewhere in the pelvic cavity. What may happen is that the inflammation results in an *adhesion*, which means that one membrane is sticking to another and causing a blockage. If the infection has been in the tubes, they themselves may be closed at either end by adhesions, but even an infection elsewhere in the region may cause the tubes to stick to other tissues or organs, preventing the passage of an egg.

A blockage can also be the result of *endometriosis*, when fragments of mucus membrane similar to the lining of the womb find their way up the reproductive tract and settle elsewhere. These fragments behave in exactly the same way as the womb itself, swelling before a period, bleeding and causing an obstruction.

One of the most important causes of infertility – and one where treatment has recently made enormous strides – is an imbalance in the body's hormone system. All the various branches of the system are closely inter-related – so problems with one can have repercussions in the other. (See the question on hormone treatment).

What will your doctor do?

To begin with, your doctor will find out as much about your medical background as possible – including details about your husband and your respective families – so that he can see whether there are any illnesses or disorders (possibly inherited) which could be preventing you from having a baby. He may well ask about your jobs – particularly your husband's since some types of work may affect male fertility.

He will certainly enquire in detail about your periods – when they first started, how long each period lasts, how regular they are and whether you experience any pain, so that he can tell if there is anything obviously wrong with ovulation. He will also want to know whether anything in your everyday life could be affecting you – stress can affect your hormone balance and if you are

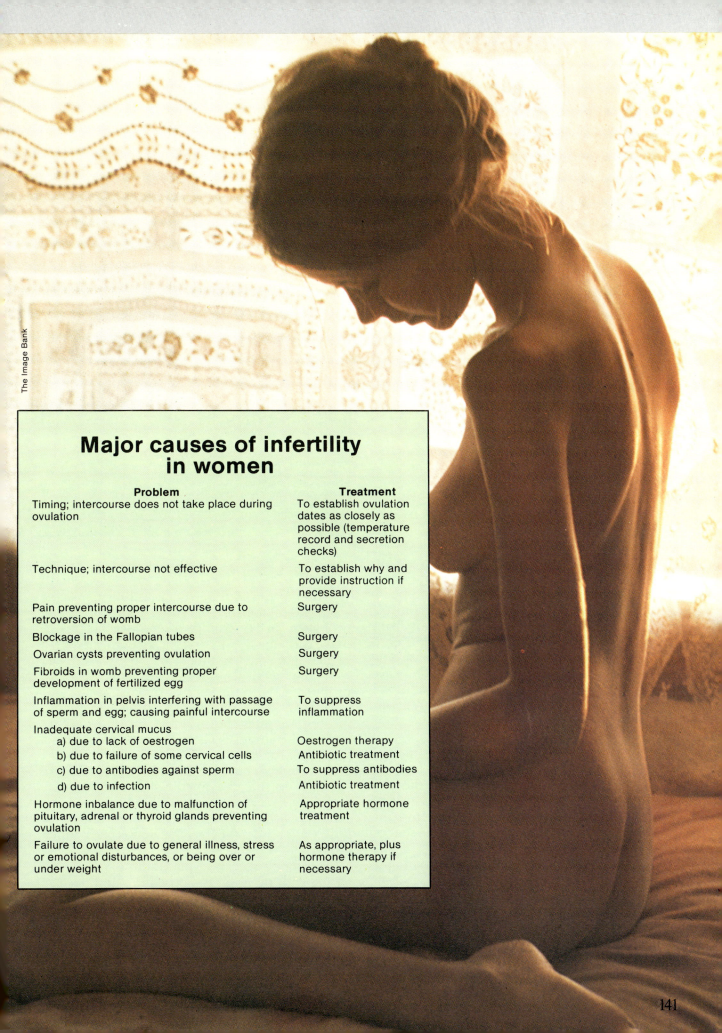

Major causes of infertility in women

Problem	Treatment
Timing; intercourse does not take place during ovulation	To establish ovulation dates as closely as possible (temperature record and secretion checks)
Technique; intercourse not effective	To establish why and provide instruction if necessary
Pain preventing proper intercourse due to retroversion of womb	Surgery
Blockage in the Fallopian tubes	Surgery
Ovarian cysts preventing ovulation	Surgery
Fibroids in womb preventing proper development of fertilized egg	Surgery
Inflammation in pelvis interfering with passage of sperm and egg; causing painful intercourse	To suppress inflammation

Inadequate cervical mucus
   a) due to lack of oestrogen
   b) due to failure of some cervical cells
   c) due to antibodies against sperm
   d) due to infection
	
	Oestrogen therapy
	Antibiotic treatment
	To suppress antibodies
	Antibiotic treatment

Hormone inbalance due to malfunction of pituitary, adrenal or thyroid glands preventing ovulation	Appropriate hormone treatment
Failure to ovulate due to general illness, stress or emotional disturbances, or being over or under weight	As appropriate, plus hormone therapy if necessary

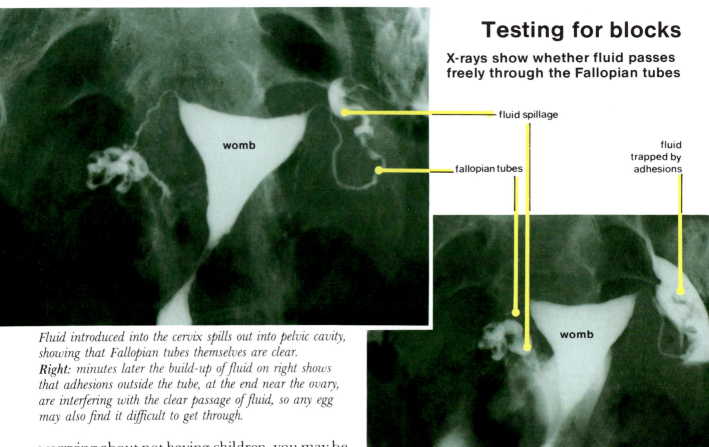

fluid spillage

fallopian tubes

fluid trapped by adhesions

womb

womb

Fluid introduced into the cervix spills out into pelvic cavity, showing that Fallopian tubes themselves are clear.
Right: *minutes later the build-up of fluid on right shows that adhesions outside the tube, at the end near the ovary, are interfering with the clear passage of fluid, so any egg may also find it difficult to get through.*

worrying about not having children, you may be making things worse. Smoking and drinking can also be contributing factors.

Of course, you will be asked about your sex life too; whether there are any problems and how often you make love. And he will want to know about your previous methods of birth control.

The next thing he will do is examine you from top to bottom. This general examination is to make sure you are not suffering from any obvious illness or disorder and to see if there are any signs of a hormonal imbalance. He will probably look at your general appearance, your skin, your reflexes and pulse and examine your breasts and abdomen.

Finally, your doctor will give you a 'pelvic' examination. This won't hurt you and is nothing to worry about. Firstly, he will examine the area around the vagina, before looking and feeling inside to check the cervix, the womb and the Fallopian tubes. He may take swabs if he sees or feels anything indicating an infection.

Before taking matters any further, your doctor may suggest that your partner's sperm be tested, so that he can check whether this could be the source of the problem. In 50 per cent of cases of infertility, there are problems with both partners, not just one, and the doctor will want to eliminate any obvious possibilities before suggesting you have any further tests.

What sort of tests are involved?

Whether or not your partner is willing to provide a sample of sperm for testing, your doctor will probably want to arrange for a post-coital test to make sure that the sperm is being deposited high in the vagina during intercourse in direct contact with the cervical mucus, and that you are producing the right kind of mucus.

You will be asked to make love the night before the test, or first thing in the morning before visiting the surgery. The doctor can then take a sample of the mucus from the canal of the neck of the womb for examination under a microscope.

If all is normal, the mucus will be rather watery and clear, like white of egg, and will contain large numbers of highly active sperm, even up to 18 hours after intercourse (and sometimes much longer).

The doctor may find that there is something wrong with the mucus. Sometimes an infection has made it too thick and sticky for the sperm to swim through, and you will need antibiotic treatment, sometimes not enough of it is being produced, and this could mean that you need extra oestrogen. Very occasionally, the mucus and the sperm won't 'mix' or the cervical cells

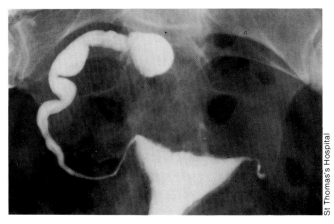

Below: both tubes are blocked. On the left at the ovary end (so tube is fluid-filled) on the right near the womb.

St Thomas's Hospital

producing the mucus are inadequate. Treatment for this is more difficult; if it doesn't work, artificial insemination (covered in a separate feature) may be the answer.

The post-coital test also gives the doctor an opportunity to test the sperm itself, should there have been any difficulty in obtaining a sample from your partner.

How can a doctor tell if there's anything blocking the reproductive tract?

There are three methods available: by a process known as insufflation, with the aid of X-rays or by laparoscopy. All require a visit to a hospital or special clinic as a rule.

Insufflation consists of passing carbon dioxide through the reproductive tract to see if the gas flows freely through or fails to do so because of blockage. Depending on the results, the doctor may want to conduct a further test to find out exactly where any blockage is occuring. He may suggest you have a *hysterosalpingogram* (or 'salp' for short). This is nothing to worry about. A narrow tube will be inserted into the cervix and a liquid which is opaque to X-rays will be syringed into the reproductive tract, filling the womb and passing along the tubes. The X-ray picks up the fluid as a solid image, so any blocks in the tubes or abnormalities inside the womb will show up.

What is a laparoscopy?

This involves a slightly more complicated procedure, since you may need a general anaesthetic, and for this reason, many doctors usually wait until after a 'salp' has been done and either failed to find any blockage, or produced an unclear result.

A special telescope known as a laparoscope is inserted into the abdominal cavity through a small cut just below the navel. Through it, the doctor can see the various pelvic organs and if a special dye is injected into the uterus (via the cervix) he will be able to check whether it passes along the tubes and emerges at the other end of them – showing that the passageway is clear. But in order to see properly, your abdomen has to be slightly 'inflated' with carbon dioxide, so you may feel a little discomfort for a day or two after this procedure.

Why do doctors run ovulation tests even if you have periods?

Even though you have periods, you may not, in fact, be producing an egg, and your doctor will first check to see whether this is your problem. One of the most straightforward ways to do this is to see whether progesterone has been released to prepare the womb, which should happen automatically once the egg has left the ovary. Since your temperature rises once progesterone has been released, a daily record of your temperature will help your doctor immensely. But the simplest way to tell is by taking a blood sample about six days before your period is due to start.

In some cases, this test will also be used to check the other hormones – from the thyroid, adrenal and pituitary glands – when no other obvious cause of infertility can be found.

Occasionally, your doctor may take a sample of the lining of your womb (an endometrial biopsy) shortly before your period is due, for examination under a microscope.

How does hormone treatment help infertile women?

First of all, hormone treatment will only be used if there is some disorder of the endocrine glands causing infertility, particularly if it's affecting ovulation. Of course, this can only work if the reproductive organs themselves (including the ovaries) are normal. Treating infertility isn't just a matter of prescribing 'fertility drugs' as if they were a magic potion.

Successful ovulation depends on all the various hormones working properly in relation to each other. That means that the hypothalamus has to give the correct signals to the pituitary gland and the pituitary gland to the ovaries.

If the body is producing too much *prolactin* (a hormone from the pituitary gland which stimulates milk production), the necessary signals will not be given. Treatment with *bromocriptine* will nearly always bring ovulation back to normal by suppressing the production of prolactin.

If the hypothalamus is failing to regulate ovulation properly and it is not sending out the right signals to the ovary, a hormone-like drug called clomiphene may be prescribed. This stimulates the pituitary gland and makes it secrete more FSH (follicle-stimulating hormone) so that the egg can ripen.

Sometimes, the problem is more complicated, and although the pituitary is responding to the clomiphene and the egg is being ripened, the hypothalamus doesn't release the hormone which will stimulate the egg's release. It may be necessary to give an injection of another hormone – chorionic gonadotrophin (HCG) to send the egg on its way – and the timing of this will, of course, be very important.

Sometimes the pituitary gland itself cannot secrete the hormones (gonadotrophins) which stimulate the ovaries, so no amount of clomiphene will be of any help. The ovaries have to be stimulated directly with gonadotrophins, initially to ripen the egg and then to release it.

The first stage is to give a series of injections of FSH in the form of HMG (human menopausal gonadotrophin) – either daily with tests to see how the ovaries are responding or three times on alternate days, again checking on results each time. Once tests show that there is a ripe follicle, an injection of HCG is given to release the egg; more than one injection may be necessary.

Why do fertility drugs sometimes cause multiple births?

Normally, once the ovaries have been stimulated and an egg begins to ripen, a complex 'feedback' system stops any further eggs from being ripened; occasionally, of course, two or even more eggs may be released, and lead to twins or triplets. But when ovulation is defective and treatment has to be given, this self-regulating mechanism may not be working, and so the ovaries may be 'over-stimulated' which means that a larger number of eggs are ripened.

When treatment involves clomiphene this is less likely to happen, but with HMG injections, the chances are much higher because this drug acts directly on the ovaries. Some women are more sensitive to these drugs than others, their ovaries responding more readily, so special precautions have to be taken to try and avoid this happening. Often the difference between an effective dose and one that will over-stimulate the ovaries is so small that it's almost impossible to make the ovaries release just one egg at a time and so a multiple pregnancy may well result.

When can surgery help?

Where surgery can be very helpful is in removing obstructions in the reproductive tract caused by adhesions or endometriosis, although there is a danger that adhesions will return. If the tubes are blocked in this way, results are often quite disappointing because even though surgery here is done with great care it can result in the formation of scar tissue, which may well block the tubes again. Modern micro-surgery has helped to improve the success rate for some (but not all) tubal operations, and future developments may give better results.

Benign growths in the womb (fibroids) or cysts of the ovaries can also be treated surgically, and certain other malformations in the womb may be tackled too. If the womb is displaced and this also pulls the ovaries down, a doctor may well suggest that surgery be used to correct this. Although the displacement doesn't in itself affect fertility, it does tend to make love-making very painful, and this of course will cause problems.

Only under one set of circumstances can surgery do anything to correct problems with ovulation itself, and that's when the ovaries are 'polycystic' (full of cysts). If they fail to respond to hormone treatment, an operation known as 'wedge resection' may help to restore egg production and release.

Can test tube babies be the answer to infertility problems?

The day when any woman can have a test tube baby is still long distant.

For the moment, the only time that test-tube babies may even be a possibility (and then only as a last resort) is if there has been a blockage in the tubes which surgery has not overcome. At the moment, doctors won't even consider it as a way of overcoming other causes of infertility – a low sperm count for instance – and the whole process is still experimental and not yet available as a practical alternative to other options, such as artificial insemination.

First a ripe egg has to be removed from the ovary (by means of a laparoscope) – a delicate operation itself – then it must be fertilized with the man's sperm in a sterile glass dish before it can be incubated in a special 'tissue culture' for some three days. If this is successful, the egg must then be replaced in the mother's womb so that the foetus can develop normally – and this is the most difficult part of the whole operation. Even if the egg is implanted successfully in the lining of the womb, success isn't guaranteed.

144

How is artificial insemination performed?

The woman lies on an examination table and an instrument called a *speculum* is inserted into her vagina, extending it to give easier access to her *cervix* (the neck of the womb). A syringe containing a quantity of semen is inserted, and the semen is expressed into the mucus at the entrance of the cervix. Alternatively, the semen may be deposited actually inside the womb by means of a fine tube. Then the syringe and speculum are removed and the woman rests on her back, pelvis raised, for about half an hour. This allows the semen to bathe the womb completely.

The timing of the procedure is critical. Insemination has to be performed at the time of ovulation, when the ripe egg is ready to be released by the ovary. This marks the peak of a woman's fertility, and is usually determined by keeping a daily record of her body temperature first thing in the morning. When ovulation is imminent there's a slight drop in temperature, followed almost immediately by a marked upward shift. Sometimes, though, the temperature chart method doesn't provide a clear enough indication of when ovulation is about to take place. If this is the case there is a simple test which can be carried out to measure the levels in the blood or urine of *luteinizing hormone* — this is known to be present in very high quantities just prior to ovulation.

How successful is artificial insemination by a donor (AID)?

Complete success can never be guaranteed. It's estimated that between 50 and 70 per cent of couples will conceive following a six-month course of treatment with AID. Over half the conceptions occur within the first two months of treatment – if a woman hasn't conceived by the sixth month then she is unlikely to do so.

There are two main reasons why this should be so. First, the woman's Fallopian tubes may be damaged, thus preventing fertilization of the egg by the donor sperm. This can be verified by an X-ray or a simple operation. Secondly, the woman's monthly pattern of ovulation may have been disrupted. Artificial insemination is quite stressful, and this frequently upsets the normal menstrual cycle. For a start, the procedure is not a natural one – many women even find it distasteful, although they are prepared to go through with it. Added to this, a number of women are conscious of the fact that AID represents their last chance of having a child; this in itself understandably creates a great deal of stress. However, regular ovulation can usually be established once more using drugs such as *clomiphene*.

The first clue that the woman has successfully conceived comes when her period following insemination doesn't arrive. If she has been keeping a record of her basal body temperature it should show a fall, followed by a rise at the time of insemination, with the temperature remaining high after the date of the missed period. A test carried out on an early morning urine sample, four weeks after the insemination, may confirm that she is pregnant.

Once it has been established that a woman has conceived following artificial insemination, then her pregnancy will progress normally, just like any conception by natural means. In other words, she runs the same risks of complications in her pregnancy as any other mother.

Is there a danger the child will be rejected by the woman's husband?

Obviously there is a theoretical risk that the child born as a result of AID may subsequently be rejected by the husband. The present legal position of AID does little to decrease this risk, because legally such a child should be registered as 'father unknown', which in effect makes him illegitimate. But because insemination is usually performed privately, with the mother's subsequent pregnancy being monitored completely separately by an antenatal clinic in the normal way, only the child's 'parents' and the AID clinic need know of the manner of his conception. Many parents, therefore, decide to keep their child's illegitimacy secret, and, as a child born within a marriage is presumed to be legitimate, no one would think of questioning this. However, to be on the safe side, many couples overcome the problem by having the child adopted by his mother's husband who then legally becomes his father.

To minimize the chances of rejection, doctors recommend that a couple continue to make love regularly throughout the treatment period, as there is just a chance that the egg will be fertilized by the husband. Alternatively, some doctors often prefer to mix donor sperm with the husband's sperm for the same reason.

However, perhaps the most important factor in reducing the risk of rejection is to give the couple thorough counselling before they embark on the treatment. It's vital that the husband and wife attend the first consultation together, so that they can discuss with the specialist just what is involved, and also voice any reservations or fears they may have. Both have to give their written consent to the insemination.

Not surprisingly, some couples decide at this

stage not to proceed with the treatment, and others will drop out once the insemination programme has started. However thoroughly a couple are counselled prior to AID, there is always the risk that, faced with what is to all intents and purposes another man's child, the father may be unable to come to terms with this fact. This may take the form of being unable to show the child affection which would cause enormous problems to all three of them. However, the couples who actually go ahead with AID form a highly motivated group.

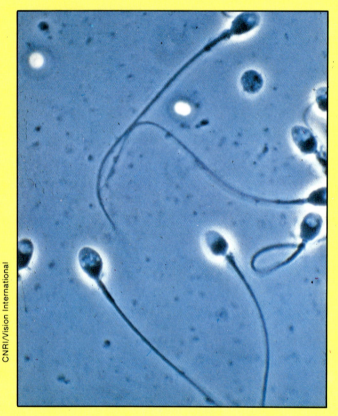

These are healthy, mobile sperm.

CNRI/Vision International

How is the donor chosen?

A donor is very carefully selected. For a start he has to be of good general health with no family history of hereditary disease. He is then screened to make sure that he is free of syphilis and hepatitis, both of which could be passed on through artificial insemination. The donor must also be highly fertile – that is, his semen must contain a large number of good quality, mobile sperm. The race of the donor and the husband must, of course, be the same, and where possible the physical characteristics of the donor – height, hair and eye colour – are carefully matched with those of the husband. The donor must also be reasonably intelligent.

Anyone can be a donor, as long as he satisfies the basic requirements, but most doctors prefer to limit the number of pregnancies fertilized by each individual donor. A large proportion of donors are medical students, since they provide a readily available supply of semen for many university-based AID centres. Probably the attraction of being a donor is the additional source of income. Men who are about to be sterilized often decide to donate their sperm.

Occasionally, relatives of a couple who have decided to have AID offer to donate their sperm, so that the resulting baby has mostly family genes, instead of 50 per cent of those of a total stranger. But most doctors would advise against this as it could cause considerable complications within the family later on.

Complete confidentiality is always maintained. Neither the donor nor the woman receiving his sperm is even aware of each other's identity. However, the doctor who arranged the artificial insemination keeps records of them both.

When can the husband's sperm be used?

Insemination using the husband's sperm, known as AIH, is used only rarely. Compared with AID, the success rate of AIH is disappointingly low – only about 10 to 15 per cent of couples conceive after six months of treatment. This is due to the considerable variation in the quality of the sperm that is available for use.

However, there is a number of situations in which AIH has proved useful. For example, a man may be producing normal, healthy sperm but is unable to fertilize his wife because her cervical mucus is too acidic and destroys the sperm before they reach the egg. Another, less common, cause of infertility – but with a similar effect – has been found to be the presence of anti-sperm antibodies in either the husband's semen or his wife's cervical mucus. In the latter case AIH has been performed by injecting the husband's sperm directly inside the womb, thus by-passing the local action of the antibodies in the mucus. When it's the husband who is affected, it's sometimes possible to 'wash' the antibodies out of the semen prior to insemination.

AIH has proved successful in bringing about conception in cases where normal intercourse is not possible – when, for instance, a husband is impotent. And a few artificial insemination centres use the technique in cases where the husband's sperm count is low, where sperm mobility is reduced, or where the volume of sperm produced is low. But the chances of conceiving are no greater than by normal intercourse, so the value of the treatment in this instance is doubtful.

Infertility in men

Are infertility and sterility the same thing?

There are, in fact, varying degrees of infertility, ranging from a slightly lower than normal number of viable sperms to a total absence – a condition known as *azoospermia* – which results in sterility. A sterile man cannot father children. An infertile man *can* father children, but his chances of doing so depend upon how far short of the ideal the quality of his sperm falls, and also how fertile his wife is. If, for instance, she has very regular periods (so that the time of ovulation can be predicted pretty accurately) and produces highly receptive mucus through which the sperms can swim easily into the womb, she may conceive with no difficulty at all. It might never even be realized that her husband is infertile. On the other hand, a less fertile woman may have just one child, or maybe none at all with such a man – although she might conceive comparatively easily with a fully fertile man.

What are the causes of infertility in men?

Infertility in some men is caused by the failure of their testes to descend from near the kidneys –

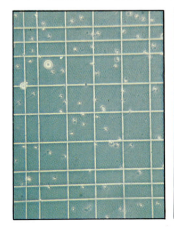 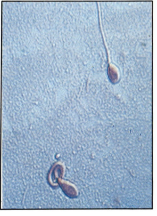

Sperms are counted by examining a sample of semen under the microscope on a specially ruled slide. Above right: contrast between a normal and deformed sperm.

Undescended testes

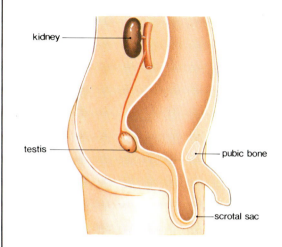

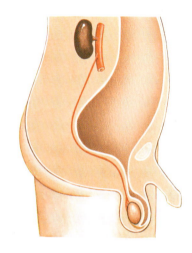

By birth, testes usually descend into the scrotal sac. In some boys, they remain in their before-birth position. If untreated, this can cause infertility because the higher temperatures inside the body damage the sperm-making capacity.

where they first develop in the embryo – to the scrotum outside the body cavity. This means that the sperms are being continually exposed to body temperature which damages them. Unless the testicles can be brought into the scrotum, by surgery if necessary, by not later than two to three years of age the patient will probably be infertile. And if the testicles remain undescended *after* puberty he will most certainly be sterile.

A common cause of infertility is a varicocele. This is an enlargement of the veins draining the testicles, quite often the left testicle. The varicocele is caused by a defect of the valves in the veins which leads to a pooling of blood. This affects the temperature regulation in the testicles, which interferes with the production of sperms.

Infections can also impair fertility. Venereal disease and tuberculosis are two extreme examples, but even a relatively common disease like mumps can present a problem, especially if contracted after puberty. The mumps virus can attack the testes, causing an acute infection known as orchitis. Large areas of the affected testicle, including the delicate seminiferous tubules where sperms are manufactured, may be destroyed by the inflammation and replaced by scar tissue, leading to permanent damage.

Sometimes infertility can be caused by a congenital or genetic defect. This can result in a severe reduction in the number of sperms developing in the testicles, or can affect the ability of the testicles to make any sperms at all. This is a permanent condition, for which there is no cure at present.

Total infertility – that is to say sterility – can result from either a failure to produce any sperms, or from a blockage of the ducts through which sperms pass to be ejaculated. In a very few cases, sterility can be caused by both these factors. This particular blockage can be caused either by defective development or infection. Where tuberculosis or venereal disease is the cause, sometimes the infection results in inflammation of one of the ducts; in the process of repairing the damage, the body forms scar tissue that can block or destroy the affected duct.

Heavy smoking, excessive drinking and obesity may be causes of low sperm count in some men, as may addictive drugs, and a number of drugs used to treat diseases such as ulcerative colitis, inflammation of the small intestine and high blood pressure.

One of the theories attracting attention is that infertility could be the result of an auto-immune reaction. In some men their bodies are manufacturing antibodies – part of the body's defence system, the function of which is to attack and destroy invading germs – to their own sperms. Doctors don't know why this happens, but they think it could be quite a common cause of otherwise unexplained infertility.

How do hormones affect fertility?

A small percentage of infertility and sterility in men is due to a hormone deficiency. Blood tests can be carried out to determine whether or not this is a factor. The pituitary gland manufactures the hormones *FSH* (follicle-stimulating hormone) and *LH* (luteinizing hormone), collectively called the *gonadotrophins*. LH stimulates the testicles to produce the male sex hormone *testosterone*, which

is essential for the manufacture of sperms; FSH stimulates the germs cells to produce sperms. Overproduction of the gonadotrophins causes severe damage to the structure of the testicles, making them incapable of responding to stimulation. A blood test will show if the gonadotrophins are present in normal amounts or, if not, whether they are deficient or excessive.

Where infertility and sterility are the result of a hormonal defect the problem can be solved by hormone replacement therapy. For instance, a patient with a defective pituitary gland which

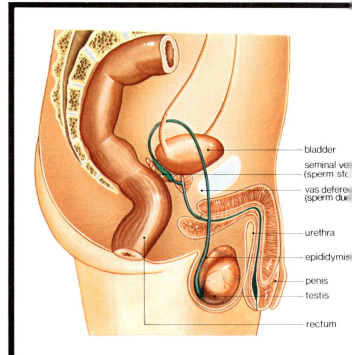

- bladder
- seminal ve (sperm sto
- vas defere (sperm du
- urethra
- epididymis
- penis
- testis
- rectum

The production line

Above and top and bottom right: details of the organs involved in producing sperm. The process can fail at several points:

☐ *if the germ cells in the seminiferous tubules which give rise to the sperms are absent or seriously reduced*
☐ *if the sperms are too few or too sluggish*
☐ *if any of the tubules or ducts through which sperms must pass are blocked*

Far right: A block in the epididymus preventing the passage of sperms can be by-passed with skilful surgery. A small incision is made in a section of the sperm duct beyond the block and this is matched to another incision made in the head of the epididymus; the two are joined together. This creates a new route for the sperm, and the blocked section becomes an abandoned loop.

isn't producing enough FSH or LH can be injected with *human menopausal gonadotrophin (HMG)* which is obtained from the urine of post-menopausal women, and *human chorionic gonadotrophin (HCG)*, obtained from the urine of pregnant women. Another hormone used to treat men with a low sperm count is *clomiphene*, which is also used to treat female infertility. This usually stimulates the pituitary gland to secrete more gonadotrophin, but in only 20 to 30 per cent of cases will it increase the sperm count. Because it takes three months to manufacture sperms, hormone therapy is a lengthy process, involving treatment over a period of many months.

Is it true that wearing very tight clothes can lower a man's fertility?

Yes it is, because infertility can be caused by keeping the testicles too warm. The ideal temperature for sperm production is 2.2 degrees lower than that of the abdominal cavity. The scrotal sac, which envelopes the testicles, acts as the thermostat. The sac is a multi-layered pouch

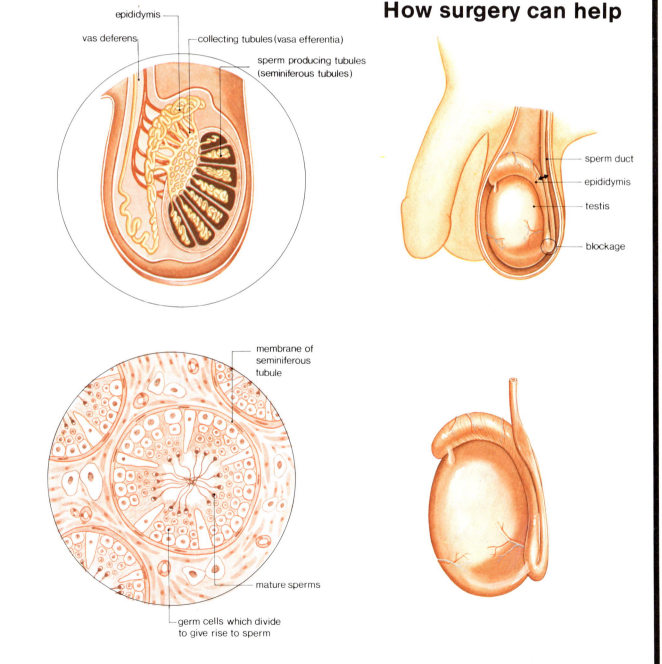

epididymis
vas deferens
collecting tubules (vasa efferentia)
sperm producing tubules (seminiferous tubules)

How surgery can help

sperm duct
epididymis
testis
blockage

membrane of seminiferous tubule

mature sperms

germ cells which divide to give rise to sperm

laced with sweat glands and muscles. When it's cold these muscles contract, pulling the testicles closer to the warmth of the body; when it's hot they relax, pushing the testicles away from the body. The sweat glands also help control the temperature. So men who habitually wear jock straps or very tight-fitting jeans, work in very high temperatures, or who sit for long periods – such as long-distance lorry drivers – can become infertile, because they are preventing these natural temperature controls from operating.

How is male infertility diagnosed?

The first stage is a fertility test. The patient has to produce a sample of semen for examination under a microscope. Because frequent ejaculation can reduce the sperm count and the volume of sperms, the patient is required to abstain from intercourse for at least three days before providing the sample. Ideally the sample should be produced by hand (masturbation). The seminal specimen has to reach the laboratory within two to three hours, otherwise it begins to deteriorate.

Its volume is measured (the average is 3.5ml – about a teaspoonful) and the number of sperms in the sample are counted on a specially ruled slide under the microscope. The shape of the sperms is also examined and the proportion of normal and abnormal sperms noted. Normal fertility probably requires not less than 20 to 30 million sperms per millilitre of fluid, but pregnancies can take place with a much lower count. However, there's little chance below one million per millilitre. Some 60 per cent of the sperms should be swimming briskly during the first two to three hours after ejaculation; if they begin to slow down rapidly this seriously reduces the chance of a pregnancy. It's possible for a man to have up to 30 per cent of abnormal sperm in his sample without his fertility being affected.

In some men the quality of their semen varies considerably from one ejaculation to another, so in some cases the fertility test has to be repeated

If the semen test shows the patient's sperms to be normal the doctor will then check the patient's state of health and his genital organs to make sure there are no problems there. He will also ask about the frequency of intercourse. If the patient and his partner are not making love during the vital couple of days of his wife's mid-cycle (when she's ovulating) then this lessens her chance of conceiving. Conversely, if the man's sperm count is already on the low side and the couple make love too often in the few days before ovulation, the frequent ejaculations will adversely affect the quantity of his sperms.

When can an operation help?

When it's suspected that an obstruction of one of the ducts may be the cause of infertility, the doctor may suggest a surgical exploration of the testicles to establish where exactly the blockage has occurred.

If there is a blockage in the vas deferens, for example, it may be possible to short circuit it through an operation called a *vaso-epididymostomy*. This involves by-passing the blockage by joining the head of the epididymus to the vas deferens at a point beyond the blockage.

Where infertility is the result of gonorrhoea there is about a 50 per cent chance that sperms may reappear in the seminal fluid after this operation. Unfortunately, in many of these so-called successful operations the patient's sperm count remains low – especially if the blockage had been present for a long time – so the chances of his partner conceiving are still not very high.

Where the blockage is due to the defective development of one of the ducts there's very little chance of curing it through surgery, and blockage due to tuberculosis can't be cured at all.

A varicocele can be treated through an operation called *high ligation*, but opinion is divided as to how effective this treatment really is. Results show that the sperm counts improve in 60 to 70 per cent of men receiving this treatment – but it can't guarantee that the patient will subsequently father a child. The operation requires considerable skill, and is carried out under general anaesthetic. The patient is in hospital for about four or five days.

Does infertility affect a man's sex drive?

In most cases, no. The majority of infertile and sterile men have a completely normal and unimpaired desire for sexual relations. They only become aware of their infertility after their semen has been examined. Unfortunately this knowledge sometimes has the psychological effect of making them feel inadequate. This in turn affects their sex drive, and in some cases even makes them impotent, so that they are unable to have an erection or an ejaculation.

But most impotent men can produce semen by masturbation, even if they can't have full intercourse, and very often their semen is found to be fully fertile. In this instance, the wife could become pregnant through artificial insemination, using the man's semen. Most men with a deficiency in their male hormone secretion do lack sex drive. In many cases their interest in sex can be fully restored through hormone therapy.

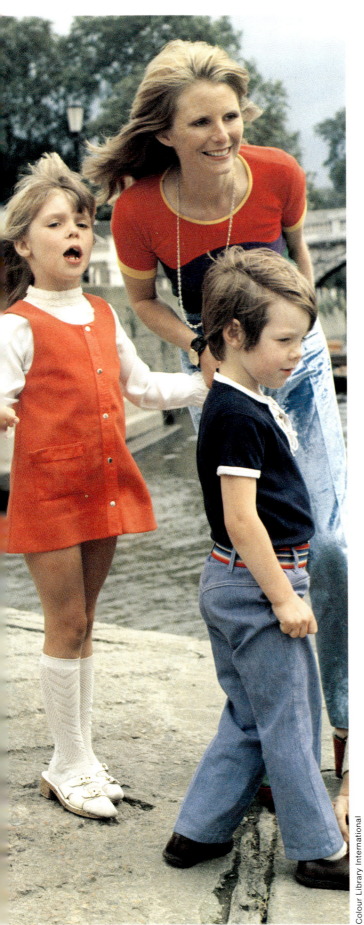

Sterilization

Why is counselling necessary before sterilization is agreed to?

The decision to be sterilized can be the most important one in a woman's life and should never be taken without very careful thought about all the possible implications. Counselling is designed to ensure that she and her partner have considered the full significance of the operation and realized the effect it will have on the rest of their lives.

Most couples are counselled first of all by their own family doctor although some family planning clinics and hospitals also offer a counselling service. He will stress the fact that sterilization is permanent and may try to make the woman aware of how she might feel once she is no longer able to become pregnant. The couple are usually asked what types of contraception they have already used to make sure that there is not an alternative method they might use for a time before making a final decision.

The surgeon who is to perform the sterilization usually expects to talk the matter over with the couple beforehand. Typically, he will describe how the operation is carried out, explain its physical and possible emotional effects, dispel the myths surrounding sterilization and answer any additional questions which the couple may have about it.

Because of the irreversible nature of the operation, no one should opt for sterilization unless they are absolutely convinced they will never want to have more children. For instance, the couple should ask themselves if they might want another child if one of their existing children dies. Or the wife could change her mind if her husband dies or they get divorced and she remarries. Unfortunately, looking into the future is extremely hard to do but the couple have to think how they would feel if circumstances should change, and weigh this against the advantages of sterilization in their present situation. Generally speaking, though, it makes sense to wait until the youngest child is over a year old before going ahead with sterilization because, even nowadays, the first 12 months is the period when a child is most at risk from serious illness.

Can you be sterilized only if you have had children?

Whether or not you have children is only one of a number of important factors a doctor will take into account before agreeing to a sterilization. There are no strict rules about what makes a woman a suitable candidate but doctors tend to keep to a set of guidelines which they apply to each couple's individual circumstances. The doctor will weigh up a combination of factors before coming to a decision.

A couple who already have a family of two or more children are probably less likely to want to add to that number at a later date, but this does not mean that couples with one or even no children – or single people – are regarded as unsuitable for sterilization.

Other considerations such as age and the stability of the marriage or partnership are just as important. A young girl in a shaky marriage is most likely to regret being sterilized as she has many years ahead of her in which to change her mind and the greatest chance of getting divorced and wanting children by a second partner. In fact it is more likely that sterilization will hasten the end of an unhappy marriage than solve any problems and it should never be carried out in these circumstances. For instance, a wife may blame an unsatisfactory sex life on her fear of becoming pregnant. When she becomes sterilized and things don't improve she loses her 'excuse' and finally has to face up to the fact that the problem is much more fundamental.

Sometimes sterilization is advisable because the mother's or any future baby's health would be in jeopardy, or because the woman is too mentally handicapped to be able to take contraceptive precautions and wouldn't be able to look after the child. Other women are offered sterilization because they or their partners have a hereditary disease which they fear to pass on.

A woman's personality and feelings about sex and her own fertility also have to be considered as part of the overall picture. Although the vast majority of women who have been sterilized say

their sex lives have improved or not changed since the risk of pregnancy has been totally removed, some are emotionally affected by the final loss of their ability to have children.

Is sterilization one hundred per cent effective?

The failure rate for sterilization is about the same as for the Pill – less than one per cent. For the very few women who do become pregnant after being sterilized the problem is usually that the clip or ring hasn't blocked off the tube completely or that the surgeon did not identify the Fallopian tubes correctly and operated on a nearby fold of tissue. It is even possible for the tubes to heal together again naturally or to develop a small opening through which the egg can pass down in

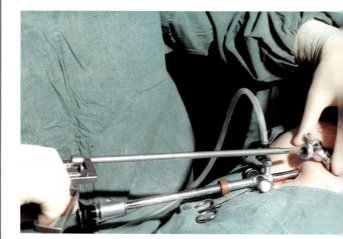
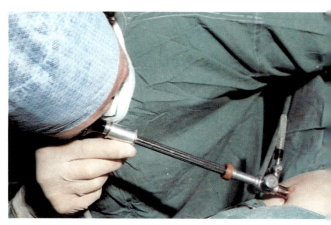

Doctors make their first incision near the navel, and then pass the laparoscope through into the pelvic cavity in order to inspect the organs. Then a second incision is made through which the special clip gun is passed. Once in the cavity, doctors can look through the laparoscope and direct the gun accordingly.

to the womb. To prevent this from happening, the surgeon often removes a small length of each Fallopian tube or buries the ends of the tubes in different layers of surrounding tissue.

Women waiting to be sterilized can be so relieved that they are finally going to have the operation that they become rather lax in using contraception. However, since they have made the decision that they definitely *don't* want any more children it is particularly important to ensure that they (or their partners) take proper precautions during this time.

Unlike male sterilization, a woman is 'safe' immediately she has had the operation. The only exception to this is if she ovulates just before the operation and the egg has travelled down the tube before it is blocked. If the operation has been carried out mid cycle then it is advisable for her to use contraception until her next period.

In the first few months following sterilization women are recommended still to look out for signs of pregnancy. This is because some women are actually pregnant when the operation is done. Pregnancy is usually detectable during a laparotomy as a pregnant uterus looks different from a non-pregnant one. When a laparoscope is used, however, the gynaecologist doesn't have a chance to see the uterus.

Either way, signs of pregnancy must not be ignored and the sooner the pregnancy is terminated the better, especially as there is a slightly increased chance that the pregnancy would be ectopic (contained within the Fallopian tubes).

All about the operation

A general anaesthetic is used in most female sterilizations. But in fact it's a relatively minor operation, and almost all can be done under a local anaesthetic (where the woman remains conscious) if the doctor and patient are happy with this.

The operation itself entails cutting or blocking the Fallopian tubes – the two tubes through which the woman's eggs pass from the ovaries to the womb. The conventional method is called 'laparotomy' or 'tubal ligation'. The gynaecologist makes an incision a couple of inches long just above the pubic hair line and then cuts each Fallopian tube and ties it with special thread. The woman can usually return

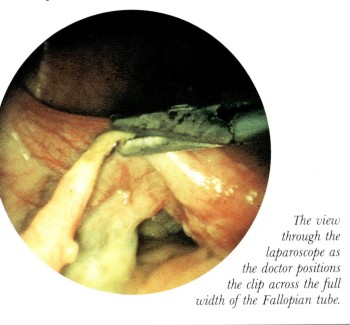

The view through the laparoscope as the doctor positions the clip across the full width of the Fallopian tube.

home after a three-to-five day stay in hospital.

A 'mini-laparotomy' can be carried out on certain (usually slim) women which allows them to leave hospital sooner – often an overnight stay is all that is necessary. A smaller cut is made below the pubic hair line and an instrument inserted through the vagina to push the Fallopian tubes into a visible position so that they can be operated on.

A newer but already widely used technique is the 'laparoscopic' method. The gynaecologist inserts a tube through a very small incision near the navel and gently pumps a harmless gas (nitrous dioxide or carbon dioxide) into the patient's abdomen. This pushes away the intestines and gives better access to the tubes. He then replaces the tube with a long narrow optical instrument called a laparoscope. Through this he can see the womb, Fallopian tubes and ovaries and can also manipulate surgical instruments. A second 'sterilizing' instrument is then inserted through another small cut near the pubic hair line. Each tube is usually blocked either by using one or two special clips or by passing a small strong rubber band (a Falope ring) round a loop or 'kink' in the tube, as shown overleaf.

The Fallopian tubes can also be cauterized (sealed off) by using a high frequency electric current but this method is less common these days because, very occasionally, it has led to other organs becoming accidentally damaged.

Whichever method is used to block the tubes, the woman usually feels well as soon as she has recovered from the anaesthetic but she should be prepared to stay one or two nights in hospital to be on the safe side.

The different forms of sterilization

Laparotomy

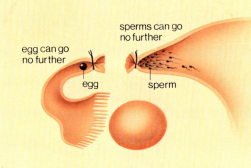

egg can go no further

sperms can go no further

egg

sperm

This is the more common method of sterilization. The Fallopian tubes are cut and tied, so that the sperm can no longer reach the egg. Once the surgeon has cut and removed a small portion of the tube, he ties each cut end and buries them in the surrounding tissue.

Laparoscopy

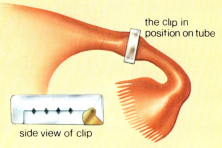

the clip in position on tube

side view of clip

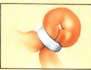

For a laparoscopy, the Fallopian tubes are not cut.
Instead they are blocked by special clips (as shown on the previous page) or by rubber bands (inset) when the tube is 'looped'.

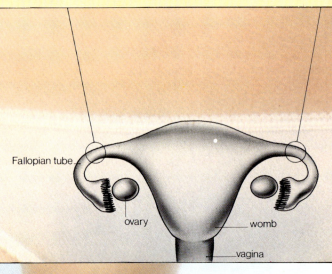

Fallopian tube

ovary

womb

vagina

Where the doctor makes his incision

incision for laparoscope

secondary incision for laparoscopy

standard laparotomy incision

mini laparotomy

Nowadays, doctors will usually try to make any scars show as little as possible. The largest incision (for the standard laparotomy) is usually about 2 in long, but is made as close as possible to the pubic hair line. For a mini-laparotomy, the incision can be smaller and lower.

A laparoscopy involves two incisions – one for the laparoscope near the navel, and the other, again at the pubic hair line, to give access to the instruments used for blocking the tubes. Both are so small, that there's barely anything visible afterwards. The second incision can be made to left or right – it's up to the doctor.

Is it true that the operation can sometimes be reversed?

Once a woman has been sterilized she continues to produce an egg every month but because it never reaches the part of the womb where it might meet and be fertilized by a male sperm, it doesn't develop and dies. Attempts can be made to unblock or rejoin the Fallopian tubes so that the eggs can once again reach the womb but the operation requires several hours of delicate, highly skilled surgery and even then success cannot be guaranteed.

A few doctors with a great deal of experience, and using a special operating microscope, have claimed that up to 70 per cent of the sterilized women they 'reverse' have become pregnant. But nobody should consider sterilization as a reversible procedure or expect even a 50/50 chance of success.

Doctors are reluctant to agree to reversal operations unless there are exceptional circumstances and the woman is desperate to have another child. The sort of things they will take into account are the woman's age, how long ago she was sterilized, the method used and how much of the Fallopian tubes were destroyed.

There are no precise figures on the number of sterilized women who request reversal but it is estimated that it runs at about one per cent. Some unforseen change in circumstances – such as divorce and remarriage or the death of a child – is usually the reason for the request. Unfortunately a large proportion of the women asking for a reversal did not fully understand what sterilization meant when they had it. They continued to believe, despite counselling, that the operation could easily be reversed.

Women who have been sterilized at the same time as having an abortion or after childbirth may regret the sterilization once they are no longer pregnant. A difficult or unwanted pregnancy is quite clearly not the ideal time to make this kind of decision. Although a woman may genuinely believe she knows her own mind at the time, it is easy to understand how she might come to regret her decision once the pregnancy is over.

How does a husband usually react to his wife's sterilization?

Since sterilization is usually a joint decision between a husband and wife it is fairly understandable that once the operation is over the overwhelming reaction of most husbands is one of relief. And because they feel grateful to their wives for solving their birth control problems the relationships are often strengthened as a result.

If, on the other hand, despite counselling, a couple are not entirely honest with themselves or with each other about their reasons for wanting the sterilization the husband may come to resent the operation, which can lead to friction within the marriage. For instance where a husband is unnaturally jealous or has reason to doubt his wife's fidelity, the apparent sexual freedom sterilization gives her can increase his suspicions and, even if they are totally unfounded, this can increase the rift between the couple. Such problems are, however, unlikely to result from sterilization if the marriage is basically sound in the first place.

What side effects does sterilization have?

Contraceptive sterilization doesn't affect the production of female hormones so there is no physical reason why a woman's normal feminine feelings or appearance should change in any way. She can resume her sex life as soon as she feels well enough and there is no pain or discomfort. This usually means in a matter of days if the laparoscopic method was used, or a week or two after the conventional operations.

Although sterilization will not physically affect a woman's sex drive or femininity, emotionally it might do. If she sees the continuing ability to have a baby as an essential part of being a woman, and vital to her own view of herself, then sterilization may not be for her and she should be quite open about her feelings during counselling. Equally, if a woman has the operation without giving it sufficient forethought she may become depressed which can lead to loss of sex drive. But for the woman who is sure she wants to be sterilized, the operation can increase sexual pleasure because the fear of pregnancy has gone.

Sterilization rarely causes any physical complications or after effects. Some women who have had the operation complain of long, heavy or irregular periods but there is no conclusive evidence that these problems are more common in sterilized women.

If a woman was on the Pill prior to the operation this would probably have made her periods lighter and more regular than they would normally be, and any increase in flow or irregularity after sterilization may simply be the effects of stopping the Pill; her menstrual cycle merely reverts back to its original pattern. Also women with severe menstrual problems sometimes find that the Pill is therefore unsuitable and are accordingly more likely to need sterilization than women with a more normal menstrual pattern.

What is a vasectomy?

A vasectomy is simply a minor operation which makes a man sterile. It works by preventing his sperm from entering the fluid he normally ejaculates during intercourse and ensuring, instead, that they are reabsorbed into the body. It's important to emphasize that a vasectomy doesn't alter a man's sexual performance in any way nor does it appreciably alter the quantity or appearance of the seminal fluid.

Male sterilization through vasectomy is achieved by cutting or blocking the two *vasa,* the thick-walled tubes about 4 mm in diameter that take the sperm from the testicles to the urethra, the tube running through the penis. You can see from the diagram that these tubes run close to the surface skin on each side of the scrotum, so they can be easily reached through one or two small incisions made in the scrotum just below the base of the penis. Either a single incision is made in the middle of the scrotal sac, or one is made on each side. The tubes are cut, a short section is removed, and the ends are usually tied with absorbable thread.

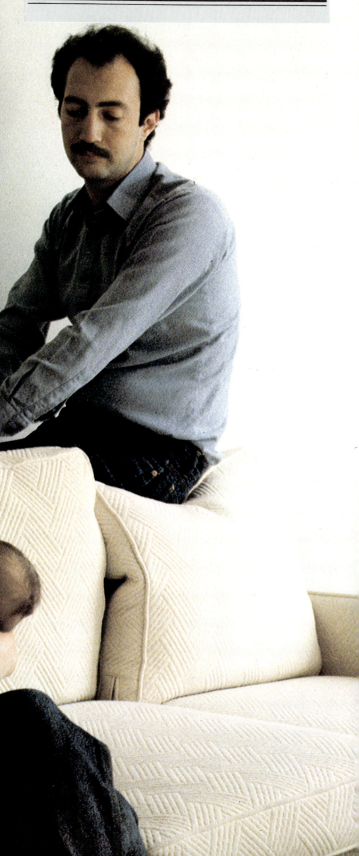

Vasectomy

A variety of techniques may be used to try to prevent the cut ends of the *vas* from rejoining: sometimes one end is doubled over and tied. Alternatively, the ends may be cauterized, or else sealed electrically or chemically. Metal clips, also, are occasionally used. The skin is then sewn up with material that can be absorbed by the body and does not need to be removed.

The whole operation takes about 10 minutes and a man can usually go home after a short rest. Healthy men rarely need to stay in hospital overnight, either before or after the operation.

Two small incisions (or alternatively a single one in the middle behind the base of the penis) are made at these sites. The vasa are cut and firmly tied, so sperm can no longer get from the testes to the urethra.

vas deferens

A man is not sterile immediately because of the sperm stored here in the seminal vesicles.

urethra

testis

Bernard Fallon

Two small incisions are made here. The vasa are cut and firmly tied, so that sperm cannot reach the urethra.

However, this may be necessary if a man has had a previous operation or problem in this region – a hernia, for example – since the vasectomy may be a little more difficult to perform.

Local anaesthetic is normally all that is necessary for a vasectomy although some men and doctors prefer general anaesthetic. Out-patient operations are still possible with either type of anaesthetic, but recovery from general anaesthetic obviously takes a few hours longer.

It is advisable for the patient to go straight home and rest for the remainder of the day, and to take things easy for the next day or two. Vasectomies are often arranged at or just before the weekend so that it's not usually necessary to take time off work (although only strenuous work is likely to cause problems).

Are some people more suited to a vasectomy than others?

Yes, although for social rather than medical reasons. There is no guarantee that the operation is reversible so a man must make his decision on the basis that he can never have any more children. Naturally this is a very big step to take,

and it's vital that he and his partner give the matter a great deal of serious consideration before making up their minds. Doctors have no hard and fast rules about those they recommend for vasectomy, but they are especially cautious when the couple is under 30 years old, if they have very young children, or if their relationship seems to be unstable.

Of course, a man chooses vasectomy so that he and his partner need no longer worry about contraception or the possibility of pregnancy, but before going through with it he must first of all ask himself three vital questions:
☐ If one of my existing children died, might I want to have another child?
☐ Is there any chance my marriage or partnership might break up, and might I then want to have children with another woman?
☐ Am I being pushed into vasectomy by my wife when I'm still not absolutely certain in my own mind that I want to be sterilized?

Vasectomy must be seen as a final and irreversible step, so it's certainly not one to be taken lightly. However, if the answer to these three questions is a definite *no,* and both you and your partner are quite sure you don't want to have any more children (or even that you don't want to have *any* children) sterilization has many advantages over other types of contraception.

The contraceptive Pill is now felt to pose a greater health risk at just the age when most women are likely to have completed their families, which makes this, the most effective contraceptive method, inadvisable. Many women are also reluctant to have intra-uterine devices (IUDs) inserted because of the possible problems associated with them. Furthermore, they are understandably reluctant about coping with the heavier, longer periods that IUDs often cause. The only male method of contraception, the sheath, like the cap or diaphragm, is not totally reliable, and can sometimes lessen or spoil sexual pleasure.

If a man has a vasectomy, neither he nor his partner have to bother with any type of contraception and the woman can allow her menstrual cycle to carry on naturally – possibly an advantage through the menopausal years.

Perhaps the single biggest advantage of vasectomy is that the couple can make love as often or as spontaneously as they like without the fear or possibility of pregnancy.

Are you sterile as soon as you've had the operation?

No, because it takes time for all the sperm stored in the tubes beyond the part that has been cut or blocked to pass out of the body through ejaculation. The amount of time it takes to clear these sperm depends on the frequency of intercourse or masturbation and also on your age, but it usually takes at least three or four months. So during this time it's important to continue to use some other method of contraception. About three months after the operation you will be asked to supply an initial sample of semen for a sperm test. A few weeks later you'll be asked to provide a further sample for testing. If both tests are clear you will no longer need to use any other form of contraception. However, if the semen is still not free of sperm you'll be given further tests every few weeks until it is certain that all the stored sperm have been ejaculated.

If sperm continue to be present, another operation may be carried out to make sure the original operation did, in fact, block the tubes.

Is it a fail-safe method of contraception?

Once his semen is found to be free of sperm, the chances of a man making his wife pregnant are very remote. However, if what appear to be symptoms of pregnancy occur in the partner of a man who has had a vasectomy, they certainly shouldn't be ignored. For it is a fact that vasectomy fails in about one in 300 men.

When this happens, the sperm fail to be prevented from passing through the penis during intercourse, and so may cause an unwanted pregnancy. In the majority of cases, this is because the two sealed ends of one of the tubes have rejoined. Indeed, the human body's amazing self-repair mechanism occasionally manages to overcome the drastic surgical intervention of a vasectomy to such an extent that the tubes are found to have regrown, and joined up again over a gap of several millimetres.

In a few very rare cases, failure to prevent sperm reaching the penis can also be due to the presence of an extra vas or tube, which was not spotted by the surgeon at the time when the first operation was carried out.

Lastly, if the ends of the tubes are not *completely* sealed off, it is just possible for sperm, despite all odds, to find their way into the seminal fluid. But this occurs in only a few cases.

Are there any side effects?

The amount of pain or discomfort men feel after a vasectomy varies enormously, lasting from a few hours to several days, but long-term side effects are extremely rare. Sexual intercourse can be resumed almost immediately, but a man may experience some discomfort at first due to tenderness and soreness.

It's a fact that every operation, however simple, carries with it some risk. However, serious complications following vasectomy are unusual. About one in a 100 men can expect to have some kind of minor complication, but these can usually be dealt with quite easily. The most common problem is infection, but this can be quickly cleared up with antibiotics. Internal bleeding in the scrotum because of damage to blood vessels can occasionally result in a painful swelling. The pain may be quite severe for a few days and can take weeks to subside completely. In a few cases, a further operation may be necessary.

Although there is no physical reason for a man's feeling of masculinity to change in any way, his emotional attitudes do sometimes alter after vasectomy. In most cases, if he has understood exactly what the operation entails and has discussed the matter thoroughly with his partner and his doctor beforehand, such problems don't arise. Sometimes however, it's not until after vasectomy has taken place that the man realizes that being fertile – capable of making a woman pregnant – is essential to his view of himself as a complete man. Mentally, he no longer feels truly masculine, and consequently his sexual performance and general attitude to life may suffer. This kind of problem is particularly likely if the man feels he was pushed into having a vasectomy by his wife. However, you can be reassured that such feelings are unusual, and normally become obvious long before the operation takes place.

Is the operation reversible?

A vasectomy operation can sometimes be reversed but the success rate is not high, and can never be guaranteed. No man should ever have a vasectomy thinking at the back of his mind that it can be reversed if necessary. This simply is not true, and it would be foolish to think otherwise.

Reversal operations take up to three hours of complicated surgery to perform and require much longer incisions than the original vasectomy. Several nights in hospital are necessary. The surgeon attempts to sew together the edges of the cut, tied or blocked ends of the tubes, leaving a clear passage through which the sperm may once again travel. This is an exceptionally difficult and delicate procedure, requiring considerable skill on the part of the surgeon. Indeed an operating microscope often has to be used.

Unfortunately, even though successful reconnection of the tubes may be possible in a fairly high proportion of men, this does not always guarantee renewed fertility. The longer a man has been sterilized the smaller are his chances of impregnating his partner because his body will begin to produce large amounts of sperm antibodies.

It's quite natural for all men to have insignificant amounts of sperm antibodies. No one yet knows why or how the male body produces them. Yet once a man has had a vasectomy his body then begins to produce these antibodies at

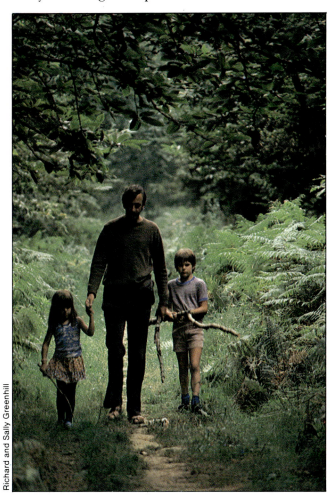

Richard and Sally Greenhill

a much faster rate than usual, and their build up, say, after five years and certainly after 10 years, will mean that the ratio of sperm antibodies to sperm is sufficiently high to make his chances of fathering a child very small. Older men, whose bodies produce low amounts of sperm, will have even smaller chances of becoming fathers since their ratio of sperm antibodies to sperm will be higher. Less than 50 per cent of reversal operations actually restore a man's fertility by ensuring a high enough number of sperm in his ejaculate.

The operating difficulties, combined with the expense of a long operation and the low chance of success, make doctors reluctant to attempt reversals except in exceptional circumstances.

Can a vasectomy affect your sex life?

There is no physical reason why vasectomy should lessen a man's sex drive and since it does not alter the production of the male sex hormone *testosterone* by the testes, it doesn't affect a man's virility either. The volume of fluid ejaculated remains unchanged – the only difference is that the fluid does not contain its normal tiny proportion of sperm.

The mechanism of orgasm is untouched by vasectomy, and some men find that not having to use sheaths or worry about contraception decidedly improves their own sexual pleasure. Vasectomy can improve a couples' sex life in several ways. For instance a couple often feel more relaxed and happy about making love when neither of them is anxious about the chance of an unwanted pregnancy. Many people also find it improves what was already a normal, satisfactory sexual relationship into something even better. It is common, too, for women to feel so relieved that they don't have to take the responsibility for contraception any longer, that they suddenly feel much more loving and affectionate towards their partners, and the marriage improves all round.

But this does not mean that vasectomy will cure sexual problems or liven up a flagging sex life. And vasectomy should certainly never be thought of as a cure for loss of *libido* or sex drive. Furthermore, sterilization can remove a woman's final excuse for not wanting to have intercourse, and reveal the truth of her feelings. Although this kind of situation can lead to the break-up of a marriage, it should be remembered that the vasectomy was not itself the cause – rather it was just the final trigger which forced the couple to face their real problems.

How do you go about getting one?

If you want to have a vasectomy it's best to go and see your doctor, and it's a good idea to take your partner along, too. (If possible, try to mention that you want to discuss vasectomy when you make the initial appointment, as the doctor may be able to arrange to give you a little more time than the patients in his general surgery.) If he is happy about recommending you for an operation, and provided that you still feel vasectomy is the best method of birth control for you after talking to him and learning the full facts, you will be referred to a local hospital consultant. If the specialist agrees, he will then make arrangements for the operation to be carried out at a local health centre, clinic or hospital.

D & C

O f all the operations performed for 'women's complaints' the D & C is both the commonest and the most simple. It can be a form of treatment in itself – often for menstrual problems – but it can also be used to diagnose some gynaecological problems by giving doctors a chance to check inside the womb and to take samples of the lining for testing.

Many 'scrapes' (as these operations are commonly called) are taken as a matter of routine for women who are experiencing annoying symptoms – very heavy periods for instance – and discomfort. Often they show no abnormality at all, or the problem can be cleared up at once as part and parcel of this minor operation.

What do the initials D & C stand for?

They stand for dilatation and curettage – which exactly describes what the operation does. It involves widening the neck of the womb slightly (dilating it) so that the doctor can scrape away the spongy surface layer of the womb lining.

The operation requires a general anaesthetic, but it leaves no scars and has no side effects. At most it means you'll have to spend a couple of days in hospital.

Removing some of the womb's lining doesn't do any harm at all. The lining is temporary anyway, building up each month under the influence of the body's natural hormones for three to four weeks before each period. When a woman has a period, she sheds this lining – and then the whole process starts again.

The opening to the womb – the cervix – is really a ring of muscle designed to stop a baby from slipping down from the womb into the vagina before its time. Until then, the opening is tiny – it looks like little more than a dimple – but it's just enought to allow fluids to pass in and out, so that sperm can reach an egg, or the womb lining can be shed each month. After you have had a baby, although the cervix contracts again, the opening is a little wider than before.

But for a doctor to be able to scrape the womb lining, the cervix has to be stretched gently with

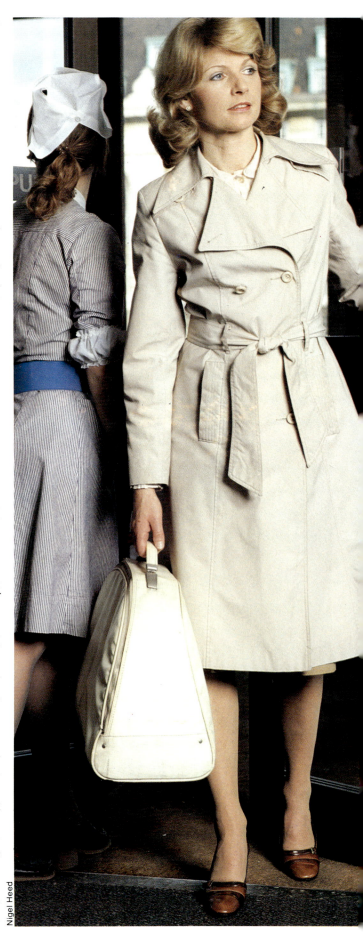

Nigel Heed

small instruments known as dilators until the muscles relax enough to admit the small scraper or *curette*. After the operation, the muscles tighten up again of their own accord.

How is a D & C carried out?

You won't feel a thing when you have a D & C because the operation is done under a general anaesthetic. Once this has taken effect, the surgeon will gently open the vagina with the aid of an instrument called a speculum, which makes it easier for him to see and reach the cervix. His next priority will be to find out the angle of the cervical canal and to establish the size of the womb itself, so that he knows how far to insert the curette. To do this, he uses a smooth metal probe called a *uterine sound* which he pushes gently along the canal into the womb until he has made contact with the far side, two or three inches from the opening.

Once he has the measure of it, the doctor can begin to dilate the cervix gently. Several dilators are used, each one fractionally larger in diameter than the one before, varying in thickness from the size of a matchstick to that of a small finger. Each has a smooth blunt head. The doctor passes the dilators, one at a time, through the cervical canal and back again, starting with the smallest and using each one in turn. Gradually, the ring of muscle begins to loosen up, just as any muscle naturally does with use, until the opening is wide enough to pass the curette through.

The doctor can now scrape the womb lining away with the curette (which looks like a long, thin spoon at the end of which is a tiny scraper that works rather like a potato peeler). He rotates the instrument so that he can reach and remove the top layer from every part.

Are there any after effects?

When the anaesthetic wears off there may be some discomfort – a little bleeding and a feeling of pain in the lower stomach similar to a period pain. Some women say this feels 'as if I had been punched'. The bleeding is only the result of the womb shedding a little extra blood in response to the scrape, and is nothing to worry about.

The pain usually lasts only a few hours and can be helped by analgesics (pain killers) and, much like an ordinary period, the bleeding only goes on for a few days. The next period should arrive within the following four or six weeks, but may be a little lighter than usual.

Since there have been no cuts made and so no stitches, there will be no scars.

Having a D&C is nothing to worry about and shouldn't cause any disruption to life at all. Only bear in mind that you shouldn't have sexual intercourse for a few days afterwards until the bleeding has stopped and, during this time, use pads rather than tampons.

When will a doctor recommend a D & C?

Whenever a woman has abnormally heavy, prolonged or irregular periods, or if she has started bleeding (even slightly) between periods, a doctor may recommend a D & C. The causes may vary, but by taking a sample from the lining of the womb, and testing it in the laboratory, doctors can find out whether there have been any changes in the cells of the womb themselves or whether the problems are likely to have a hormonal basis.

Sometimes the problem may be very obvious – it may be that a polyp or fibroid has developed. These benign (harmless) growths are very common, provoking heavy, prolonged periods or even causing bleeding midway through a cycle. If a doctor finds either of these growths during the course of a D & C he may remove them straight away.

But many women have irregular or heavy periods from time to time, and a doctor may not always recommend a D & C. Age certainly comes into it. A doctor is far less likely to recommend a 'scrape' for a 19-year-old girl, who complains of heavy, painful periods than for a 55-year-old woman who has begun bleeding slightly some years after her periods have stopped.

Can a D & C help in treating painful periods?

Yes, in certain cases, but only the dilatation part of the operation is used, and it's only effective in stopping the pains in about half the women who have the operation. Although it is not known exactly why a D & C works for painful periods it seems likely that stretching the muscles of the cervix allows the menstrual blood to flow more freely. Doctors usually prefer, though, not to stretch the neck of the womb in women under 20, rather waiting to see whether the problem clears up of its own accord. Above that age, if periods continue to be painful and don't respond to other treatments, a D & C may be an effective answer.

Periods are generally most painful for younger women but get progressively less discomforting once women begin to have regular sex. Certainly after a woman has a baby, she usually finds the problem eased.

In fact, nowadays painkillers or 'hormone' tablets like the Pill are often used in preference to a D & C to treat period pains. The results of this treatment are usually very good.

Is it true that the operation is used to detect cancer?

Unexpected or heavy bleeding from the vagina can be a sign of cancer of the womb – or any one of the other disorders already mentioned. But because older women (between 45 and 60) are more at risk, a doctor will almost invariably recommend they have a D & C in order to establish the cause. Of course, this is bound to be worrying, but the chances are that the symptoms have a much simpler explanation. After menopause, some women do have 'flooding' periods which suddenly occur out of the blue as a result of some hormonal imbalance, which can easily be treated.

Once a scrape has been taken, the tissues can quickly be analysed in a laboratory and the doctor can then start appropriate treatment. Fortunately, even if the results do indicate a cancer, this is a type which responds well to treatment, and the chances of a complete cure are high, particularly if it's caught in the early stages. For this reason, it's obviously sensible to consult your doctor, whatever your age, if you do experience any of these symptoms.

Is the operation sometimes used as a method of abortion?

Before the tenth week a D & C can be used to terminate a pregnancy. However, it is far less common than the D & E operation (dilatation and evacuation) which involves the use of suction rather than a scraping action.

The reason is that in early pregnancy the womb lining is richer and softer than normal and a surgeon has to take special care not to damage the soft and thickened muscle wall of the womb which could tear and bleed easily.

Sometimes a pregnancy fails during the early weeks but instead of miscarrying, the foetus, though no longer living, remains inside the womb. This is called a 'missed abortion' and a D & C will usually be required to clear the womb completely.

Similarly a D & C may take place just after childbirth if, as sometimes happens, part of the afterbirth (placenta) is left behind. This may cause heavy bleeding and bad pain and can lead to infection, so a D & C may be necessary to remove the fragments.

What a D & C can do

Broadly speaking, the reasons for having this operation fall into two groups:

Diagnostic
● for investigating heavy and irregular periods
● to establish why there is breakthrough bleeding mid-way between periods
● to find the cause of any bleeding after menopause
● as a routine investigation for infertile women to test for ovulation and check for any deformity

Therapeutic
● for removing any fibroids or cysts found in the womb
● as a treatment for painful periods
● to terminate an early pregnancy
● to clear the womb after a 'missed' abortion
● to remove any fragments of placenta left after childbirth

What other reasons might there be for recommending a D & C?

There are several other reasons for a D & C – all of them less common than those already mentioned.

It's often part of a routine series of tests for women suspected of being infertile. By taking a sample of the lining for testing, doctors can tell whether an egg has been released. If a woman isn't ovulating properly, the body will not have released the oestrogen and progesterone which normally stimulates the development of the womb's lining; the 'scrape' analysis will be able to reveal this.

Of course, this will only be undertaken once the more straightforward reasons for a couple's infertility – problems with the man's sperm, for instance – have been ruled out. There are other ways of telling if a woman isn't ovulating (from blood tests, for example), but a D & C can also give doctors an opportunity to see if there is any obvious deformity of the womb which could be preventing her from conceiving.

Curettage

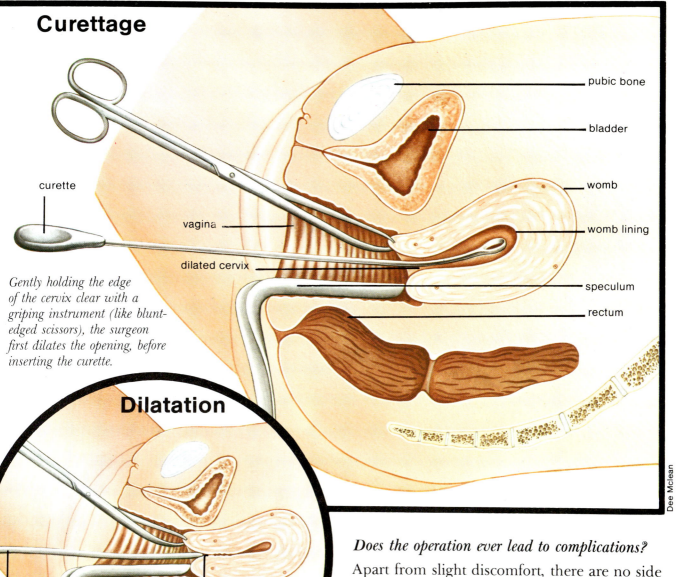

curette

pubic bone

bladder

vagina

womb

dilated cervix

womb lining

speculum

rectum

Gently holding the edge of the cervix clear with a griping instrument (like blunt-edged scissors), the surgeon first dilates the opening, before inserting the curette.

Dilatation

dilator

cervix

Dee Mclean

Is there a particular time of month when the operation should be done?

Generally a D & C would not be done while a woman is having a period; though this will depend on the urgency of the case.

But sometimes more exact timing is necessary; when checking on ovulation for instance. Then it is important that the D & C is done *after* the woman would normally have ovulated, about a week before her next period is due.

Does the operation ever lead to complications?

Apart from slight discomfort, there are no side effects, and it is very rare that a complication arises afterwards. On the whole, a D & C is the safest operation carried out by gynaecologists.

But every operation carries a slight risk and it is possible that the wall of the womb could be perforated by the surgeon's instrument or that, if the cervix is dilated too quickly or too far, the muscles can tear. This could cause problems during a subsequent pregnancy, since it could mean the neck of the womb opens prematurely, when the weight of the baby presses down on it. The woman may then miscarry. This is called 'incompetence' of the neck of the womb. It is a rare condition but can be overcome quite easily once diagnosed.

Occasionally, the operation could lead to an infection, but this is very rare indeed. Usually women feel quite well within a few days of the operation and quickly resume their normal activities. There's no need to be nervous of having a D & C.

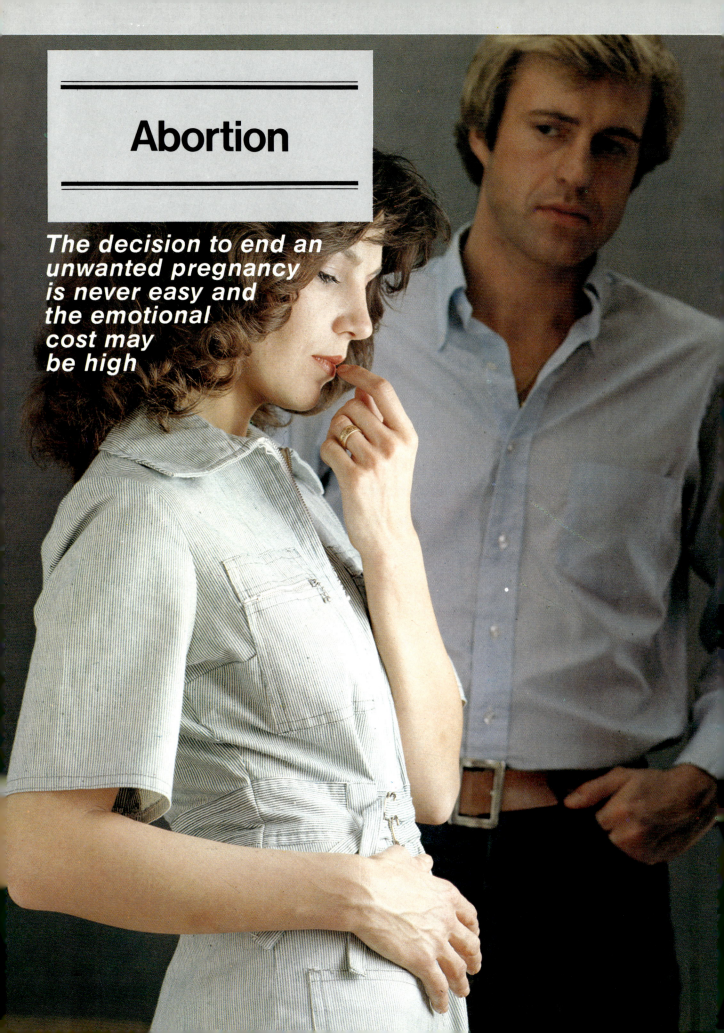

Abortion

The decision to end an unwanted pregnancy is never easy and the emotional cost may be high

A woman faced with an unwanted pregnancy is presented with an agonizing choice. Despite the fact that in many countries abortions are now relatively easy to obtain, making the decision to have one is still a very difficult and personal dilemma. It's a subject that many people have strong emotional views about – sometimes moral and religious beliefs – all of which can bring a lot of pressure to bear on the individual woman. In the end, however, it's her decision, and the best insurance she can have against feeling depressed about an abortion afterwards is to be sure she is making the choice that feels right for her.

Why do women ask for abortions?

Every woman's reasons are slightly different – after all, an unwanted pregnancy can be the result of anything from a simple contraceptive failure to an incident of rape. Nor is there any one 'type' who is most likely to seek an abortion; it might be a careless, promiscuous girl who takes no precautions and is uncertain of the father, but it could just as easily be a careful married woman whose coil has failed.

However, the fact that a pregnancy is 'unplanned' is generally not sufficient reason for seeking an abortion – there have to be stronger motivations, which are usually financial or social. A woman may well want the *child* as such, but have very strong career or family pressures which mean the baby would cause a great deal of disruption and unhappiness.

Money problems are often a major consideration. A young couple who haven't got their first home organized may feel, quite realistically, they simply can't contemplate the idea of looking after a tiny baby. Nowadays the woman of the family is an important source of income, so her pregnancy not only adds another mouth to feed but cuts down quite considerably on the money coming in to the household. Even if a couple already have children, it may be living conditions are already cramped or that they are living on a very low income.

Young, single girls usually have other priorities when it comes to an unwanted pregnancy. The social stigma attached to being an unmarried mother is much less nowadays, but the practical and emotional problems of bringing up a child without the support of the father are very daunting indeed. And, even if they get help from their families, many single girls are not prepared to have a child ruin their training or career.

Sometimes, of course, a doctor will recommend an abortion on medical grounds, when he has reason to believe the child will be abnormal or carry an inherited disease. There are also occasions when an abortion is suggested because the mother's psychological health is at risk. If someone has been mentally ill as a result of a previous birth, it may be better for her to have an abortion than suffer the same problem again, and there are some women who become so severely depressed during pregnancy as to be suicidal. As a rule doctors will always place the health of the mother and her existing family as their highest priority in such cases.

What happens if the man involved disagrees about the abortion?

As a potential parent, the man can, and often does, have strong feelings about the situation. Legally the man's attitude cannot affect the situation. If a woman wants to terminate the pregnancy then she does not have to ask the father's permission. On the other hand the father can influence the decision by threatening to break off the relationship, or just by making her life hell, if she goes ahead with an abortion against his wishes.

A woman has to balance her desire to continue the relationship with her need to end the pregnancy. A woman who gives in to the father may in fact enjoy and love the baby, once it is born. On the other hand, it can be disastrous if the mother goes on with the pregnancy for the sake of the father and dislikes the child intensely on arrival.

Unwanted children can cause untold stress in a marriage, and the relationship may well break up over a child who is loved and wanted by one party, but rejected by the other.

An abortion rarely causes a basically sound relationship to break up, although it may put it under severe strain. Perhaps the woman feels she has to conceal the pregnancy from her partner and have an abortion without telling him, or there may be recriminations about who was responsible for the pregnancy in the first place, resulting in quarrels or repressed resentment.

Why do some people object to abortion on moral grounds?

Many people today believe that no woman should be forced into motherhood simply because she finds herself unexpectedly pregnant. This is a view that has been reinforced by the 'legalizing' of abortion in many countries. There are some, however, who have serious reservations about a woman's right to do what she likes with her own body in these circumstances, and consider abortion to be little better than a form of murder. These views may be a deeply held religious belief or simply a serious moral objection to the idea of 'taking a life'.

Theoretically, an abortion is the removal of a foetus from the mother before it can sustain an independent existence but, when abortions are performed later on in a pregnancy, this fact isn't always easy to establish. This is because it is sometimes difficult to determine accurately the age of the foetus. Even using advanced techniques such as ultrasound, a theoretical 28 week pregnancy may in fact be 32 weeks, with an increasing danger of a live baby.

As a pregnancy goes on, termination becomes more and more like a normal birth. With some methods the mother has something like a mini-Caesarian, or is brought into labour and delivers a palpably live foetus that just doesn't go on living. This can be very traumatic for the patient and medical staff alike. Certainly it seems ironic that in one hospital ward the staff may be fighting to save the life of a premature baby of 26 weeks, while in another doctors are operating on a woman to remove a foetus of the same age.

Is it usual for a woman to feel depressed after an abortion?

When an abortion is over, the overriding feeling for the woman is usually one of immense relief. It is natural that this relief should be mixed with a certain amount of guilt or resentment and be tinged with sadness for the baby that might have been, but this mild depression does not usually last for more than a couple of weeks.

The operation will temporarily affect a woman's hormone balance, and this in itself can produce emotional changes. Even in the early stages, the mother's body responds to pregnancy by producing increasing amounts of certain hormones. An abortion alters these levels and the sudden change may well bring on depression. Some abortion methods also involve the mother taking high doses of hormones, which further interfere with her body's delicate chemistry.

It's also important for everybody's peace of mind that the abortion should take place as quickly as possible. This means the woman should go to her doctor or a pregnancy advisory centre early on, particularly as there may be administrative delays.

Although in many countries abortions can be carried out up to the 28th week of pregnancy, most abortions take place at 12 to 14 weeks or earlier. In practice, doctors are reluctant to terminate a pregnancy beyond the 16th week;

physically, the danger of haemorrhage is then greater, but the chances of emotional damage are also increased. Around this stage of pregnancy the baby starts to move and to have the abortion after this is likely to be a much more upsetting experience for the woman.

Unfortunately, some women postpone seeking advice because they really feel in two minds about having the operation. They may even refuse to accept their pregnancy is real in the vain hope that, if they ignore it, it will somehow cease to exist. As the weeks go by the situation can only worsen – the baby in fact becomes more real and the decision is much more difficult.

A woman's age is another important factor in how easily she can accept an abortion. For an older woman, the pregnancy may have been her last chance of having a baby, so she is likely to grieve longer than a young woman.

Does abortion ever cause long-term emotional problems?

It's unusual for a woman to suffer from serious psychological effects after an abortion but there are some women who find it more difficult to accept the loss on a long term basis.

Sometimes a woman gets pregnant again soon after an abortion. This can be a conscious decision because she has rearranged her life and feels able to cope with a child. Or it can be in response to a dimly recognized need, and only lead to a further abortion. Perhaps she is a very lonely person who – without realizing it – is seeking a child of her own as someone to love and who will give her the love she needs.

Recent research has shown that women who have had an abortion are more likely to become depressed during a subsequent wanted pregnancy. This seems to be a kind of delayed emotional impact – it's more likely to affect a woman who failed to face up to her real regrets at the time of the abortion. Occasionally an abortion can cause miscarriages in later pregnancies or even sterility. When this happens a woman can feel terribly guilty about what she has done to her body and to her marriage.

If a woman is having real difficulty coming to terms with the idea of abortion, she should seek advice from her doctor, or from a pregnancy advisory service – this can be just as important *before* an abortion as after. A professional counsellor can do a great deal to help someone sort out the conflicting emotions she is experiencing and face up to taking responsibility for her own actions. The important thing is for the woman to arrive at the decision that is right for *her*.

CHAPTER 6

Medical Guide

Period problems

It's the lucky few – just 20 per cent of women – who pass through the years between puberty and menopause without some trouble with their periods.

Unfortunately normal periods do cause normal women a certain amount of discomfort and pain (although that doesn't mean they have to grin and bear it). It's when there's a radical change of some kind in the menstrual cycle that medical help may be advisable.

Painful periods

It's estimated that one in every two women suffers from some discomfort during menstruation. The pain may begin a few hours before the bleeding starts and lasts for a maximum of 12 hours; it's uncomfortable but bearable and can be dealt with by simple measures – taking aspirin or lying down with a hot-water bottle.

But for some women, the pain can be agonizing, accompanying almost every period. Although this condition, known as *dysmenorrhoea*, does tend to get easier with the passage of time – often once a woman has had a baby – this knowledge doesn't make the intervening years any easier to bear.

The root of the pain lies in the muscles of the uterus, which go into cramps under the influence of prostaglandins – hormones produced in the muscle tissues. It seems that the higher the levels of prostaglandin, the more forcibly the walls of the uterus contract.

Most women evolve their own techniques for dealing with the miserable days of pain, and certainly there's no shortage of suggested remedies. Some women find that exercise helps. Acupuncture, meditation, even a change of diet to include less meat and more vegetables have their enthusiastic exponents, while for some women having sex seems to be an effective pain-reliever. Simple aspirin is one of the most effective pain killers to use, as long as it's taken in good time. It works because it's an anti-prostaglandin but, like all drugs, the body needs time to absorb it, so it's important to take one or two before the pain sets in, repeating the dose every four hours, as directed.

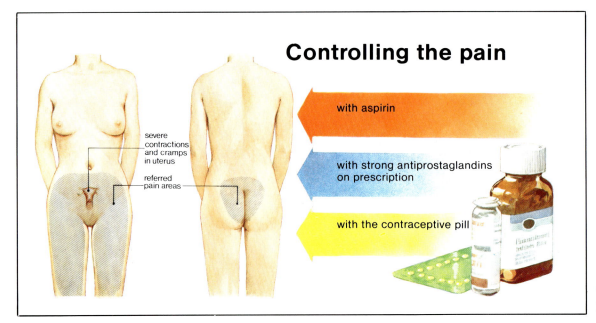

Controlling the pain

severe contractions and cramps in uterus

referred pain areas

with aspirin

with strong antiprostaglandins on prescription

with the contraceptive pill

John Fraser

If none of these remedies help, do consult your doctor, who may be able to offer a number of alternatives. There are drugs called *mefenamic acid* and *flufenamic acid*, both of which are antiprostaglandins, but slightly stronger than aspirin. These are still relatively new so, as yet, there's no long-term research into their effects.

The contraceptive Pill has also proved to be very helpful with period pains. It may succeed in banishing the problem altogether, even after women stop taking it, but this isn't always a viable alternative, particularly for young girls.

For older women, a simple D and C operation can be the solution. Why this operation, (which involves stretching the neck of the womb slightly and gently scraping away its lining) should work isn't at all clear. It's possible that by stretching the cervix the uterus has to contract less forcibly to expel the lining in the future.

Disorders that cause 'period' pain

If a woman starts experiencing pain when she menstruates, having never had any discomfort before, there's usually a very specific cause and she should always see her doctor about it so that tests (including a smear) and an internal examination can be made. It's reassuring to know that pain is rarely a sign of cancer, but some of the conditions which do give rise to pain can cause infertility if they are neglected.

Frequently, as well as becoming painful, the periods are also heavier than usual. One rather curious condition which produces these symptoms is *endometriosis*; small spots of the womb's lining (the endometrium) appear quite inappropriately elsewhere in the abdomen. Every month, the hormones which stimulate the womb also stimulate these spots of tissue, making them swell and bleed – and causing pain which can be agonizing in intensity, and often lasts much longer than the normal period pain.

Hormone preparations can do a great deal to quieten these spots, and a six-month course of the Pill or progesterone hormone is often the answer. But if these fail to work, surgery may be necessary.

Chronic infection of the womb or Fallopian tubes also provokes pain and heavier bleeding because it increases the flow of blood to the organs, making the tissues hot, red and swollen – with increased throbbing and cramps in the lower abdomen. As a rule, there's a discharge too, and the pain isn't necessarily associated with menstruation – it may be more or less constant, but is often worse during intercourse.

Infection needs immediate treatment with antibiotics and since it's not always easy to diagnose, let alone eradicate, treatment may go on for several months. If the infection is allowed to go on unchecked, there's a danger that it will cause infertility or reach a stage where the only cure is surgery.

Pelvic congestion

Muscular cramps in the abdomen are very common, but, if they are accompanied by backache and a feeling of pressure in the pelvis, the problem could be *pelvic congestion syndrome*. This is often associated with heavy and too-frequent periods. What happens is that the womb becomes too congested with blood, as a result of a hormone imbalance. Emotional stress or unhappiness, particularly marital or sexual problems, are often at the back of this, but if it doesn't settle of its own accord, the doctor may prescribe hormone therapy in the form of progesterone tablets.

Loss of periods

In itself, going without periods can't do any harm – all it means is that the womb is not building up its lining each month. This happens quite naturally after having a baby, or following a miscarriage or an abortion, because the hormones controlling menstruation are temporarily disrupted. But a number of other factors can disrupt the chain of hormone-producing glands (the hypothalamus, the pituitary and the ovaries) and their 'target organ', the womb.

Certain chronic diseases can produce loss of periods: tuberculosis (though this is now rare), anaemia, thyroid disease and other disorders which affect the hormone system. Some tranquillizers, anti-depressive drugs and those used to control blood pressure can provoke the same results. If you are in any doubt about any drugs you are taking, check with your doctor. For the most part, though, loss of periods has a simple cause. Being pregnant is the commonest – but sometimes overlooked – reason for loss of periods. It is also very common not to have periods for several months after coming off the contraceptive Pill – but they invariably return in time.

Sometimes, though, girls go through their teens without starting their periods. Often, menstruation is simply delayed, but occasionally there's a physical abnormality or a glandular disorder responsible which will need investigating. But there's no need to consult a doctor, usually, unless the girl has not menstruated by the time she is 16.

Emotional factors

Being seriously over-or under-weight (nearly all girls suffering from anorexia lose their periods) often leads to this kind of disruption, and stress or emotional disturbance is an extremely common cause. This is because the hypothalamus also contains the centres that control appetite and metabolism and is influenced by the 'higher centres' in the brain connected with our emotions. A change of job, a death in the family, moving house or a broken marriage can all cause periods to stop for a while.

treatment Often the disruption is very short-lived. Indeed unless more than four months pass by without a period, it's not even considered to be a problem. Although a doctor will conduct various tests at this stage to check for any serious disorder, provided none is found, he may well be reluctant to start any treatment to induce the cycle to start again until at least six months have gone by. If a specific disease is causing loss of periods, treatment to clear it up will usually restore the monthly cycle.

Disorders affecting the hormone balance

Although the timing of the periods is principally controlled by the hormones produced in the pituitary gland and the ovaries, other hormonal changes in the body can, indirectly, affect the hormone balance, and cause loss of periods. An underactive thyroid gland results in the slowing down of many of the body's systems – and the periods may stop as a result. As soon as the condition is diagnosed and treated with thyroid hormone, the periods will return. Problems with the adrenal glands may have a similar effect.

Sometimes the problem lies within the pituitary gland itself. Over-production of a hormone called *prolactin* may cause a constant milky discharge from the nipples and also a loss of periods. Occasionally, the excessive production of prolactin comes from a small benign growth in the pituitary, and this can be removed surgically.

The hormones produced by the ovaries may be upset by the presence of cysts. If these cysts lead to the over-production of certain hormones, they may have to be removed. On the other hand, under-production of hormones from the ovaries occurs in a condition called the Stein-

Leventhal syndrome. A woman with this condition tends to be heavily built and to have high blood pressure, and will often have more body hair than usual.

Heavy periods

Finding that their periods suddenly become very heavy can be of much concern to women. It is important to see a doctor if this happens, but often it's the result of something as simple as a temporary hormonal imbalance due to an emotional upheaval, or a reaction to an IUD internal contraceptive.

Anything which enlarges the surface area of the womb will increase the flow of blood each month; after each pregnancy, the womb is slightly larger than before, leading to heavier periods than previously experienced.

Fibroids in the womb or endometriosis will have the same effect, and a prolonged imbalance of the two ovarian hormones progesterone and oestrogen can eventually make the womb swell. Certain blood disorders, when clotting is defective or the blood capillaries are excessively fragile, may cause heavy periods, and disruption to any of the glands – an underactive thyroid or disease of the hypothalamus – can have the same result. Occasionally heavy periods are accompanied by bleeding between periods as well. If this occurs more than once, it is important to see a doctor without delay as it can be an early sign of cancer of the womb or cervix.

treatment The most effective drug treatment is hormonal – the high dose combined contraceptive Pill or alternatively a synthetic progestogen. The Pill prevents the lining of the uterus getting too thick and eventually makes it flat. Progestogen also stops the lining thickening.

Of course, any fundamental disorder will need medical attention. Only if the condition fails to respond to other treatment will an operation be considered; initially this may be just a D and C. As yet the only treatment for fibroids is to remove them. In older women who have had children, a doctor may recommend a hysterectomy, but this is never something to take lightly. It is usually only recommended if the symptoms are seriously disabling.

Women who suffer from naturally heavy periods right from the start can benefit from hormone treatment; other than that there's little that can be done, except to rest during the period and eat plenty of iron-rich food to avoid the risk of anaemia.

Vaginal problems

Whatever their cause, vaginal problems can be very distressing, not only because they concern such an intimate part of the body, but also because they can be very painful and may interfere with sexual enjoyment. But these troubles are really quite common. About one woman in every two experiences some such disorder in the course of her life.

Vaginal secretions

To keep the vagina and womb clean and free of germs the body secretes a protective mucus, so a certain amount of discharge from the vagina is absolutely normal. You have probably noticed how it varies in consistency and quantity during the course of the month, becoming heavier mid-way between your periods or just before one is due.

The discharge is quite bland – it doesn't smell unpleasant or itch – although it leaves a slight stain on underwear. But if you have contracted an infection you may notice the first signs when the secretions change and perhaps give off an offensive odour. Often this is accompanied by itchiness or tenderness.

Vaginal thrush

One of the most common infections of the vagina is caused by a tiny organism called *Candida albicans,* which often lives on the skin, quite harmlessly. But this tiny germ, related to the yeast family, grows well in any warm, dim and moist area, so the vagina is particularly inviting. Once it takes hold here it quickly becomes a nuisance, causing intense irritation round the vagina and changing the normal mucus into a thick, white discharge which can be very profuse. If the infection is mild, there may be irritation with very little discharge, but if it gets worse and is left untreated, the discharge takes on a curd-like consistency and yellower hue and the irritation can spread down the inside of the legs and even to the buttocks.

The inside view

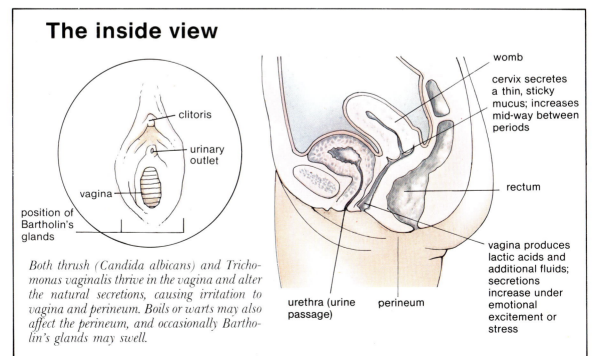

clitoris

urinary outlet

vagina

position of Bartholin's glands

womb

cervix secretes a thin, sticky mucus; increases mid-way between periods

rectum

vagina produces lactic acids and additional fluids; secretions increase under emotional excitement or stress

urethra (urine passage)

perineum

Both thrush (Candida albicans) and Trichomonas vaginalis thrive in the vagina and alter the natural secretions, causing irritation to vagina and perineum. Boils or warts may also affect the perineum, and occasionally Bartholin's glands may swell.

Mike Tregenza

What causes thrush?

Thrush affects both men and women, and even children (since it lives happily in the mouth as well) and although it may appear quite spontaneously, it's also sexually transmitted. So if your partner has this infection, you may also get it, and if you don't receive treatment you may keep re-infecting each other.

The environment inside the vagina is always attractive, but it becomes more so if the acid/alkali balance of the secretions changes and become too alkali. This is why many women tend to develop thrush just before they menstruate, when they are on the Pill or during pregnancy. A prolonged course of antibiotics may also lay you open to this organism. This is because the antibiotics can affect the harmless bacteria in the vagina which form part of the body's natural defences against infection.

The fact that men can carry the germ responsible for thrush is a fairly recent discovery. They often have no symptoms at all, but the infection may show itself as a slight irritation around the fore-skin or even a discharge. Men who have not been circumcized are much more vulnerable to thrush.

treatment ▷ Thrush may give you trouble just once, and never return, but often it recurs again and again. If you have it in a mild form, paying special attention to vaginal hygiene may be enough to banish it. A daily soak for 15 minutes in a bath containing a handful of cooking salt will help the irritation, while a coating of natural yoghurt may prove very effective in getting rid of it altogether.

If the thrush doesn't clear up within a couple of days, or if the discharge is very heavy, go and see your doctor. He will give you an internal examination, and may take a sample of the discharge from the inside of your vagina for laboratory testing.

Treatment consists of an antibiotic specially formulated to attack the thrush and it comes in the form of creams or 'pessaries'. These are cone-shaped tablets which are inserted as high into the vagina as possible. It's quite safe to push these up with your fingers, but often there's a plastic inserter to help you position them correctly. If the infection is confined to an area round the opening of the vagina, the cream may be all that's necessary. But often, both the cream and the pessaries are used together. The pessaries are usually put in at night but in some cases they may be prescribed for day-time use as well.

During the day ordinary sanitary pads will protect your clothes from any staining. The treatment can last for anything from two to 14 days, depending on the type of antibiotic.

Because thrush can be transmitted sexually from one partner to another, it's important that both of you receive treatment, so that you're not constantly passing the infection backwards and forwards between you; men should use the antibiotic cream on the penis. As long as you're both receiving treatment, there's no need to abandon sex at all, although you may find you are too sore to enjoy it for a couple of days until the irritation dies down.

Vaginal trichomoniasis

Commonly known as 'trich' or 'TV', the germ *Trichomonas vaginalis* also causes an intense irritation in the area around the vagina, and you will notice that secretions then take on a rather unpleasant odour and a greenish tinge.

The infection is usually spread by sexual contact, but an old infection can sometimes become active again for no particular reason. This germ can actually survive outside the body for a short time, so it's possible to pick it up by contact with infected articles, such as unwashed towels – but this is quite unusual. Although men are infected – and so pass it on – they seem to escape any symptoms.

Unless the proper treatment is given, the condition will not clear up, so doctors have to be careful to make an accurate diagnosis. If your doctor has any doubts – and vaginal infections tend to share similar characteristics – he will take a sample 'swab' for testing in the laboratory.

treatment ▷ Treatment is with tablets – usually of a drug called metronidazole – and it's essential that both partners are treated at the same time to prevent re-infection. It's best to avoid intercourse until the treatment is complete; usually about a week.

Cervical erosion

Sometimes a discharge that is heavier than usual can be a sign of cervical 'erosion'. This is not nearly as alarming as it sounds, and in fact the so-called erosion is quite harmless. It's only the discharge which may be a nuisance, especially as you become more prone to infections.

What happens is that the normal smooth covering of the neck of the womb is replaced by roughened skin which 'moves' downwards from its normal position in the cervical canal. This roughened

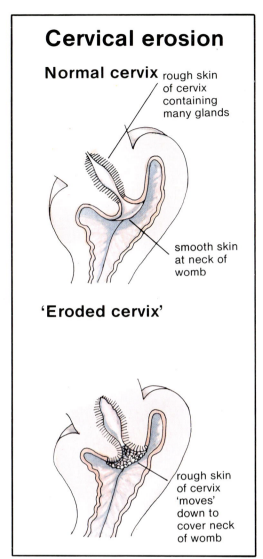

Cervical erosion

Normal cervix
rough skin of cervix containing many glands

smooth skin at neck of womb

'Eroded cervix'

rough skin of cervix 'moves' down to cover neck of womb

Mike Tregenza

skin secretes much more mucus than the smooth skin, so the discharge increases. The shift of skin covering may be completely spontaneous, but pregnancy or the Pill can increase the tendency.

If infection does set in, the discharge will take on a yellower hue, and may give off an unpleasant odour. You may notice some spotting or bleeding.

treatment Your doctor will prescribe any necessary creams or pessaries if an infection is present, but often the erosion rights itself of its own accord. However, if it's severe or the infection doesn't clear up, your doctor may suggest surgical treatment. This consists of 'freezing' the area, so that the skin can shed its old lining and build a new one. The process is very straightforward, and may not even need a general anaesthetic.

Swellings in the vagina
Sometimes, ordinary skin conditions, such as eczema, can affect the vagina.

There may also be infections which may cause little boils around the vaginal opening which are tender and painful. As a rule, they settle down without any specific treatment, but if they become rather large, you should visit your doctor for an examination.

treatment He will probably prescribe a course of antibiotic tablets, or, in extreme cases may recommend surgery, but this is unusual.

Occasionally, one of the glands on either side of the vagina called 'Bartholin's Glands' becomes infected and swells up like a very large boil. A simple operation is all that's necessary to put this right.

Small painless lumps may be caused by warts. These are transmitted by a virus and you can catch them from a sexual partner. Unfortunately, they tend to spread very rapidly, and it's wise to see a doctor fairly quickly.

treatment If there are only a few, he can treat them with special caustic 'paint' which has to be applied very carefully so as not to damage the surrounding skin. They may need one or more sessions until they disappear. Larger warts may need surgery in order to remove them.

Prolapse of the womb
A large painless swelling in the vagina may be due to a prolapse, when either the side of the vagina or the neck of the womb drops down into the vaginal entrance, see *Womb Disorders*, but this can be corrected by surgery.

Vaginal dryness
Many women find that vaginal dryness becomes a problem after menopause, the reason being that the hormones which keep the vagina moist are no longer present in such high quantities once your periods stop. If there isn't enough of the secretion to keep bacteria at bay, infection and an irritating discharge may follow.

treatment It's well worth consulting the doctor, since the condition is easy to cure with the aid of creams or pessaries containing the hormone oestrogen.

If you find that vaginal dryness is a problem during intercourse, use an artificial lubricant to help, available from any pharmacist.

Bleeding from the vagina
Periods can vary enormously from one woman to another. Many women have them regularly every four weeks, but some will have one every three weeks while others once every three months or

173

so. As long as the periods are fairly regular, there is no need to worry. But irregular periods may be a sign that something is wrong – an infection of the vagina or an inflammation in the womb or around the neck of the womb. Occasionally, it may indicate a growth (usually quite harmless).

The signs to watch for are:
☐ bleeding after intercourse
☐ bleeding or 'spotting' between periods
☐ bleeding after the menopause.

treatment Go to your doctor if any one of these occurs. He will take a smear test and give you an internal examination. Often the cause will turn out to be quite simple, but otherwise further tests in hospital may be arranged.

Any bleeding from the vagina during pregnancy may be a sign of complications. In this case it is best to go straight to bed, and ring the doctor for advice rather than waiting for an appointment or walking long distances to the surgery.

Of course, spotting or break-through bleeding may occur if you are on the Pill. This is quite common and there is usually no cause for alarm, but it is still worth checking with your doctor if it happens more than a couple of months running.

Internal tampons

Forgotten tampons are a common problem. If they are left in for more than a day or two, you may have a very unpleasant discharge.

See your doctor as soon as possible, so that he can remove it, and it should quickly clear up. If you leave it longer, a more serious infection may build up.

Vaginal problems in children

In small girls, the area round the vagina can easily become sore and inflamed, and this may be due to irritation from soaps used for washing, or to the fact that bacteria has been allowed to build up instead of being washed away.

treatment A cream prescribed by the doctor and simple attention to cleanliness should clear this up, although it can be very painful while it lasts.

If you notice any kind of discharge, always see your doctor. No child should have a discharge before puberty. It may be caused by an infection, but sometimes by something in the vagina. Unfortunately small girls sometimes push beads or other little toys into their vaginas, but a visit to the doctor should get this sorted out.

How to keep problems at bay

There's no question that regular washing with a mild soap helps keep infections at bay. But if you're over-enthusiastic, you may actually do more harm than good. There is no point in putting household antiseptics into bath water; they do nothing to stop infections. But they can cause soreness, and some people can be allergic to them. Bubble baths and vaginal deodorants should also be used with caution – especially if you are already prone to infections such as thrush.

In the past, many women used douches – which squirt water into the vagina and 'rinse' it out – in the hope that this would help prevent infections. But this routine can actually be the cause of trouble, since it removes the vagina's natural protective secretions.

If you suffer from recurrent thrush, following a few basic rules may help prevent it.

☐ Avoid tight-fitting jeans or trousers, which don't allow air to circulate.

☐ Always wear cotton underpants and use stockings or 'one-leg' tights instead of normal tights. Avoid nylon underpants.

☐ Wash twice a day using plain soap and water only.

☐ Do not use bubble baths, vaginal deodorants or perfumed tampons.

☐ If you develop itching around the vagina, take a daily salt bath or try a 'coating' of natural yoghurt around the area. If the itching doesn't settle, see your doctor.

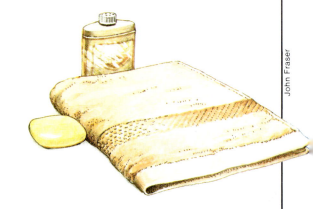

John Fraser

Sexually transmitted diseases (STD) are a group of infections passed on from one person to another by sexual contact. This may be genital to genital, mouth to genital or *vice versa*, or genital to anus. STD can also be transmitted by kissing, but this is rare.

Detecting STD

Sometimes a STD will produce warning symptoms such as discharge from the vagina, penis or anus, or there may be irritation or soreness in these areas. A sore lump or rash may develop on the genitals, around the anus or in the mouth. But some men and most women with a STD have no symptoms at all.

If you hear that a sex partner has recently had one of these diseases, or if you have had sexual intercourse with someone you know to be promiscuous, or with more than one partner within a short time, it is vital to consult a doctor or go direct to the STD clinic at your local hospital so that the necessary examination and tests can be carried out. If you do have one of these infections, it can then be treated and cured before it can do any damage.

The address of your local STD clinic can be found by looking in the telephone directory under 'venereal disease' or 'VD', by asking at the casualty department of any hospital, or by ringing the Citizen's Advice Bureau in your area.

In Britain today, most STD are treated in hospital clinics which are staffed by doctors and nurses with special training and experience in the subject. The necessary examinations and laboratory tests are done as quickly as possible, and any treatment required is given immediately.

Non-gonococcal (or non-specific) urethritis

This is referred to as 'non-gonococcal' to distinguish it from gonorrhoea. It is also known as 'non-specific urethritis', and is the most common STD in Britain and many other countries. It is caused by several different bacteria, including *Chlamydia*, responsible for nearly half of all NGU infections, and believed to cause all the serious complications arising from them.

When they occur, NGU symptoms in men are similar to those of gonorrhoea – discomfort in passing urine and a discharge from the penis – but they are usually less severe. They appear, if at all, one to two weeks after contact with the infection. Some men with NGU are un-

aware that anything is wrong, and women with a NGU infection rarely have symptoms.

Doctors diagnose non-gonococcal urethritis in men in much the same way as they diagnose gonorrhoea – by examining a specimen of any discharge from the urethra under a microscope. Other laboratory tests are also used to confirm the diagnosis. The lack of symptoms makes it difficult for a woman to realize when she is infected with NGU, but it can be diagnosed by special tests.

treatment NGU needs thorough treatment with a one- to two-week course of *tetracycline* or some similar antibiotic. Penicillin and the other single-dose antibiotics prescribed for gonorrhoea won't cure NGU. Both men with NGU and women who have had intercourse with them are treated with the same antibiotic to stop to-and-fro infection, and to prevent complications.

Follow-up tests to determine whether the disease has been cured are very important, and every effort should be made to find and treat any sexual contacts of patients with NGU. It is sensible for patients to avoid sexual activity of any kind until they are completely cured of the illness. It is also important to avoid alcohol for two weeks after the start of treatment as taking alcohol can cause the infection to recur.

Complications resulting from NGU

As with gonorrhoea, epididymitis in men and salpingitis in women are the most serious complications that can occur as a result of NGU. Babies born to women infected with *Chlamydia* often develop an eye infection called *inclusion conjunctivitis*, and they may also get chest infections.

Some men get NGU many times, sometimes even without a change of sex partner. The reasons for this are not clearly understood, but fortunately complications seem to be unusual in men with recurrent NGU. However, they may infect or re-infect a partner, who should have a proper examination and treatment without delay to prevent complications developing.

Genital warts

These are painless, irregular lumps which can appear on the vulva or penis or round the anus. They are caused by a sexually transmitted wart virus, and it takes from one to nine months for them to develop. Although they are unpleasant and a nuisance, they aren't serious. Usually

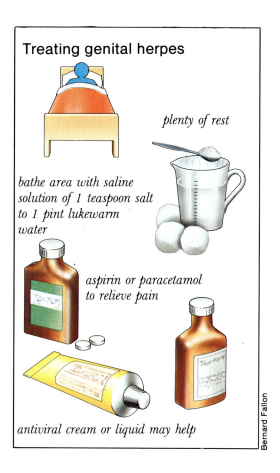

Treating genital herpes

plenty of rest

bathe area with saline solution of 1 teaspoon salt to 1 pint lukewarm water

aspirin or paracetamol to relieve pain

antiviral cream or liquid may help

Bernard Fallon

several of them form in a particular area. They are usually small to begin with but they may grow quite large if they are left untreated. Sometimes they get bigger during pregnancy, but decrease in size again after the baby is born.

There are several ways of treating genital warts. The most usual is to paint each individually with a preparation of *podophyllin* which destroys the wart cells. As this compound may cause skin irritation in some people, it must be applied by a doctor or nurse. If podophyllin doesn't work, the warts can be removed by freezing them with liquid nitrogen.

Genital herpes

This is a very unpleasant complaint which has recently become much more widespread. It is caused by a virus usually transmitted by sexual contact – vaginal or anal intercourse or through oral sex. A few days after such contact, a group of tiny blisters appears on the vulva or penis and sometimes around the anus: these burst and form shallow painful sores.

These are often accompanied by pain on passing urine, particularly in women, and by enlargement and tenderness of

glands in the groin. The sores heal in 10 to 14 days, leaving the genital area normal. However, in a number of people the virus persists even though they feel perfectly well.

Some people get recurrent attacks of genital herpes. These may occur only twice a year, but can happen as frequently as every few weeks. The attacks continue because the virus responsible for them lies dormant under the skin until it is reactivated and causes another attack.

While the virus is dormant, it is unlikely to infect others, but once reactivated it can do so, and the patient is often unaware when a new attack of genital herpes is starting.

The infection is diagnosed by taking swabs from the sores to see whether the virus is present. At the same time other laboratory tests are carried out to discover whether any other germs are present.

There is no point in prescribing antibiotics for genital herpes because it is a viral, as distinct from a bacterial infection, and no existing antibiotic will kill the virus.

Generally the best treatment is for the patient to rest as much as possible, to bathe the sores with a saline solution (one teaspoon of salt in a pint of lukewarm water), and to take aspirin or paracetamol to relieve the pain. Some patients benefit from antiviral drugs in the form of a liquid or cream to apply to the sores. Although these drugs may reduce the length of time an attack lasts, they do not prevent the sores recurring.

Danger of genital herpes during childbirth

Women who have genital herpes may, during childbirth, pass the infection on to the baby. This can have very serious consequences, as the virus may invade the child's bloodstream or central nervous system, occasionally causing death. For this reason a doctor will watch very carefully a woman with recurrent herpes who becomes pregnant, or who develops herpes for the first time just before the baby is due. A Caesarian operation may be advised for the small number of women who are infected, just before or when labour begins, as the outlook for the baby is much improved by this form of delivery.

In Britain only a very small number of women encounter problems with herpes during childbirth, but it is important for a doctor to know if his patient has a history of this disease. Fortunately the infection doesn't damage the baby in the womb.

Problems with the womb

Diseases and disorders affecting the womb and other reproductive organs such as the ovaries and Fallopian tubes can be particularly worrying. As well as causing considerable pain and discomfort which may sometimes interfere with your sex life, there is always the anxiety that they may prevent you from having a baby or make becoming pregnant more difficult.

Some women are reluctant to consult a doctor about these problems, perhaps because they are afraid he will dismiss their symptoms as being purely psychological.

But fibroids, prolapse and endometriosis – all fairly common disorders affecting the womb – have physical causes which can be treated, and even if these disorders cannot always be completely cured, many of the more unpleasant symptoms can be alleviated.

(Details of common vaginal problems, disorders of the ovaries and Fallopian tubes and painful periods are dealt with in separate chapters).

Fibroids

Fibroids are swellings in the wall of the womb consisting of muscle and fibrous tissue. They develop into lumps that can be smaller than a pea, or very rarely bigger than a football. They can protrude into the womb, or out into the pelvic region and then into the abdomen if they get very big. Apart from taking up space, they do no direct harm and the chances of them developing into cancer are very, very small. Around 20 per cent of all women have fibroids at some time in their lives, often without even knowing they have them, and only around a quarter have problems with them.

When do fibroids cause trouble?

When fibroids push into the womb, they enlarge it, stretching and indenting the endometrium, the lining of the womb that is shed every month during a period. The more lining there is, the more there is to shed and more bleeding there will

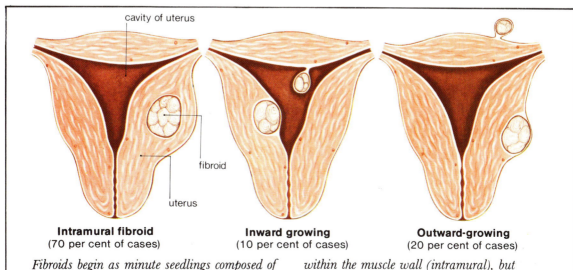

cavity of uterus

fibroid

uterus

Intramural fibroid
(70 per cent of cases)

Inward growing
(10 per cent of cases)

Outward-growing
(20 per cent of cases)

Fibroids begin as minute seedlings composed of muscle and connective tissue. Sometimes there's just one, but more often they are scattered in the body of the uterus. The seedlings grow gradually, developing into tumours. Usually they remain within the muscle wall (intramural), but sometimes they start moving inwards and may even end up suspended in the cavity. More often, if they do move, it's towards the outside, although these, too, can become pendulous.

Dee McLean

177

be. So fibroids can cause heavier and longer periods.

Fibroids don't usually prevent you becoming pregnant, but if there are several sitting under the womb lining, the fertilized egg may have trouble finding some healthy muscle in which to grow, and the risk of an early miscarriage is therefore increased. If the egg does succeed in becoming properly embedded, and you become pregnant, the baby may not be able to get into the ideal head-down position before birth because fibroids are in the way. In this case, a Caesarean delivery is sometimes necessary.

treatment Because no one knows how or why fibroids grow, there are no drugs available at the moment which will effectively prevent or cure them, although some anti-oestrogen drugs may shrink them a little. If the fibroids are small, they are usually best left alone, but once they have made the womb large enough to be felt above the brim of the pelvis – about equivalent in size to a three months' pregnancy – they are usually dealt with by surgery because they are beginning to get in the way.

Where just a single fibroid has developed, one, say the size of a tennis ball hanging on the outside of the womb, it can easily be removed on its own by an operation called a *myomectomy*.

If, however, you have several fibroids so that removing them individually would involve a great deal of intricate surgery with the risk of considerable blood loss, doctors often recommend a *hysterectomy*, an operation to remove the whole of the womb. This not only gets rid of fibroids that have already developed, but ensures that any tiny seedling fibroids that are also present but difficult to detect will not have a chance to grow.

It also means you won't be able to have children, so doctors won't insist on a hysterectomy if you want to start or add to your family, unless the fibroids show signs of abnormal growth. This is extremely unlikely.

Prolapse

Causes of prolapse

In some women, if the muscles supporting the womb are naturally weak or have become weakened through childbirth, particularly if labour was lengthy or the baby large, the womb or part of it may drop into the vagina. This is called a prolapse (which means 'falling through').

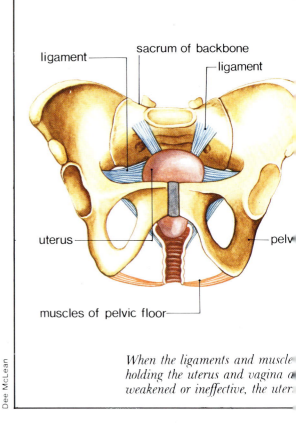

When the ligaments and muscle holding the uterus and vagina a weakened or ineffective, the uter...

labels: ligament — sacrum of backbone — ligament — uterus — pelv... — muscles of pelvic floor

Dee McLean

It tends to occur more often in the 30-plus age group than in younger women, especially after the menopause when the muscles lose their elasticity because of hormonal changes.

In the past, women were often left for hours in the second stage of labour with the baby's head pushing into the vagina. The result was flabby, devitalized muscles around a stretched vagina and damaged womb supports, making a subsequent prolapse almost inevitable. To help deliver a baby which is otherwise going to take over two hours, doctors nowadays often perform an *episiotomy*, a small cut in healthy muscles which can easily be repaired and quickly returns to normal.

How to prevent prolapse

The best preventive measure for prolapse is to do the post-natal exercises that get the vaginal muscles back into shape. Often after a second baby, you feel you really haven't got the time to bother with them, but it is worth it. You need to squeeze and relax the muscles in the base of the pelvis up to 100 times, as many times a day as possible. The exercises can be done while watching television or waiting for a bus, so you shouldn't need too much will power to do them.

If the muscles of the pelvic floor are weakening, the first sign is usually 'stress

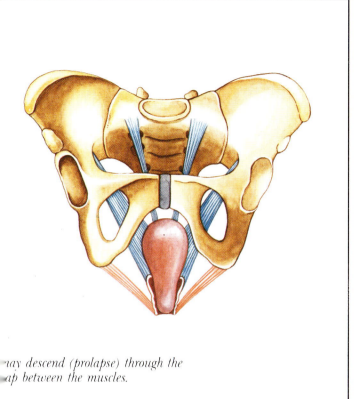

...may descend (prolapse) through the ...ap between the muscles.

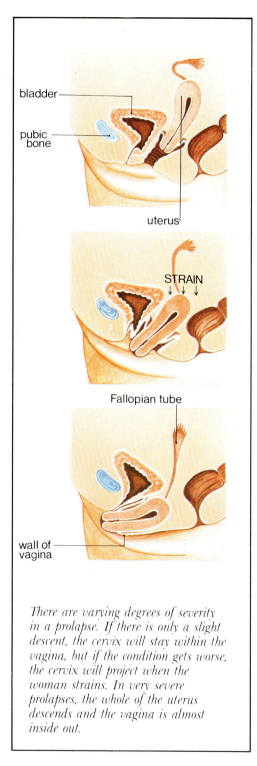

bladder

pubic bone

uterus

STRAIN

Fallopian tube

wall of vagina

There are varying degrees of severity in a prolapse. If there is only a slight descent, the cervix will stay within the vagina, but if the condition gets worse, the cervix will project when the woman strains. In very severe prolapses, the whole of the uterus descends and the vagina is almost inside out.

incontinence'. Urine leaks from the bladder when pressure inside the abdomen is increased by coughing, sneezing, laughing or running.

This can be treated by special exercises under the guidance of a physiotherapist. Done regularly, they not only secure the incontinence, but can prevent a prolapse.

What does a prolapse feel like?

As the womb drops, it may pull on the ligaments attached to the lower part of the back bone, resulting in a dull ache or a dragging sensation in the lower abdomen, as if something was trying to get out between your legs. Some women describe it as being like a baby's head waiting to be pushed out. The womb can also drag the back of the bladder down and cause problems of incontinence later on.

treatment By the time the symptoms of prolapse appear, surgery is the best treatment. Women who don't want any more children, usually have a hysterectomy. The operation is done through the vagina, so there's no scar, and at the same time a tuck is made in the skin on the front and back walls of the vagina and the underlying muscles are tightened.

If you want more children it is possible to do the repair to the vagina only and to leave the womb. Since another full scale labour is likely to undo the repair the

baby will usually be delivered by Caesarean section before labour starts. Even if you don't become pregnant the womb may pull down again, so the repair operation may not be a permanent cure.

Where surgery isn't suitable the alternative is to insert a hard rubber ring, a pessary, which hitches up the womb by supporting it at the top of the vagina. The ring does, however, have to be changed every few months for reasons of hygiene.

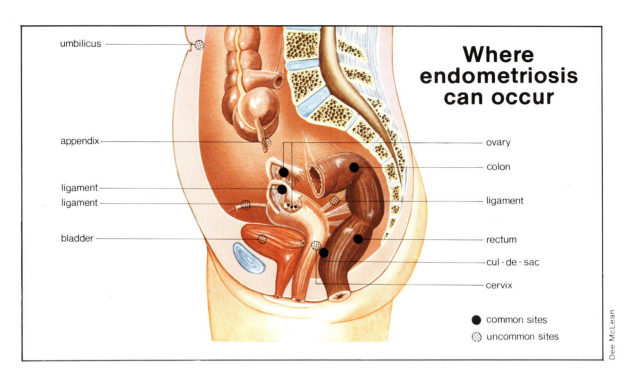

Where endometriosis can occur

umbilicus

appendix

ligament

ligament

bladder

ovary

colon

ligament

rectum

cul-de-sac

cervix

● common sites

⊛ uncommon sites

Dee McLean

Endometriosis

No one knows exactly what causes this. Sometimes cells from the endometrium, the tissue that normally lines the womb, become displaced and grow somewhere else. They may move up the Fallopian tubes to the ovaries, or even into the gut. This disease is called endometriosis. It's more common in women over the age of 30, especially if they haven't had any children.

Just as the normal lining tissue of the womb bleeds each month, so do the endometrial deposits which have developed in different places outside the womb. If the bleeding occurs inside the abdomen, for example, scar tissue will form between the deposit and other nearby organs

Endometriosis and infertility

This scar tissue often adheres to the nearest organ, sometimes restricting or interfering with its function. If one or other of the Fallopian tubes is affected, the adhesion often hinders the movement of the tube. As a result, it may be unable to pick up the egg released from the ovary each month and direct it down the tube towards the sperm moving in the opposite direction. So although endometriosis doesn't necessarily make you infertile, it can make becoming pregnant very difficult.

Symptoms of endometriosis

The usual symptoms of this disorder are very painful periods – the pain being

caused by the build up of blood from the endometrial deposits in areas from which it cannot escape. Sexual intercourse is usually painful as well.

Endometrial deposits may form as small, hard, tender bumps in the tissue behind the womb and in front of the rectum – your doctor will probably be able to feel these during a vaginal examination. If, however, endometriosis develops in the wall of the womb, the whole of the womb will become enlarged and feel tender.

If there is any doubt as to whether or not you have endometriosis, then your doctor will arrange for you to go into hospital for a *laparoscopy*. This involves examining the womb and other reproductive organs while you are under a general anaesthetic by inserting a lighted telescope-like instrument into your abdomen via a small cut made just below your navel.

treatment The first course of action is usually hormonal treatment. Your doctor will probably prescribe progestogen which quietens the activity of the womb lining and all its displaced cells. A new, very expensive drug called Danazol, has recently been developed which can in some cases completely cure the disease. Both types of drug are usually taken for six months. They may cause your periods to stop and will prevent you from becoming pregnant during that time.

If medical treatment is not successful then your doctor may suggest an operation to clear out the active spots of endometriosis and their deposits.

Breast cancer

As the commonest form of cancer among women living in Western countries, breast cancer strikes one woman in every 14 at some time during their lives. It is also responsible for more deaths among women in the 35 to 55 age group than any other disease, killing in total each year more than 12,000 women in the United Kingdom and 34,000 in the United States. There is evidence to suggest that even these high figures are on the increase.

It's little wonder, then, that breast cancer has become a subject of so much concern and often over-emotional discussion.

But the high levels of publicity serve an essential purpose, for by drawing attention to the problem, they increase the chances of a woman with early symptoms seeking treatment. Like all cancers, the earlier the growth is diagnosed, the better the chances of a cure.

What researches reveal

Although a great deal of research has gone into the causes of breast cancer, the evidence is still inconclusive.

At one time doctors thought that the part of the world a woman lived in or the race she belonged to might affect her chances of developing breast cancer. This was because a much higher proportion of women living in Western Europe and the United States developed the disease than, for example, their contemporaries living in South East Asia.

But in the past 10 years it seems that the rate for the disease among Japanese women living in their own country has been increasing to the same rate found among expatriate Japanese living in the United States. Furthermore, second generation Japanese women living in the USA now run the same risk of getting breast cancer as their American compatriots.

This suggest that it's environment and way of life rather than geographical or racial considerations that are the determining factors.

Some doctors believe that there may be a link between diet and the occurance of breast cancer, but this hasn't been proved as yet.

What research has shown is that having a child at an early age appears to give a woman a certain amount of protection against developing breast cancer at a later date, and that the degree of protection is the same whether the woman breast or bottle-feeds her baby. It has also been suggested that the younger the woman when she first becomes pregnant (or more precisely the fewer the number of monthly cycles she has experienced between the start of menstruation and her first pregnancy) the smaller the risk she is likely to run.

Breast cancer, the Pill and HRT

The Pill has come under a lot of suspicion in the past and there have been claims that it contributes to the development of breast cancer, but the latest studies seem to have given it an all-clear in this respect. Incidentally, one research project actually came up with results that showed a reduction in the incidence of *non-malignant* breast disease among women on the Pill.

But the connection between hormone replacement therapy (HRT), used to treat certain 'change of life' symptoms, and breast cancer is slightly more suspect. Although a number of studies have revealed no link between HRT and breast cancer, one large American survey does suggest that there is a slightly higher risk than usual of the disease developing among women who have been receiving HRT for more than 10 years.

Effects of radiation

Certainly exposure to radiation can increase the risk of breast cancer – the larger the quantity and the more frequent the exposure, the higher the risk of developing the disease. Unfortunately this creates something of a dilemma, since standard 'screening' procedures to detect cancer (among other things) do involve X-rays. Because no one knows how low the level of radiation has to be before the risk becomes insignificant, some doctors are afraid that repeated breast X-rays result in build-ups sufficient to cause cancer.

Most doctors, however agree that the benefits of screening outweigh the small risk that may be involved, and certainly doctors won't recommend X-rays unless they are absolutely necessary.

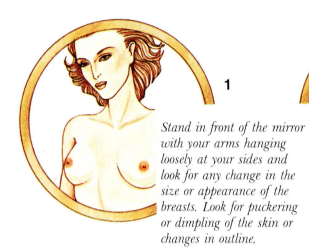

1

Stand in front of the mirror with your arms hanging loosely at your sides and look for any change in the size or appearance of the breasts. Look for puckering or dimpling of the skin or changes in outline.

2

Now raise your arms a your head and look at yourself from varying angles, by turning from to side, to see if there h been any changes. Look down at your breasts, t and make sure there's unusual discharge or bleeding from the nippl

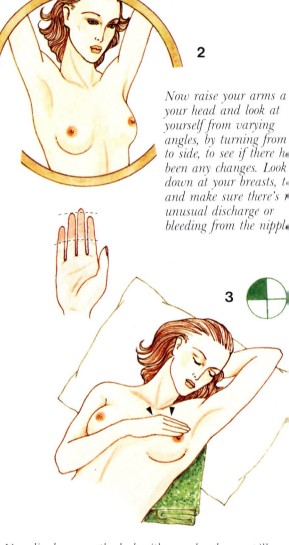

3

How to examine your breasts

Giving yourself an examination once a month will ensure that you discover any change as early as possible. The best time to do so is just after your period, when the breasts are usually at their softest. (If you are no longer having periods, you can choose any day – but try to stick to the same one each month).

When you first start examining your own breasts, you may well be surprised at their 'lumpiness'. What you are feeling is a mixture of fat and milk-producing glands which should be soft and lumpy. It will take several sessions for you to get used to your own breasts – remember that it's quite normal for one breast to be bigger than the other – what matters more is that they should feel the same. The breasts do change in size in the course of the month and become 'lumpier' just before a period. It's because they change that it's important to choose the same point in the menstrual cycle to check your breasts each month.

If you think you have found something during the course of an examination, feel the same part of the other breast, just to make sure it's not just the way both breasts are made. If there is something unusual, do not hesitate to check with your doctor – he would far rather see you and set your mind at rest, even if it is a false alarm, than have you neglect an important early symptom. Arrange to see him at the next surgery and, in the meantime, try to leave the breast alone.

Now lie down on the bed with your head on a pillow; place a pillow or folded towel under your left shoulder. This helps to spread the breast tissue and makes it easier to examine. Put your left hand under your head and use the right to examine your left breast. With fingers together, use the flat of your fingers (not the tips) to gently, but firmly, feel the breast to check for lumps, thickenings, or anything unusual.

Think of the breast as being divided into four quarters of a circle, and begin by examining the upper, inner quarter as shown. Start from the ribs above and from the breastbone, working towards the nipple.

Women most at risk from breast cancer

According to the statistics, the women most likely to get breast cancer are those living in highly developed Western countries who are over the age of 30, and who haven't had any children.

But irrespective of her age, environment, diet, racial characteristics, and whether or not she has had children, a woman whose mother, grandmother, daughter, sister or other close blood relative has already developed breast cancer, is herself at slightly greater risk from the disease than a woman with no family history of this form of cancer.

Signs to watch for

One of the earliest signs of breast cancer is the presence of a hard, rather ill-defined lump in one of the breasts. The lump is nearly always painless, and may occur anywhere in the breast. To begin with it moves freely, being unattached either to tissue beneath it or to the overlying skin.

As the tumour gets larger it pulls in the skin over it to produce a characteristic 'dimple' and may also affect the milk ducts causing these to shrink and the nipple to become inverted.

If the tumour continues to spread, it may attach itself to the overlying skin, sometimes causing skin ulcers. It may also invade the tissue beneath, eventually becoming fixed to the underlying muscles. If the cancer spreads into the lymphatic glands under the arm, obvious and hard lumps will appear in the armpit.

Importance of early diagnosis

Cancer of the breast alone is not fatal; the danger lies in the fact that it has the capacity to spread by shedding cells which can be carried by the bloodstream all over the body. Cancer may develop in the bones, liver, lungs, brain or elsewhere. Women patients with symptoms as different as jaundice or spontaneous bone fractures may in fact be suffering from secondary growths, in the liver or bones, of an original breast cancer.

The cancer can spread and form these new growths almost from the moment it first develops, so the earlier it is diagnosed, the better are the patient's prospects of halting the disease, whatever form the treatment takes.

If you find you have a lump, however small, in your breast you should see a doctor without delay. Fewer than a quarter of these lumps turn out to be malignant – often they are harmless cysts or benign tumours known as *fibroadenomas*, which are also more easily dealt with, if they need any treatment, while they are still small.

Since early detection of breast cancer is so vital to a patient's subsequent recovery, in some countries (such as the United Kingdom) special clinics have been set up

---

4

In the same way, examine the lower, inner quarter, again starting from the breast bone and also from the ribs below the breast. Examine the area all round the nipple as well.

5

Move your left arm down to your side and start examining the lower, outer quarter. Start from well out at the ribs below and at the side of the breast.

6

In exactly the same way, examine the final quarter. Bear in mind that there is a little extra section of breast tissue between this upper, outer quarter and the armpit. Make sure you feel across the top of the breast again, towards the armpit, to include this part.

7

Finally, feel in the armpit itself, looking for any lumps.
Repeat the whole process, for the right breast, but using your left hand, of course.

in certain areas. These provide free medical examinations to screen women for breast cancer as well as other illnesses. Women attending these centres are taught how to examine their own breasts regularly to check whether any lumps have developed so that these can be reported to a doctor and diagnosed promptly.

Diagnosing a lump in the breast

To find out whether a lump is cancerous or not the doctor consulted will carry out a thorough examination of both of the patient's breasts. He will ask her to sit up straight facing him, first with her arms by her sides, and then with her arms above her head so that he can see whether the nipple has become inverted or if there is any dimpling or lack of symmetry in one of the breasts. Then, while the patient is lying down with her head and shoulders propped up by pillows, the doctor will examine each breast carefully, section by section, with the flat of his hand. If he detects an isolated lump not attached to other parts of the breast tissue, he will either carry out a *needle aspiration* himself, or refer the patient to a specialist.

This is a simple and virtually painless test whereby the doctor can draw off fluid from the lump, by means of a thin, hollow syringe. If the lump is a harmless cyst, drawing out the fluid content will cause it to disappear so the test is in effect, both the means of diagnosing and curing the condition.

If no fluid is drawn off and the lump proves to be solid, the doctor will probably follow this up right away with a *biopsy* to obtain a small sample of the suspect tissue for more detailed tests. This will probably involve spending a few hours in the outpatient department of a hospital.

The minute piece of tissue taken from the lump (via a very small incision in the breast) can then be examined by a pathologist to see if it contains cancer cells. If the breast tumour is found to be malignant, the patient can be checked immediately, to see whether she has any secondary growths.

An *open biopsy* is sometimes carried out when the patient has an isolated, unattached lump in her breast. If the other tests (needle aspiration or outpatient biopsy) fail to yield satisfactory results or cannot be undertaken. The patient is admitted to hospital to have the whole lump removed under a general anaesthetic, so it can then be analyzed for any signs of cancer.

If breast cancer is diagnosed, the doctor will discuss with the woman concerned and with her husband or family the most suitable kind of treatment for her particular condition so that she knows exactly what's going to happen to her before she undergoes surgery or other forms of treatment.

Treating the disease in its early stages

If breast cancer is diagnosed early on, while the tumour is still small, the surgeon usually carries out a mastectomy, an operation to remove the whole, or part of the breast. He will probably treat the glands in the adjoining armpit too, as the disease often spreads rapidly to this area. The glands may be removed surgically as an extension of the mastectomy operation, or they may be dealt with after the operation by a course of radiotherapy lasting for approximately six weeks.

Surgery is not necessarily the only answer to early breast cancer. For patients who feel that they are unable to face a mastectomy, it may be possible to treat the disease by modern radiotherapy techniques but this option is not usually recommended. Although these techniques are still largely in the experimental stage, most surgeons are willing to discuss and consider this alternative method of treatment.

Follow up

After the initial treatment, doctors follow up their breast cancer patients indefinitely so that if the disease recurs, either in the original area of the operation or elsewhere in the body, it can be detected as soon as possible. If the cancer does reappear, it can often be successfully controlled either by radiotherapy or drugs.

Although most women adjust very well to a mastectomy over a 12-month period, and quickly get used to the 'false' breast form with which they are provided, many doctors continue to monitor carefully their breast cancer patients' psychological reaction to the operation to see whether it might be better to reconstruct the breast by inserting a plastic implant under the surface layer of skin, although this is not always possible or advisable.

Treatment of advanced breast cancer

If the disease is too far advanced for surgery, patients are usually treated by a combination of radiotherapy and anti-cancer drugs. Good teamwork between surgeon, radiotherapist and cancer treatment specialists are helping to prolong and improve the life of many breast cancer patients.

Cancer of the cervix and the womb

In Britain each year around 8,000 women develop cancers of the womb and the *cervix* (neck of the womb). In spite of the amount of publicity they often receive, these are two fairly rare types of tumours – they affect far fewer women than, for example, breast, lung or stomach cancers.

Together, cervical and other uterine tumours account for only about 10 per cent of all cancers which occur in women in the UK. But the fear that they may develop cancer of the cervix or womb often causes a great deal of unnecessary suffering to some women, who may put off consulting a doctor when they have symptoms such as vaginal bleeding. If these cancers are diagnosed and treated promptly enough, they can, however, often be effectively treated and sometimes completely cured. This is especially true of cervical cancer for which there is a very efficient early screening programme in most Western countries.

Where the tumours form

The healthy womb is roughly the shape and size of a small inverted pear, lying behind the *bladder* and in front of the *rectum*. At the lower end of the womb is the *cervix,* a narrow canal connecting the vagina with the main part of the womb. Together they form the *uterus*. Both the womb and the cervix are made of many layers of muscle fibres covered on the inside by a thin lining – the *epithelium*. It is the epithelium which is usually the site of cancer of the cervix or womb.

How cancers of the uterus develop

The uterus, like other organs in the body, is made up of millions of tiny cells. These cells are continually dividing to produce new ones to replace those which are worn out. As they multiply, cells from the deeper layers of tissue surrounding the uterus move upwards to replace the cells in the epithelial layer which die and flake off as they mature. This process of replacement is controlled partly by the balance of hormones such as *oestrogen* and *progestogen* in a woman's blood, and partly by the fact that each cell has a built-in mechanism which regulates how quickly it must divide in order to keep pace with the loss of the cell it is replacing.

If a cell's control system breaks down, perhaps because of an imbalance of hormones, then that cell can give rise to a whole host of other abnormal cells, all out of control and dividing more rapidly than usual. It is this group of uncontrolled cells, spreading haphazardly in all directions and displacing normal cells, that forms the malignant tumour. As it develops the cancer spreads into adjoining tissue, first into the muscle layer of the uterus and then outside the uterus into the surrounding organs such as the bladder and rectum. If untreated, the tumour may invade nearby lymph glands and eventually cancerous cells may be carried in the bloodstream from their original site to more distant parts of the body such as the lungs or liver, where they may form secondary growths.

Women most at risk

So far no single factor has been identified as causing cancers of the uterus, but researchers have found a number of circumstances which may contribute to the risk of developing these tumours.

Women most at risk from developing cancer of the womb are those in the 45 to 60 age group who have never had children. Over half the women affected by this form of cancer are childless.

Cervical tumours, on the other hand,

occur mainly in 35- to 50-year-old women who have had children. About 95 per cent of all women with this form of cancer have had families.

It is very rare for virgins to develop cancer of the cervix, and the risk of doing so seems to be increased if you start having sexual intercourse at a comparatively early age, and also if you have a large number of sexual partners. The reason for this is not clear, but it may be that a long and varied sex life causes a certain amount of inflammation of the cervix, and that this in turn tends to result in the epithelial cells becoming cancerous over a period of years.

Cancer of the cervix seems to be rarer in those women whose partners have been circumcised. Again, the reason is not clear, but it is thought that the foreskin of uncircumcised men may trap viruses or other germs which in some way contribute to the risk of their partners developing cancer.

Women with a very high oestrogen level are at greater risk of developing cancer of the womb. One of the main functions of oestrogen is to make the cells lining the uterus divide more rapidly but in women with normal hormone levels, this effect is balanced by the progestogen in the bloodstream. A few women do, however, have a very high oestrogen level. This may happen if, for example, they have a tumour on one of the ovaries which is abnormally increasing the output of this hormone. The chances of these women developing cancer of the womb is further increased if they are also taking a form of contraceptive Pill or HRT drug containing a high proportion of the female hormone oestrogen.

Since a balance of oestrogen and progestogen is found in most types of the contraceptive Pill or HRT drugs, there is virtually no danger that these will cause cancer in healthy women.

Symptoms of cancer of the uterus

The most common symptom of cancers of the uterus is a discharge from the vagina which may consist of a thin watery liquid, sometimes tinged with blood or sometimes amounting to a loss of pure blood. The discharge may have an offensive smell, and is likely to be brought on or increased either by sexual intercourse or vaginal douching.

Bleeding from the vagina, except at times of menstruation, should always be taken seriously, and any woman, particularly if she's above the age of 35, should consult a doctor at the first sign of any abnormal blood loss. Sudden vaginal bleeding in a woman who is well past the menopause should be investigated without delay by a specialist. Also if a woman going through the menopause experiences an irregular pattern of bleeding, she should consult her doctor as soon as possible.

If the tumour has progressed to the stage where the bladder or rectum have become involved, there may be additional symptoms: passing water may be more frequent or painful, or the patient may suffer from diarrhoea or discharge from the rectum. Pain is usually only a symptom of advanced cancer so if you experience, for example, a pain in your pelvis during intercourse you should consult your doctor. In most cases, he'll probably find that it is caused by infection or inflammation rather than by any cancerous cells.

Diagnosing a tumour

The doctor will examine your abdomen externally. He will then perform a gentle internal examination in order to detect any abnormality of the cervix, womb or ovaries. This examination will almost certainly involve taking a smear from the cervix (see box on page 47) and some fluid from the vagina for a laboratory analysis. You may also need to have some simple blood tests.

If your own doctor cannot find a simple explanation for your symptoms – for example a vaginal infection – or if any of the tests show some abnormality, he will probably arrange for you to see a *gynaecologist* at a nearby hospital. The gynaecologist may arrange for some more detailed tests to be carried out in hospital over a period of a few days.

If the specialist suspects a problem in the cervix, he will do a *cone biopsy* (see box on page 47).

When cancer of the uterus is suspected, the gynaecologist will arrange for the patient to have a *dilatation and curettage* (often referred to as a *D and C* or a *scrape*) under a general anaesthetic. This involves scraping the lining of the womb to obtain further cells for analysis. It should be remembered that the D and C is a very widely used method of treatment for all kinds of gynaecological problems, and is not used only in diagnosing suspected cancer. It will take a few days for the results of these tests to become available to the patient.

Cone biopsy and a D and C are both very minor operations and most patients are able to go home the following day.

Cervical smear test

Your own doctor can perform this simple test, or you can have it done as part of your regular check-up at a family planning clinic.

Before taking a cervical smear, the doctor will first examine you internally and will then gently pass a *speculum* (a tube-like instrument) into the vagina so that he can see the cervix. Having inspected the cervix carefully, he will then rub a wooden spatula across the neck of the womb to remove some of the surface cells. These cells are then placed on a microscope slide and sent to a local laboratory for analysis. The whole procedure takes but a few minutes.

The result of the smear will usually take a week or two to come from the laboratory and if it indicates any abnormality, your doctor will get in touch with you. If you are called back, don't be alarmed as this test can detect many conditions other than cancer, including common vaginal infections such as thrush. One of its major advantages is that by showing the existence of pre-cancerous cells it can predict the possibility of cancer up to 20 years in advance. At this early stage, a cone biopsy can be performed to remove any abnormal cells which may be present before a tumour develops.

Cone biopsy

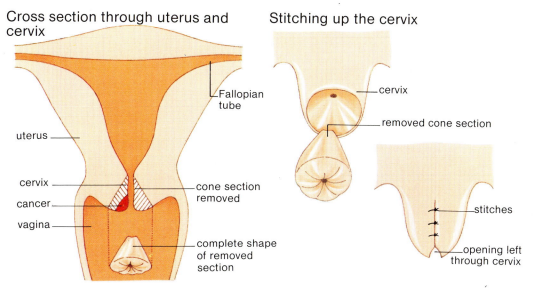

Cross section through uterus and cervix

- Fallopian tube
- uterus
- cervix
- cancer
- vagina
- cone section removed
- complete shape of removed section

Stitching up the cervix

- cervix
- removed cone section
- stitches
- opening left through cervix

Terry Evans

This is performed under a general anaesthetic, and involves the removal of a cone-shaped piece of tissue from around the part of the cervix that protrudes into the vagina. In some hospitals, cone biopsy has been replaced by a technique using a laser beam which is controlled by a periscope-like instrument placed in the vagina. This allows an even smaller amount of tissue to be removed from the edge of the cervical canal.

The tissue is then analyzed. The biopsy may reveal the presence of pre-cancerous cells or the existence of an early tumour. If, however, the cut-away surface of the cone is free from abnormal cells, then there is a very good chance that the biopsy has cured the patient and she will need no further treatment.

This is because in its initial stages cancer of the cervix is confined to one specific area and affects only superficial layers of cervical tissue. It is also a type of cancer which spreads only very slowly and is, therefore, unlikely to have invaded other parts of the body. Once the tumour has been removed, so that the remainder of the cervix is quite clear of abnormal cells, no problems should remain.

Treating cancers of the cervix and womb

If a tumour of the cervix or womb is diagnosed, a number of tests will be done to determine the nature and extent of the cancer to help the specialist decide on the most suitable course of treatment in each case. X-rays of the patient's kidneys and abdomen will show whether the cancer has spread to these sites.

Treatment of cancers of the cervix and womb may involve surgery, radiotherapy or drugs, or a combination of these. Sometimes there is more than one form of suitable treatment in a particular case, and the specialist concerned will usually discuss the various possibilities with the patient so that she can also be involved with the choice of treatment.

Surgery

Some patients will need an operation to remove the womb or cervix and sometimes other organs, such as the ovaries, if these have also been affected by the tumour. Although much depends on the condition of the individual patient, surgery is usually performed when the tumour is not too far advanced and is confined to a fairly specific area, so that it can be removed completely.

After an operation there will, of course, be an abdominal scar, though its size will vary according to the site and extent of the cancer – often a bikini-line incision is all that is required. Following surgery, the patient will probably have to stay in hospital for a couple of weeks and will then be allowed to go home.

Radiotherapy

Sometimes surgery is preceded or followed by a course of radiotherapy, or this may be given as a treatment on its own.

Radiotherapy for cancer of the cervix may be given by inserting an *isotope* containing radiocrive material such as radium into the vagina under general anaesthetic, so that the treatment is concentrated at the site of the tumour. The capsule containing the radioactive substance is left inside the patient and removed at a later date – usually after about three days. For some early stages this may be all that is required, but patients with more advanced tumours which have sometimes spread to other organs may also need external radiotherapy. This is given by a machine similar to that used for taking ordinary X-ray pictures, but which emits far more powerful rays capable of destroying cancer cells.

External radiotherapy usually lasts from four to six weeks, during which time the patient lives at home and visits the hospital daily for treatment. During treatment the patient may feel rather tired and may also suffer from some nausea, sickness or diarrhoea. However, once the treatment is finished, these reactions should disappear. Long-term side effects from radiotherapy are extremely rare.

Chemotherapy

Hormones or *cytotoxic drugs* may be prescribed for some patients, either as a complete treatment on their own or following surgery and/or radiotherapy. At certain stages, cancer of the womb is sometimes very responsive to treatment with hormones such as progestogens, which are usually given in tablet form.

After all these treatments, a cancer patient should be able to continue a perfectly satisfactory sex life, although if the ovaries have been removed some hormonal treatment, such as the insertion of oestrogen cream, may be needed to keep the lining of the vagina healthy. Radiotherapy may cause the vagina to thicken and contract some months after the treatment. Again, the application of oestrogen cream can help, but the best way to stop this happening is to have regular intercourse. This helps to stretch the tissue in and around the vagina and so prevents any long-term damage from developing. For this reason many doctors recommend that gentle love-making should begin as soon as the immediate effects of any treatment have worn off, to keep the vaginal tissues elastic.

Preventing cancer of the uterus

Apart from the impractical and unattractive solution of having the whole womb and cervix removed at an early age, there is no foolproof method of avoiding cancers of the uterus. The risks can, however, be reduced by sensible behaviour.

If you do have frequent changes of sexual partner, use a barrier contraceptive, such as a cap or sheath, which prevents any potential cancer-causing viruses from entering the cervix. If your husband or regular lover is not circumcised, encourage him to make sure that the head of the penis beneath the foreskin is kept clean and free from infection by regular washing. Above all, make sure you have a regular cervical smear at least once every three years, especially if you're over 35, and even if you have recently had a normal smear do not ignore symptoms such as unusual vaginal bleeding — consult your doctor as soon as possible.

Cystitis

Cystitis can make life a misery. Instead of visiting the toilet three or four times a day, to empty your bladder, it's more like three or four times an hour – and each time it may be a painful and uncomfortable experience. A very high proportion of women have cystitis at some point in their lives (about one in four all told).

A one-off attack, whether mild or severe, can usually be cleared up very quickly with the help of your doctor, if necessary, though home treatments may prove very effective. But for some women, cystitis is a long-term problem returning again and again over the years, perhaps only for a few hours at a time, but often for months on end. Nobody is clear why some women seem to be so much more vulnerable, but for them preventative measures which may ward off attacks are crucial.

Identifying cystitis

Just because you feel a frequent urge to empty your bladder, doesn't mean that you've got cystitis. It's well known that people who are anxious about something – whether they're awaiting a job interview or going through a difficult time – suffer from 'frequency'. And, of course, if you drink more liquid than you need, you will have to go to the toilet more often. But what distinguishes cystitis is the discomfort involved.

Usually when you empty your bladder, it's quite painless; you feel full and afterwards a pleasant sense of relief. But with cystitis, you have that full feeling much more often, though you may find that only a few drops pass when you try to 'go'. When you do empty your bladder, it's very uncomfortable, ranging from a mild scalding sensation to agonizing pain which may well reduce you to tears.

The constant dash to the toilet doesn't stop at night (unlike the sort of urge that's the result of emotional excitement or upheaval), and if you do not respond to the promptings of your bladder, there is a danger of incontinence (bed-wetting).

In severe attacks (and these seem to happen especially in women who are long-term sufferers) the combination of lack of sleep and the infection can affect general health, making them look drawn and haggard.

The more severe the attack, the worse the pain, and it may be constant, affecting the lower stomach and back as well as the sexual organs. You may notice changes in the urine as well; often there's a little blood and other debris in it (turning it pink and cloudy) which may make it smell rather unpleasant. Occasionally the last few drops are fairly heavily blood-stained.

Common causes of cystitis

Essentially, cystitis means an inflammation of the bladder, which stores the urine. Being elastic, it can stretch to hold a whole day's output from the kidneys, but if the lining becomes inflamed, the bladder loses its elasticity – hence the need to empty it more often.

The inflammation makes you feel full, even when you aren't, and of course, makes it painful to go to the toilet, especially if the urethra, the passage down which the urine passes, is also involved.

Bacterial infection

A common cause of cystitis is germs finding their way into the urine where they multiply, irritating the bladder and inflaming it. Normally, urine in the body is quite sterile, but if bacteria find their way in from outside, they can take hold in the bladder, despite the body's efforts to get rid of them.

The germs usually responsible are the bacteria *E.coli* which live in and around the rectum. Normally they cause no trouble, unless they find their way from the back passage up the urinary tract.

In women, the opening of the urethra is much closer to the anus than in men, so it's much easier for the bacteria to move across, especially if 'helped' on their way with toilet paper.

treatment If you have an attack of cystitis, the best thing you can do is drink plenty of water to try and 'flush' the bacteria out.

The bacteria thrive in an acid environment, so taking an alkaline substance like baking powder (sodium bicarbonate) will help (see panel).

You should avoid drinks and foods which contain acid or produce acid in the body; coffee, tea, lemon drinks, carbonated soft drinks, oranges, grapefruits, highly spiced dishes, etc, are all potential trouble-makers. Another good reason for avoiding stimulants (tobacco, alcohol, coffee etc.) is that they tend to stimulate the muscles in the wall of the bladder, so that it contracts making you feel the need to 'spend a penny' even more.

Smoking tends to 'concentrate' the urine and therefore stopping the habit will increase the flow and help to clear the system.

In severe cases, some sufferers find passing water becomes less painful if a towel-wrapped hot-water bottle is held close to the sexual organs for a while before urinating; others find it easier to pass water while sitting in a warm bath.

Consulting your doctor

If the attack lasts for more than just a few days, or if you are in pain and passing a little blood in the urine, you should see your doctor. He will not only be able to prescribe tablets to relieve the discomfort, but will also be able to check that it is indeed cystitis and that there are no other problems (see below).

When you make an appointment, he may ask you to bring along a sample of your urine in a small, clean, screwtop jar, since he will need this for testing.

Your doctor will question and examine you to rule out other possible causes. He will feel the lower part of your tummy and around the areas where the kidneys are located to check for tenderness. He may also take your temperature and feel your pulse.

treatment If the symptoms are mild, you may be given tablets to reduce the acid in the urine, thus killing off the bacteria.

But in severe cases, your doctor may prescribe a course of suitable antibiotics (remember to tell him if you have been allergic to any antibiotic in the past). The course will usually last from 10 to 14 days and *should be completed*. Even if your symptoms soon disappear, the infection may flare up again. Taking your tablets or capsules at mealtimes will reduce any tendency for them to upset you.

Recurrent cystitis

There are several theories as to why some women seem to suffer from repeated attacks of cystitis. It may be that the bacteria remain dormant, even after antibiotic treatment, and flare up again at the slightest provocation. Or the acidic content of the urine may be much higher in

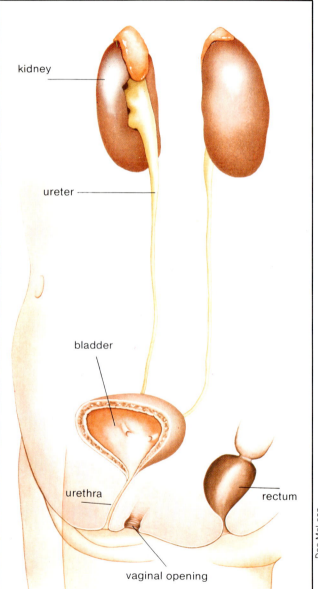

kidney

ureter

bladder

urethra

rectum

vaginal opening

Dee McLean

Cystitis – sources of infection

● *external – carried forward from opening of rectum to urethra*
● *internal – carried down from kidneys in urinary tract, or in bloodstream*

certain women, and this may be aggravated by eating acid-producing foods, and by worry or stress.

Other doctors believe that the recurrent cystitis might not be caused by an infection at all. They suggest that the problem is a sensitive urethra and bladder, that the bladder itself is not inflamed but is responding to pain nearby; for example after a woman has had a baby, when the area around the genitals may be quite sore.

Some doctors are more sympathetic than others when it comes to recurrent cystitis. You may find women doctors are more helpful, as many will have had some experience of cystitis themselves.

Cystitis and sex

Many girls seem to get cystitis when they first make love, and this can be for a combination of reasons. It's possible that an influx of 'new' germs may provoke the problem, or it could be that the friction and chafing during love-making sets it off. This may irritate the opening to the urethra itself, but any rubbing – even from clothing like close-fitting underwear or trousers – will irritate the skin, making a little fluid seep through from the blood. And this fluid is a very rich environment for bacteria to grow in.

> **treatment** Apart from the usual treatment, a brief respite from love-making will allow the inflammation and soreness to die down. Using a water-based lubricant, obtainable from any chemist, will also help to prevent dryness during intercourse and the risk of chafing in the future.

Cystitis and kidney infection

In some cases, the germs which start an infection may get in from above, reaching the bladder from the bloodstream or the kidneys, if there is an infection there.

For this, as for other forms of cystitis, antibiotics should quickly clear up the infection at its source.

Cystitis in children

The most common cause of cystitis in young children is through a kidney infection, and can result when one (or both) kidneys are not properly formed.

It can be a difficult thing to spot because children tend to show signs of general illness – fever, vomiting, fretfulness – rather than obvious bladder pain and a frequent need to go to the toilet.

But many small girls suffer from cystitis, due to a simple bladder infection transmitted from the lower bowel – often because the child has not been taught always to wipe her bottom from the front to the back.

> **treatment** Always seek a doctor's advice if a child shows frequency or pain on passing water; neglected cases can go on to become kidney infections. Many adults today who suffer from kidney disease do so because their childhood infections were ignored.

Your doctor may well want to tackle the cystitis with acid-reducing tablets first before resorting to antibiotics if necessary.

Cystitis and pregnancy

During pregnancy and after birth, women often find that emptying the bladder becomes more difficult, because the changing shape of the womb has affected the other organs in the abdomen. If you are pregnant and suspect you have cystitis see your doctor, as early treatment is especially important in pregnancy.

Tips on prevention

- Avoid anything acidic and highly spiced (coffee, tea, carbonated soft drinks, citrus fruits, curries)
- Restrict intake of other stimulants (tobacco or alcohol)
- Give up smoking (it concentrates the urine)
- After a bowel movement, always wipe from front to back
- Wash the area around the vagina with a plain soap (not perfumed or medicated)
- Drink plenty of water
- When making love, use a lubricant
- Choose open-crotch tights and cotton underpants rather than nylon
- Avoid tight jeans and trousers which could chafe

Home treatment

Try drinking the following mixture every two hours during the day for a couple of days: Add one or two heaped teaspoonsful of baking powder (sodium bicarbonate) to a glass of preferably warm water, sweetened with a teaspoonful of honey.

If simple home treatment fails to bring relief, consult your doctor as soon as possible.

Complications in pregnancy

Pregnancy is a natural event, and it usually ends with a healthy mother and normal baby. While the great majority of women have no major problems, there is a degree of risk involved – about 20 per cent experience some kind of complication. However, modern antenatal care now does a great deal to spot potential problems and deal with them before they put the life of the mother or baby at risk. (This section deals with the range of major complications, but see also the sections dealing with *Cystitis* and *Anaemia* for information on these conditions in relation to pregnancy).

Toxaemia (pre-eclampsia)

This happens to one in 10 women in the last weeks of pregnancy. The blood pressure is raised, protein substances leak into the urine, and the retention of water in the tissues leads to swelling of the body or a sudden weight gain. It is commoner in a first pregnancy than in later ones, and in an older mother than a younger. It also occurs more frequently if the mother is carrying twins. Nobody knows its precise cause, but it is probably related to cells from the placenta leaking into the mother's circulation, causing damage to the kidney filtering mechanisms and the walls of the small blood vessels.

If the condition is allowed to proceed unchecked, the blood pressure slowly creeps up to levels that are dangerous to the baby. The baby, living on the other side of the placenta, depends entirely upon the flow of blood from the mother that reaches the placental membrane. If the blood pressure is raised, there may be some damage either to that membrane or the blood vessels supplying it. The baby is then at risk because the exchange of nutrients and oxygen from the mother's blood is poorer than normal. Additionally, in labour the condition may lead to an acute shut-off of oxygen.

The mother is affected too. Her fluid retention increases so that there may be sudden weight gain or puffiness of the ankles, the hands and the face. If the condition is not checked it could lead to a more dangerous state; she could have eclampsia – a series of dangerous fits – recurring every few minutes. It's very rare for the problem to get this far nowadays, because the toxaemia is usually diagnosed and treated early on.

Because of the large load they are carrying around, many women in later pregnancy have swollen ankles – this is particularly noticeable in the afternoon. But if the swelling occurs in the morning, it should be reported to the doctor. Some pregnant women may also notice that their hands are becoming puffy.

Tests to diagnose toxaemia

A rise in the blood pressure reading – taken at a regular antenatal visits – will bring the problem to the attention of the doctor. This does not usually happen until the last four or five weeks of pregnancy, but in rare cases it may be earlier. In addition to checking blood pressure, a sample of early morning urine can be tested at each antenatal visit. This will show if the kidney filters are damaged.

If the doctor diagnoses toxaemia he can do certain tests to check that the baby is progressing well. He may investigate the growth of the baby by ultrasound scans, or he may check the baby's well being by estimating oestrogen production. This hormone, made mainly by the baby and the placenta, is passed into the mother's body, then excreted in her urine. Checking urine samples to assess the full 24-hour production of oestrogen is a good guide to the health of the unborn child.

treatment The best treatment for toxaemia is bed rest. This allows a reduction in blood pressure and a slight increase in the blood supply to the uterus and growing baby. In the earlier stages a woman can rest in bed at home, provided it's fairly

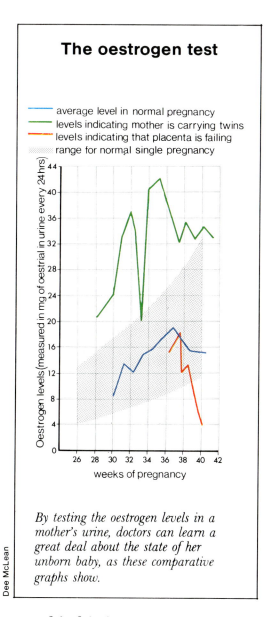

The oestrogen test

— average level in normal pregnancy
— levels indicating mother is carrying twins
— levels indicating that placenta is failing
▒ range for normal single pregnancy

Oestrogen levels (measured in mg of oestrial in urine every 24hrs)

weeks of pregnancy

By testing the oestrogen levels in a mother's urine, doctors can learn a great deal about the state of her unborn baby, as these comparative graphs show.

Dee McLean

Rhesus incompatibility

A woman with a rhesus negative blood group who conceives a rhesus positive child produces a potentially dangerous situation. Blood from the rhesus positive baby can pass across the placenta into the mother's circulation and 'sensitize' her natural defence mechanism to make antibodies. These antibodies will destroy rhesus positive cells. Fortunately, this passage of the blood from baby to mother occurs most commonly at the time of delivery and so there is not enough time to affect the first baby. But if his mother is sensitized into producing the antibodies, these will damage the blood cells of any rhesus positive baby she carries in future.

The antibodies may cause the red cells in the baby's blood to break down so the baby becomes anaemic – and makes increased amounts of a bile substance from the breakdown of iron pigments in his red cells. Whilst the baby is in the uterus, the excess bile is shunted across the placenta, but once the baby is born his own liver is too immature to cope with this heavy load, so he rapidly becomes jaundiced. In extreme cases, this might cause brain cell damage, so without treatment, the baby could be spastic.

There are no symptoms of rhesus incompatibility that the mother will notice. It is one of the hidden conditions which is only detected by proper antenatal care and testing. The doctor detects rhesus incompatibility by checking the mother's blood group early in pregnancy. If she is rhesus negative, he then examines her blood further for rhesus antibodies. These will not be present in the first pregnancy, but if he finds them in a later pregnancy he will do further tests to assess the degree of the problem.

treatment The whole treatment of rhesus incompatibility depends upon blood tests, and tests of the fluid around the baby. Blood tests will show whether the baby is being affected by rhesus incompatibility, and the doctor will want to assess the speed at which the antibodies build up to see how serious a problem it is for the baby. Once 20 weeks of pregnancy have passed, some of the fluid surrounding the baby in the uterus can be removed and checked for bile breakdown products. If the rate of bile breakdown is very rapid, the doctors may give the baby a blood transfusion.

A very fine needle is passed into the uterus and through the baby's stomach wall. Via this needle a transfusion of compatible blood is given to the baby to tide him over for a few weeks when his

peaceful. If she has an active young child to look after this could be difficult, but pre-eclampsia is commonest in a first pregnancy. Should the condition become worse, she may be admitted to hospital for more rest, and drugs can be given to help reduce the blood pressure level further. If the tissue swelling becomes painful, other treatments can be given to cause the kidneys to excrete more water, so reducing the tension.

If, despite this, the toxaemia persists, most doctors advise that the baby should be delivered as soon as it reaches full term. They usually recommend inducing labour when the neck of the womb is ripe, or if the condition worsens very sharply, performing a Caesarean section. This will remove the baby from the hazardous environment of raised blood pressure inside the uterus, and produce good results for mother and baby.

193

own red blood cells are being broken down by the antibodies. The transfusion may have to be repeated several times, until the baby is delivered.

Once the baby is delivered, special blood tests are done immediately to check the degree to which he is affected. If this is serious, an exchange transfusion takes place – the baby's blood is slowly removed in small quantities, each fraction being replaced by compatible blood that will not break down. Any rhesus negative mother who gives birth to a rhesus positive baby is now routinely given a special injection soon after delivery to prevent sensitisation. This usually prevents rhesus problems with the next baby. Since this technique became widespread, 'rhesus babies' are now rare.

Severe vomiting

About two thirds of women have some vomiting in early pregnancy, but they are quite able to continue their usual activities. About one in 1000 have such severe vomiting that the woman becomes de-hydrated and, unless this is controlled, her levels of fluids, nutrients and vitamins are greatly reduced.

This excessive vomiting can happen at any time of the day or night, often going on continuously for many hours at a time. The woman can retain no food or fluid and loses weight. She may obviously be ill, and if the condition is left untreated for some time she may develop jaundice.

treatment Hospital treatment is advisable. An intravenous drip is usually required to bypass the overactivity of the intestine; this will restore fluid and salt balance and provide essential vitamins. Anti-vomiting drugs are also given.

Vaginal bleeding in early pregnancy

Any bleeding in pregnancy after the last menstrual period is abnormal and needs to be investigated. The blood might not look bright red, for if blood stays in the upper vagina for a few hours before leaking out, it looks more dark brown in colour. If there is only a small amount of brown blood loss, contact the doctor the next morning. If the bleeding is more rapid and accompanied by pain, ring the doctor immediately and retire to bed.

Sometimes bleeding in early pregnancy is due to a polyp or erosion of the surface tissue of the cervix – the neck of the womb. But in both of these cases, the bleeding is actually quite slight and often no more than a brown discharge. Usually a polyp or cervical erosion will be left alone until the pregnancy is over, as they are not a serious threat either to the mother or to her baby.

Miscarriages

The commonest cause of bleeding is a threatened miscarriage. The egg has been implanted in the uterus for some weeks but is not secure, and so when the uterus makes a few contractions it causes bleeding. If the condition worsens and there is more bleeding, the cervix starts to open and the embryo is passed out – a complete miscarriage. In a few cases the embryo dies at this early stage, but the bleeding and miscarriage don't actually occur until a few weeks later.

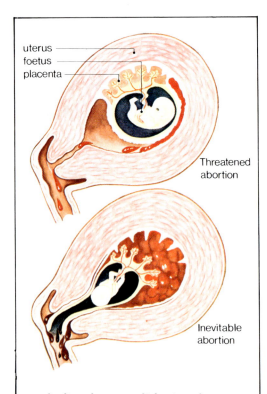

uterus
foetus
placenta

Threatened abortion

Inevitable abortion

Bleeding, however slight, is a danger signal for a pregnant woman because it could indicate that the foetus may miscarry. If the bleeding is slight and settles quickly, and if the uterine contractions are very minor, the chances are the pregnancy will continue, provided the mother stays in bed for a few days.

But, if there are strong uterine contractions, giving the pregnant mother severe pain, the cervix may well be dilating, and in this case abortion becomes inevitable.

When the doctor examines the woman he checks to see if the cervix is open. If it is closed, there is only a threat to miscarry at this stage. The best treatment for this is bed rest. By resting the whole body, the uterus is rested too, and in most cases the threat recedes, and a normal pregnancy follows. The doctor may prescribe a mild sedative to help the woman sleep.

If the cervix is open, a miscarriage is inevitable, and the woman will be admitted to hospital because the bleeding can be very severe. As nothing can be done to save the pregnancy, an operation is carried out to evacuate the lining of the uterus (similar to a D and C).

Ectopic pregnancy

If the embryo is implanted in the Fallopian tube instead of in the uterus, there may be a small amount of bleeding accom-

Vaginal bleeding in late pregnancy

This can be a sign of a serious threat to the mother and baby. Any bleeding in the last months of pregnancy should be reported immediately to the doctor. It's important to note the amount of bleeding and whether there is any pain associated with it; also, keep any pad which has been soaked in blood, as this may prove useful to the doctors when they are diagnosing the problem.

As with bleeding earlier in pregnancy, a local cause such as cervical erosion or polyps could be responsible, and very rarely it can be a sign of a generalized blood disease in the mother. More often, however, it's caused by a problem with the placenta either becoming detached or being in the wrong position.

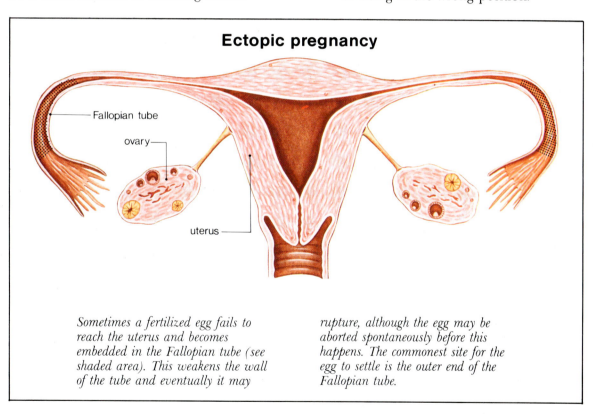

Ectopic pregnancy

Sometimes a fertilized egg fails to reach the uterus and becomes embedded in the Fallopian tube (see shaded area). This weakens the wall of the tube and eventually it may rupture, although the egg may be aborted spontaneously before this happens. The commonest site for the egg to settle is the outer end of the Fallopian tube.

panied by symptoms of pain and a tender area on one or other side of the uterus. The embryo will not develop because the Fallopian tube cannot support a baby.

treatment This is an urgent matter, requiring immediate surgery, for there is a risk that there will be heavy bleeding, and the woman may become very ill. The surgeon has to remove the embryo and the tube in which it is implanted. Most women recover from the operation very well and go on to have a normal baby – the other Fallopian tube is still intact.

Detached placenta

The placenta is the exchange station between the blood supply of the mother and the unborn baby. Sometimes it develops quite normally, but then prematurely separates from the wall of the uterus, causing bleeding. This is a very rare occurrence, but when it does happen it presents a major threat to the baby, because its oxygen supply is disrupted. There is also a serious threat to the mother from severe shock.

Urgent hospital treatment is required.

Detached placenta

wall of uterus — placenta

If the placenta separates from the wall of the uterus prematurely, emergency treatment is essential for the safety of both mother and unborn child since the oxygen supply is cut off.

Dee McLean

Occasionally, if the uterus is tense and the mother is very shocked, a doctor may call out a team of hospital doctors to perform an emergency blood transfusion before moving her. Once in hospital, an ultrasound monitor will be used to check the baby's heart rate. If the baby is mature a Caesarean section may be performed to avoid further risk to the mother and baby. If the bleeding is less severe, it may be a case for hospital rest for a short time followed by an induced delivery when the mother is in better condition.

Placenta praevia

Normally the placenta is situated on the upper part of the uterus, lying above the baby's head. But sometimes, if the fertilized egg implanted lower down in the uterus, the placenta develops below and in front of the baby's head. This is known as *placenta praevia*. During the last two months of pregnancy, the stretching and softening that takes place in the lower part of the uterus and the cervix causes some degree of separation between the placenta and uterus – resulting in bleeding.

> **treatment** The mother will be admitted to hospital. If the symptoms suggest it is not a detached, normally sited placenta, the doctors will carry out tests, such as an

ultrasound scan, to see precisely where the placenta is lying. Every effort is made to carry on the pregnancy until the baby is mature (beyond 36 weeks). Then, if the placenta is very low lying, the doctors may deliver the baby by a Caesarian operation, because a normal vaginal delivery would involve a great deal of bleeding and the loss of the baby. If the placenta is lying low, but to one side, a normal delivery may be all right, but the doctor will usually first examine the woman under anaesthetic in the operating theatre to make sure this is the position. The membranes surrounding the baby will then be burst so that a vaginal delivery can go ahead.

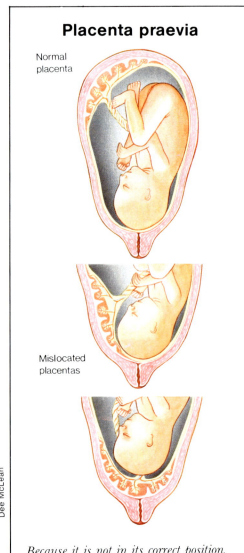

Placenta praevia

Normal placenta

Mislocated placentas

Dee McLean

Because it is not in its correct position, the mislocated placenta shown here might well stop the head from 'engaging' in the pelvis and there can be very heavy bleeding as the placenta is separated from the uterus.

Problems in labour

Giving birth is a natural event, and the vast majority of women have trouble-free labours. In fact three-quarters of all women produce their babies through normal deliveries. The problems which can occur for the remaining quarter are largely guarded against by good ante-natal care and by continued monitoring during labour itself.

What can go wrong

A baby's four-inch journey through its mother's pelvis is potentially the most dangerous trip he will ever make. The mother, too, may be put at risk during labour so a careful watch must be kept at all times. When problems occur during labour they often do so very quickly and unexpectedly, and need prompt attention if they're not to become grave hazards.

Breech deliveries

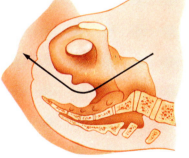

The path that a baby has to negotiate at birth can be awkward if the baby is in a breech position.

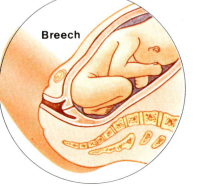

Foetal distress

Sometimes strong contractions to the uterus may squeeze the arteries taking blood to the placenta (the organ supplying the unborn baby with oxygen and nourishment). When this happens the unborn baby's vital oxygen supply is diminished, and it responds by first increasing its heart rate, then dropping it to a lower level. If the heart beats too fast or if the rate drops too low, then this means that the baby is being stressed by lack of oxygen and the heart can't cope. *Foetal distress*, as this is called, happens in between five and 10 per cent of labours.

The midwife can check the heart rate by listening in with a special stethoscope, but many hospitals now use electro-cardiography to continuously monitor the baby's heart. A tiny electrode is safely attached to the baby's scalp and electrical impulses from its heart are picked up, analyzed and displayed on a dial as well as on a paper trace. To check for diminished oxygen levels a bead of the baby's scalp blood can be taken quickly and examined.

> **treatment** If there is concern for his safety, rapid action must be taken. A Caesarean section will be performed (see further on) if the cervix is not fully opened, or a forceps delivery carried out (see next page) if the cervix is open, and the baby's head can be drawn through the vagina.

Maternal distress

A choice of pain relief is available fairly readily, and most women manage to get through labour with no real problems. But if, for example, the baby's head is slightly too big for the mother's pelvis, or if contractions are not co-ordinated, she may become *distressed*. She'll be exhausted and thoroughly fed up with labour.

Depending on how far the labour has advanced, the obstetrician may decide on a Caesarean section or a forceps delivery, so avoiding any further strain or exhaustion in the mother.

197

Forceps delivery

push down with left hand

pull on handles with right hand

Forceps curved to fit around foetal head.

Vacuum extraction

chain for pulling

tube to apply vacuum

line of pull

A vacuum extractor with tube to apply vacuum and chain for pulling.

Dee McLean

Malpresentation

The space in the mother's pelvis through which a baby makes his journey is not a perfect cylinder. The baby has to negotiate the space rather like an armchair being taken through a doorway that's a shade too narrow – the manoeuvring must be just right.

For normal delivery, the baby should lie with his head down and his chin tucked against the chest. This ensures that the narrowest part of the baby's head arrives first, forging an easy route for the rest of the head and body.

If the baby is in the wrong position, the top of his head or his face may be the first to appear, and the head sometimes gets jammed into the pelvis.

The mother may be able to continue unaided, but some help from the obstetrician is usually needed especially if the baby's face is presented first. With malpresentation, labour is more difficult and so it takes longer.

Breech presentation and transverse position

Rather than having the head ready to be born first, about 3 per cent of babies present themselves bottom-down with their heads high in the stomach; this is called a *breech presentation*. The feet only very rarely come first – usually the baby is squatting like a tiny gnome with knees and hips bent up in front of him.

A baby's soft buttocks don't fit the *cervix* (neck of the uterus) as well as his head would, so labour is often slower. The baby starts to descend down the vagina once the cervix has dilated fully, helped by controlled pushing on the part of the mother. The buttocks and body usually come fairly easily, but the shoulders might get held up in the pelvis. Then the head, the largest and hardest part of the baby to deliver, comes last.

> **treatment** If the breech baby is expected to weigh between 5½ and 7½ pounds, and the mother's condition is normal, then a breech delivery – with the aid of an experienced obstetrician – usually presents no problems. But if the baby is very small or very large, a Caesarean section may be advised to avoid any hazards. Since complications may arise, the labour should always take place in a fully equipped maternity unit.

On extremely rare occasions a baby may lie across the uterus so that the head and body are in a horizontal line across the mother's body. A baby in this transverse position is impossible to deliver via the normal vaginal route, so the obstetrician usually performs a Caesarean section.

Ways of assisting childbirth

To get round the problems of foetal distress, maternal distress or malpresentation of the baby, several courses of action are open.

Forceps delivery

If the cervix is fully open, forceps can be used to aid delivery. Forceps have been around in Britain for 300 years. They are shaped like large serving spoons with a part of the bowl cut out. The 'spoons' fit together around the baby's head and guard it against pressure while the baby is being gently removed. The baby is then led from the pelvis through the vagina to the outside world.

From the mother's viewpoint, forceps tend to look rather big and clumsy, but most of the instrument stays outside the body. Only the slim blades are inserted to guard the baby's head and guide it out.

A local anaesthetic at the base of the vagina is nearly always given with a forceps delivery. (However, if the woman is already anaesthetized with an epidural this won't be necessary). The forceps are then cupped around the baby's head and the doctor skilfully draws the baby down the birth canal. Once the head is born the forceps are removed and the rest of the delivery can proceed normally.

Vacuum extraction

If the cervix is partly, but not fully, dilated then it's not safe to use forceps to help out a stressed baby. A special vacuum cap can be used instead to bring the baby's head quickly down against the cervix to stimulate full dilation, allowing the baby to be delivered more rapidly. The method has been in use for 250 years.

A vacuum extractor is usually used in the last part of the first stage of labour. A small flat cap is passed through the vagina and partly dilated cervix to lie against the baby's head. The air is extracted from the inside of the cap through a tube so that the soft, loose skin on the baby's head is gently sucked against the cap. When the vacuum is just right, the doctor gently pulls down and brings the head into contact with the cervix. This makes the cervix dilate and within a few minutes the head is usually in the vagina. A few more gentle pulls combined with the mother's pushing, deliver the baby.

Caesarean section

When it is dangerous to speed up delivery via the vagina, an abdominal delivery of the baby may become necessary. This is called a Caesarean section.

An *elective* Caesarean section is one which is decided on and performed in the last weeks of pregnancy before labour even starts. This might happen if the mother's blood pressure had risen too suddenly or if the baby's head and mother's pelvis are known to be a tight fit.

Sometimes a Caesarean section in labour is decided upon because prolonged labour may be dangerous to the child or the mother. The most common reason for this is foetal distress, when the baby might die if left in the uterus.

Some form of anaesthesia is always needed. A general anaesthetic is the most common type, but sometimes an *epi-*

dural anaesthetic, which numbs only the lower part of the body, is used so that the woman can stay completely conscious. Occasionally a local anaesthetic is given in the stomach wall.

The most common incision is a low one close to the pubic mound. This results in a small scar which is hidden by the pubic hair, when it regrows. The baby is taken out through the incision and handed over to a paediatrician who ensures that the baby starts to breathe properly. The umbilical cord is cut and the placenta can then be removed from the uterus. The uterus then contracts and the surgical wound in its wall closes up. The stomach wall is closed in layers using sutures (stitches) which dissolve after a few days. The whole procedure takes about 45 minutes.

Induction

Sometimes, late in pregnancy, the obstetrician thinks it unwise for the baby to stay in the uterus any longer, and may induce labour, because, for example, toxaemia has occurred.

Induction methods vary according to the hospital in which they are done, but first the cervix is checked to see if it is ripe and ready for labour. Then the membrane around the baby is punctured (it's not painful) so that some fluid escapes and the baby's head comes down into contact with the cervix.

A labour-stimulating hormone may be given as well. An *oxytocic* hormone may be given as an intravenous drip put into one of the veins on the back of the wrist. Alternatively, *prostaglandin* may be given in the form of a pessary or paste inserted into the upper vagina. Both methods cause the uterus to start contracting within a few hours, and so labour commences.

Acceleration of labour

This is *not* the same as inducing or starting off labour even though similar methods are used. Sometimes, when labour has already started quite spontaneously, the obstetrician may feel that the baby is not progressing well, and decide to speed up its arrival. Either labour-stimulating hormones are used to hurry things along, or the membrane is snagged via the cervix once dilation has started.

For most women, labour is a safe event and a happy one, too. As long as the woman is thoroughly prepared, and provided adequate care is available for the few who may run into trouble, then labour can be kept safe and pleasant.

Miscarriages

A miscarriage is always a very distressing experience and can have a profound psychological impact on a woman. It's common to suffer feelings of remorse at losing the baby and to worry unduly about the reason for the miscarriage.

However, if you've recently gone through all this it may be some small comfort to know that you're certainly not alone. In fact at least 20 per cent of all pregnancies end in miscarriage, and the figure may well be much higher than that. This is because many early miscarriages are confused with a slightly delayed period and are therefore either not noticed at all, or else not reported to the doctor. After a miscarriage, it's also vital that the mother reassures herself with the knowledge that the most difficult part of achieving motherhood is becoming pregnant, and having demonstrated this ability to conceive, the outlook for finally achieving a full-term pregnancy and having a healthy, bouncing baby is very good.

Miscarriage, or to use its medical name, *spontaneous abortion,* is defined as the expulsion of a pregnancy or part of a pregnancy from the womb before the 28th week of pregnancy (or in some countries before the 24th week). This length of pregnancy is chosen because it is considered that a baby is incapable of living an existence separate from the mother before that time.

Miscarriages occurring within the first three months of pregnancy are called *first trimester* miscarriages. These are by far the most common, with the majority taking place in the second month of pregnancy, and relatively few in the third month. Those in the middle three months are known as *mid trimester* miscarriages. The reasons for losing the foetus tend to vary according to the trimester in which this loss occurs.

Regardless of timing, miscarriage may either be complete or incomplete. Most women have what are called *incomplete miscarriages*. This means that although the amount of bleeding may have been considerable some of the pregnancy still remains within the womb. Others have *complete miscarriages*, when the entire contents of the womb are expelled.

It is a fact that some women have a tendency to miscarry during the first three months of pregnancy. There is no known reason for this and doctors stress that there is no cause for alarm. Indeed, up to three first trimester miscarriages in succession are considered to be absolutely 'normal', and little will usually be done to investigate possible reasons until a woman has had her third miscarriage. On the other hand, any miscarriage in the second trimester is considered more significant and investigations may be started soon after the miscarriage.

First trimester miscarriages

These can be divided roughly into *threatened miscarriages* or *inevitable miscarriages.*

Threatened miscarriages

These usually start with bleeding from the vagina. The blood lost can vary from slight brown staining to heavy bleeding with blood clots. At this stage a threatened miscarriage is similar to a period and the bleeding is not severe enough to terminate the pregnancy. The outcome of a threatened miscarriage is unpredictable but in most cases, if the bleeding stops, pregnancy is likely to continue.

Bleeding may occur during the first three months for reasons entirely unrelated to threatened miscarriage. A few women tend to bleed slightly at the time the first, second and third periods are missed. Bleeding may also be caused by cervical erosions, or vaginal infections. Unfortunately, there is no way the bleeding due to these causes can be distinguished from the bleeding due to a threatened miscarriage.

This is why it's essential for a pregnant woman who has *any* vaginal bleeding to report to her doctor. If the bleeding is very heavy she should go to bed and ask the doctor to visit her at home. It's also important to save any blood clots or heavily stained pads or clothing so that he can check that none of the developing embryo or placenta has been lost.

treatment ▷ The doctor will examine you to ensure the cervix is still closed, and that the size of the uterus corresponds to the dates of the pregnancy calculated from the last period. Provided that this is the case, he will usually advise bed rest until the bleeding has stopped.

When it has, he will check to make sure there is a continuing pregnancy, and, where facilities are available, will arrange for an ultrasound test on the womb. This will help to confirm that all is well.

If the size of the uterus doesn't correspond to the date of the last period then the doctor is alerted to the following possibilities: either simply that the woman has got her dates wrong (this is extremely common – about 70 per cent of women who say they are sure about the date of their last period are in fact proved wrong!) and the baby is due either earlier or later than previously estimated; or, if the womb is smaller than expected, it's possible that the foetus has died (see 'delayed' miscarriage).

Apart from bed rest there is no specific treatment for a threatened miscarriage. Indeed, even the value of bed rest is hotly debated among many doctors. Surveys have shown that women who continue to go about their normal daily duties (provided they avoid strenuous exercise and sexual intercourse) have just as much chance of continuing the pregnancy as those who are confined to bed in hospital. In the last analysis, doctors say that only nature can decide the final outcome of a threatened miscarriage.

Injections of pregnancy hormones, such as *progesterone*, rarely prevent miscarriages. They are now used only in a few unusual cases as some of them have been found to cause abnormalities in the baby, and they are generally aborted.

Inevitable miscarriage

A miscarriage tends to become inevitable when the bleeding is accompanied by tummy cramps similar to period pains, and/or low backache in which the pain may be quite severe. This indicates that the womb is making miniature contractions, similar to labour contractions, in an effort to expel the pregnancy from the womb. The cervix becomes dilated and quite soon after the onset of the symptoms the miscarriage usually occurs, and may be complete or incomplete.

Sometimes the whole thing happens quite quickly with none of the warning symptoms of a threatened miscarriage. On other occasions the sequence of events may occur more slowly. In these cases, the symptoms of a threatened miscarriage are usually found on examination to be accompanied by a dilated cervix. If this is so, then eventual miscarriage is considered inevitable, even if neither the developing embryo or placenta have yet been lost. The doctor will advise the woman to rest in bed until miscarriage 'proper' occurs.

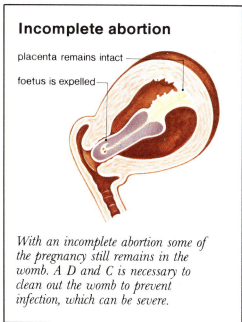

Incomplete abortion

placenta remains intact

foetus is expelled

With an incomplete abortion some of the pregnancy still remains in the womb. A D and C is necessary to clean out the womb to prevent infection, which can be severe.

Dee McLean

In some cases, this may not be until a couple of days later.

treatment ▷ It is very difficult for a doctor to be sure that all the contents of the womb have been expelled unless he has been able to examine everything that has been lost from the vagina. In practice this happens very rarely, so he will usually err on the safe side and advise a D and C operation to clean out the uterus.

This is a very important procedure as any remaining parts of the developing pregnancy may become infected and give a woman a high temperature, or cause prolonged period-like bleeding and pain.

Common causes of early miscarriages

Chromosomal abnormalities in the developing embryo are by far the most common causes of miscarriages which occur during the first three months of pregnancy.

Chromosomes are minute chemical packages contained within each cell of the body and they are inherited equally from both parents to determine all bodily characteristics of the developing baby. Sometimes mistakes occur in the structure of these chemical packages. This is very serious, as even minute mistakes can have disastrous effects on the bodily shape and characteristics of the baby. It would seem that in the case of a foetus having chromosomal abnormalities, miscarriage is simply nature's way of reducing the number of abnormal or defective babies being born.

Any illness which causes a high temperature like 'flu or malaria may result in a miscarriage. It is vitally important that a pregnant woman with 'flu asks her doctor to visit her immediately, so that he can make every effort to lower her temperature as soon as possible.

A woman expecting twins or triplets is more prone to miscarriage than a woman with a single pregnancy. This could possibly be due to the womb cavity not being able to stretch quickly enough to accommodate the babies' rapidly increasing size.

Severe kidney disease, disease of the thyroid gland and diabetes also increase the risk of miscarriage. This may be due to the increased physical stress that these diseases inevitably place on the woman during pregnancy.

Very rarely, unusual infections may enter the womb and induce miscarriage. Unfortunately, the discovery of these unusual germs by special testing often occurs too late for any effective treatment. However, such infections tend not to recur in subsequent pregnancies.

Contrary to popular belief, it would seem that shock or emotional upset play little part in causing miscarriage.

Delayed miscarriage

Sometimes, after the symptoms of a threatened miscarriage have disappeared and all seems well, the signs of pregnancy such as morning sickness or breast tenderness disappear, and the mother no longer 'feels' pregnant. In this situation the doctor may then notice that the uterus is too small for the expected duration of pregnancy.

A pregnancy test usually reveals that the baby has died, and this is then termed a 'missed abortion'. After some time – often several weeks later – the symptoms of miscarriage return, and the pregnancy

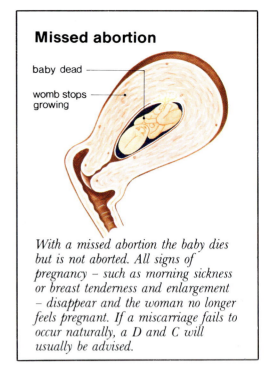

Missed abortion

baby dead

womb stops growing

With a missed abortion the baby dies but is not aborted. All signs of pregnancy – such as morning sickness or breast tenderness and enlargement – disappear and the woman no longer feels pregnant. If a miscarriage fails to occur naturally, a D and C will usually be advised.

Dee McLean

is then finally expelled from the womb. If miscarriage fails to occur of its own accord, the doctor will usually advise a D and C to clean out the womb.

Mid trimester miscarriages

These are rare and are usually due to an abnormality of the mother's womb – in particular a weakness of the neck of the womb *(cervical incompetence)*. They may also be caused by irregularities in the shape of the womb due to *fibroids* or the presence of a *septum*.

Why cervical incompetence causes miscarriage

Normally the circular muscle fibres of the cervix remain tightly closed throughout pregnancy and act as a barrier to prevent the baby 'escaping' from the womb. However, if the cervix is weak it is slowly stretched open by the weight of the developing foetus until it's no longer efficient enough to contain the contents of the womb. Most miscarriages due to cervical incompetence take place at about the 16th week of pregnancy, when the cervix has become so dilated that the developing baby simply 'falls through'.

An incompetent cervix is almost impossible to predict in advance and is usually only discovered after a miscarriage has occurred. The most common cause is overstretching of the cervix muscles, either during a previous D and C or termination of pregnancy operation, or during a particularly difficult or rapid labour when the baby is unduly large. Very occasionally it can simply be that a woman is born with an inherent weakness of the neck of the womb. However, it's a fact that very few women suffer from an incompetent cervix where there is no history of previous operation or pregnancy. In the case of a woman carrying twins, however, the weight of the babies can be enough to dilate the cervix and so cause miscarriage.

Recognizing a mid-trimester miscarriage

Regardless of cause, miscarriages in the second three months of pregnancy often occur rapidly and without much warning. Bleeding may sometimes occur beforehand, but often the first a woman knows about the miscarriage is when the membranes surrounding the baby rupture and the waters break. This can happen anywhere and at any time and is often extremely embarrassing for the woman. Wherever she is, it's important that she finds somewhere to lie down and a doctor is called. If this isn't possible then someone should call an ambulance and get her to hospital. Unfortunately, once the waters break, the miscarriage is virtually inevitable.

The foetus is often expelled quite quickly, usually within a matter of hours. Although stomach cramps may sometimes accompany it, the miscarriage is normally relatively painless.

treatment In most cases a D and C will be carried out and the womb will be carefully explored in order to find a possible cause for the miscarriage. If it doesn't reveal an obvious cause, your doctor will probably test the strength of the cervix a few weeks later when things have settled down again. This will be done by gently attempting to insert a rigid rod of a certain critical diameter into the cervix. If it passes easily down the cervical canal it indicates that the cervix is weak.

If this is the case, treatment is straightforward and future prospects for achieving a full-term pregnancy are very good. When the woman becomes pregnant again the doctor will advise that the cervix is strengthened by placing what's called a 'purse string stitch' around it. This is then pulled tight to keep the cervix firmly closed. The stitch is put in under general anaesthetic when the woman is about 14 weeks pregnant. It is removed at about the 38th week of pregnancy by a simple, painless procedure which does not require a general anaesthetic.

A D and C after a mid trimester miscarriage may reveal, or lead the surgeon to suspect, that the woman has an abnormally shaped uterus. This is commonly due either to a septum, or to fibroids. Either possibility may subsequently be confirmed by a special X-ray test of the womb, called a *hysterosalpingogram*. This involves injecting a special radio opaque dye through the cervix into the womb

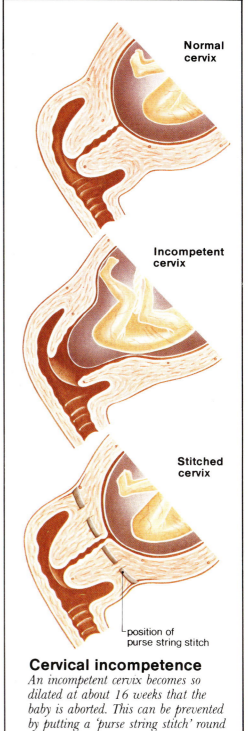

Normal cervix

Incompetent cervix

Stitched cervix

position of purse string stitch

Cervical incompetence

An incompetent cervix becomes so dilated at about 16 weeks that the baby is aborted. This can be prevented by putting a 'purse string stitch' round the neck of the cervix.

Dee McLean

cavity. When the X-ray is taken, the dye casts a shadow outlining the shape of the womb cavity on to the X-ray plate, thereby revealing any abnormalities.

Fibroids

These are swellings of muscle and fibrous tissue in the wall of the uterus which may sometimes protrude into the womb and distort its shape. They do not necessarily cause miscarriage; indeed many women who suffer from fibroids achieve full term pregnancies, but their existence does increase the risk of miscarriage. This can be because unequal stretching of the womb wall tends to induce contractions and the early expulsion of the baby. Alternatively, the distortion of the womb wall may cause the placenta to become detached and so induce miscarriage.

If the fibroids cause miscarriage they can later be dealt with by an operation called a *myomectomy*, whereby each fibroid is removed individually. There is then no reason why subsequent pregnancies should not run to full term.

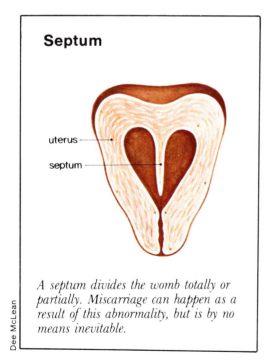

Septum

uterus

septum

A septum divides the womb totally or partially. Miscarriage can happen as a result of this abnormality, but is by no means inevitable.

Dee McLean

Septum

This is a wall which either partially or completely divides the uterus in two. As in the case of fibroids, this uterine abnormality does not necessarily mean abortion is inevitable. However, if a septum causes a miscarriage, treatment is much more difficult since extremely complicated surgery is required to correct this condition. In fact, the operation is rarely performed, and is usually only considered

after three mid-trimester miscarriages have occurred in a woman with this unusual feature.

Placental insufficiency

There is also a condition, known as *placental insufficiency*, which may affect a small proportion of babies. It usually begins to develop in the 24th to 26th week of pregnancy, but does not become an obvious problem until after the 28th week – during the last three months or *third trimester* of pregnancy.

If a normal healthy baby is to be produced it's obviously vital that the placenta functions efficiently. In the case of placental insufficiency the placenta grows slowly and fails to mature properly. It is therefore unable to provide adequate nourishment and oxygen for the developing baby.

Although the foetus matures normally it is much smaller than it should be after 28 weeks of pregnancy, simply due to lack of nourishment. Placental insufficiency may in some cases become so severe that it can no longer supply the baby's basic requirements. The foetus may then die in the womb and be expelled as stillbirth.

However, in many instances placental insufficiency is recognized and may be treated in time to prevent the foetus being lost.

Smoking is a common cause of placental insufficiency and in this case obviously the best treatment is to try to give up the habit. It may also occur in pregnant women suffering from toxaemia, or alternatively it may occur for no apparent reason at all. In these last two instances, bed rest may help the pregnancy run to full term and prevent a miscarriage.

Becoming pregnant again

It's usually advisable not to try for another pregnancy until at least three menstrual periods have elapsed. (The first menstrual period usually occurs four to six weeks after a miscarriage although a larger interval is not uncommon.) This will ensure that the lining of the womb is suitable to receive a fertilized egg, and it will also establish a definite date for the last period, from which the expected date of delivery can be accurately calculated.

If a woman conceives directly after a miscarriage it may be difficult to calculate the ovulation date and so virtually impossible to give an accurate expected date of confinement.

Index

Page numbers in **bold type** refer to
complete chapters on a particular topic.